90

Ergonomics in
Health Care and
Rehabilitation

Ergonomics in Health Care and Rehabilitation

Edited by

Valerie J. Berg Rice, Ph.D., OTR/L, C.P.E., FAOTA

Colonel, U.S. Army

With 27 Contributing Authors

Butterworth–Heinemann

Boston   Oxford   Johannesburg   Melbourne   New Delhi   Singapore

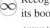

Library of Congress Cataloging-in-Publication Data

Ergonomics in health care and rehabilitation / edited by Valerie J. Rice.
    p. cm.
    Includes bibliographical references and index.
    ISBN 0-7506-9714-8 (alk. paper)
    1. Rehabilitation technology.   2. Human engineering.
3. Physically handicapped--Services for--Equipment and supplies.
I. Rice, Valerie J.
  [DNLM: 1. Human Engineering. 2. Equipment Design.
3. Rehabilitation.   4. Delivery of Health Care.   5. Biomechanics.
WB 26 E67 1998]
RM950.E74   1998
620.8'2'08861--dc21
DNLM/DLC
for Library of Congress   97-34808
                                                           CIP

British Library Cataloguing-in-Publication Data

A catalogue record for this book is available from the British Library.

The publisher offers special discounts on bulk orders of this book.
For information, please contact:

Manager of Special Sales
Butterworth–Heinemann
225 Wildwood Avenue
Woburn, MA 01801-2041
Tel: 781-904-2500
Fax: 781-904-2620

For information on all Butterworth–Heinemann publications available,
contact our World Wide Web home page at: http://www.bh.com

10 9 8 7 6 5 4 3 2 1

Printed in the United States of America

This is dedicated to the ones I love (or at least some of them):
My husband, Donald Michael Rice, and my son, Elia Edward Berg Rice,
who suffered my absence and long discourses during this process
My brother, Copy Berg (alias Vernon Edward Berg III), who is always and
forever an inspiration. All of us, his family and friends, visit him whenever we
want to feel competent or be given permission to succeed
My mother, Vera Lee Cornell Berg, who is, after all . . . my mother

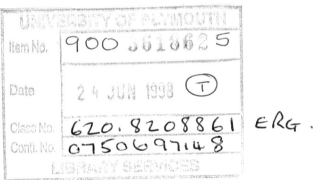

Contents

Contributing Authors

Laura W. Abed, M.A.

Laura W. Abed received her Master's degree in Speech and Language Pathology from Indian University in 1982. She has since worked as a freelance writer and editor, focusing on various education and design themes. She is coauthor, along with Wm. L. Wilkoff, of *Practicing Universal Design: An Interpretation of the ADA*.

Donald S. Bloswick, Ph.D., P.E., C.P.E.

Donald S. Bloswick is an associate professor in the Department of Mechanical Engineering at the University of Utah where he teaches and directs research in the areas of ergonomics, safety, occupational biomechanics, and rehabilitation engineering. He is Director of the Ergonomics and Safety Program at The Rocky Mountain Center for Occupational and Environmental Health and holds adjunct appointments in the Department of Family and Preventive Medicine, Department of Bioengineering, and Division of Physical Therapy. He is a registered Professional Engineer and Certified Professional Ergonomist with 10 years of industrial experience. For the past 15 years he has served as an ergonomic and safety consultant to industry, the Occupational Safety and Health Administration, and the legal community throughout the United States.

Bloswick received a B.S. in Mechanical Engineering from Michigan State University, an M.S. in Industrial Engineering from Texas A&M University, and an M.A. in Human Relations from the University of Oklahoma. He earned his Ph.D. in Industrial and Operations Engineering at the University of Michigan, where he studied at the Center for Ergonomics.

Marilyn Sue Bogner, Ph.D.

Marilyn Sue Bogner is President and Chief Scientist of the Institute for the Study of Medical Error. In that capacity, she directs and conducts research using her systems approach to identify factors that contribute to or induce error.

She edited and contributed to the book *Human Error in Medicine*. She has also contributed chapters to four books and was the editor of the special health care section of the journal *Human Factors,* for which she serves on the editorial board. She initiated and is senior editor of the *International Journal on Human Error*. She reviews manuscripts and journals for five journals and three publishers.

Bogner has made more than 100 presentations to national and international professional meetings. She is active in numerous professional organizations and an officer of many of them, including Past-Chair of the Medical Systems and Rehabilitation Technical Group of the Human Factors and Ergonomics Society.

Bogner is a Fellow of the Human Factors and Ergonomics Society and the Washington Academy of Sciences. Her Ph.D. is in Psychology from the University of Kansas.

Susan Brakefield, P.T.

Susan Brakefield graduated with a B.S. degree in Physical Therapy from the University of Washington in 1969 and has continued to specialize in manual therapy and ergonomics. She is President and cofounder of Professional Therapy Associates, a private practice physical therapy clinic in Montana.

Brakefield has drawn on her clinical expertise as well as postgraduate instruction to act as ergonomic consultant for both large and small industries since 1988, offering work-site analysis and modification as well as teaching injury-prevention classes in upper body and spine-related injuries. She also treats workers with early signs of injury. She has worked extensively with engineers and employers to develop an accurate post–job offer employee assessment.

Bryan Buchholz, Ph.D.

Bryan Buchholz received a B.S.E. in Chemical Engineering (1979), an M.S.E. in Applied Mechanics (1983), and an M.S. and Ph.D. (1989) in Bioengineering, all from the University of Michigan. He is currently an associate professor in the Department of Work Environment at the University of Massachusetts, Lowell, teaching graduate courses in Occupational Biomechanics and Ergonomics. His research focuses on two major topics: ergonomic exposure assessment and hand biomechanics. He is currently examining various ergonomic aspects of construction work to reduce the incidence of work-related musculoskeletal disorders in that industry. He also is studying the biomechanics of prehensile activities to better understand how stresses that cause chronic hand and wrist injuries can be reduced.

Marilyn J. Bull, M.D.

Marilyn J. Bull is a professor of Pediatrics and Medical Director of Automotive Safety for Children at Riley Hospital for Children in Indianapolis. She continues her leadership as a national advocate for occupant protection for all children through a variety of responsibilities with the American Academy of Pediatrics and as a member of the Blue Ribbon Panel on Child Passenger Safety for the National Highway Traffic Safety Administration. She has been instrumental in the development of several policy statements pertaining to safe transportation of children with special needs through the American Academy of Pediatrics. She is a leading voice for the development of policies and resources for transportation safety of preschoolers and children with special needs on school buses.

Pascale Carayon, Ph.D.

Pascale Carayon has an Engineer Diploma from the École Centrale de Paris and a Ph.D. in Industrial Engineering from the University of Wisconsin, Madison. Since 1989, she has been an assistant professor, then an associate professor of Industrial Engineering at the University of Wisconsin, Madison. Since 1995, she has also been a visiting professor at the École des Mines de Nancy, France. Her research interests include occupational health and safety; office and video display terminal ergonomics; job stress and work-related musculoskeletal disorders; management of quality, and technological and organizational change. Her research has been funded by the

National Science Foundation, the National Institute for Occupational Safety and Health, and other public and private organizations. She has published more than 150 journal articles, conference proceedings papers, book chapters, and books. She is a coauthor of *Work-Related Musculoskeletal Disorders (WMSDs): A Reference Book for Prevention.* She is a member of the editorial board of the International Journal of Human-Computer Interaction and Behavior and Information Technology. She has participated in the scientific committees of more than 12 conferences.

Sara J. Czaja, Ph.D., C.P.E.
Sara J. Czaja is a professor of Industrial Engineering at the University of Miami and the Director of the Miami Center on Human Factors and Aging Research at the University of Miami School of Medicine. The Center is one of the six Edward R. Roybal Centers for Research on Applied Gerontology funded by the National Institute on Aging/National Institutes of Health. She received her Ph.D. in Industrial Engineering from the State University of New York at Buffalo. She is a fellow of the Human Factors and Ergonomics Society and of the American Psychological Association and is a certified professional ergonomist. She has done extensive research in aging and cognition with an emphasis on computer and information technologies. The focus of Czaja's work is on designing systems so that they can be successfully used by older adults.

Biman Das, Ph.D., P.Eng.
Biman Das is a professor of Industrial Engineering at the Dalhousie University, Canada. Recently, he served as Visiting Professor, Centre for Biomedical Engineering, Indian Institute of Technology. He has had extensive and diversified industrial experience in Canada, the United States, Germany, and India. His current research and teaching interests are in the areas of industrial ergonomics, production systems, and manufacturing. He serves as an industrial consultant. He has authored more than 150 publications. He obtained a Ph.D. degree in Industrial Engineering with specialization in Ergonomics from North Carolina State University. Recently he served as President of the International Society for Occupational Ergonomics and Safety. Currently he serves as Editor-in-Chief of *Occupational Ergonomics.* He is a Fellow of the Institute of Industrial Engineers and Institution of Electrical Engineers (Manufacturing Division).

Mark Dumas, M.S.
Mark Dumas received his Bachelor's of Science degree in Biology and his Master of Science, Public Health, degree from the University of Utah, where his studies focused on ergonomics and industrial hygiene. He has served as a consultant in industrial hygiene and ergonomics and spent several years in the workers' compensation area providing industrial hygiene, ergonomic, and loss-control services to a wide variety of industries. Altogether, he has been addressing occupational health issues for more than 8 years. He is currently the Manager of Health, Safety, and Environmental Quality for a neutriceutical manufacturer in Spanish Fork, Utah.

Janet Stout Everly, M.S., OTR
Janet Stout Everly is an associate professor of Occupational Therapy at Indiana University, Indianapolis. In her former position as staff therapist at the James Whitcomb Riley Hospital for Children, she worked with the hospital's safe transportation multidisciplinary team. In addition to safe transportation, her research interests include playground safety and accessibility and occupational therapy student stress and coping styles.

Marla C. Haims, M.S.

Marla C. Haims is a Ph.D. candidate and a research and teaching assistant in the Department of Industrial Engineering at the University of Wisconsin, Madison. She received her B.A. in Psychology from Miami University in Oxford, Ohio, and her M.S. in Industrial Engineering at the University of Wisconsin, Madison. Her degrees are specialized in the areas of human factors and ergonomics and sociotechnical systems.

Haims is currently president of the University of Wisconsin, Madison, student chapter of the Human Factors and Ergonomics Society and serves on the executive committees of the University of Wisconsin, Madison, Society of Women Engineers and the American Society for Engineering Education. Her research interests include occupational stress and work-related musculoskeletal disorders in office and computer work, organizational change, and community quality. She is especially interested in conducting longitudinal intervention research.

Dana C. Jefferies, B.S., C.S.P.

Dana C. Jefferies is the corporate safety director for Plum Creek Manufacturing, L.P., a progressive forest products company manufacturing lumber, plywood, and medium-density fiberboard for specialty markets. He received his B.S. in Occupational Safety and Health from Utah State University in 1976. His 21-year career has been split between nuclear process engineering and forest products manufacturing. He has successfully implemented ergonomics programs for his employers and demonstrated the benefits of proper workplace design and matching human performance to the work task.

One-Jang Jeng, Ph.D.

One-Jang Jeng is an assistant professor in the Department of Industrial and Manufacturing Engineering, New Jersey Institute of Technology. He received his B.S. degree in psychology from the National Cheng-Chi University, Taiwan, in 1984. He received M.S. (1991) and Ph.D. (1994) degrees in Industrial Engineering from the University of Wisconsin, Madison, majoring in human factors and ergonomics. His research emphasizes the evaluation of functional performance associated with cumulative trauma disorders. He is interested in the design and evaluation of workstations and work tasks and evaluation of human performance.

Eric King, M.S.

Eric King is the Operations Manager for Medron Inc., a company specializing in the design and manufacture of medical devices. He received his B.S. degree in Mechanical Engineering from Brigham Young University in 1991. He received an M.S. in Mechanical Engineering majoring in ergonomics and human factors from the University of Utah in 1993. His research was centered around the design and testing of rehabilitative equipment for children with cerebral palsy and the elderly. He has worked in research and development for companies in the medical device industry and has brought several innovative medical products to market.

Barbara L. Kornblau, J.D., OTR, FAOTA, D.A.A.P.M., A.B.D.A, C.D.M.S., C.C.M.

Barbara L. Kornblau is a professor of Occupational Therapy and Public Health at Nova Southeastern University in Fort Lauderdale, Florida. She is also a practicing attorney, a certified case manager, a disability management specialist, and a rehabilitation specialist. She assists business, industry, hospitals, insurance companies, local governments, and universities in complying with the Americans with Disabilities Act (ADA) and implementing injury-prevention programs. Her current law practice focuses primarily on disability discrimination legislation.

Kornblau has presented papers, workshops, and training sessions in the area of work rehabilitation and authored more than 60 publications, including book chapters addressing the ADA, work rehabilitation, ethical and legal issues in practice, and the role of the expert witness. She authored and prepared the videotape "The Path to ADA Compliance: The Job Interview." She also writes a recurring legal column, "Legalines," on legal issues in occupational therapy practice in *Advances for Occupational Therapists*.

Kornblau is the current chair of the American Occupational Therapy Association's (AOTA) Standards and Ethics Committee and a former chair of the AOTA's Work Programs Special Interest Section. She received her B.S. in Occupational Therapy in 1977 from the University of Wisconsin, Madison, and her J.D. from the University of Miami in 1984. She is board certified in pain management and disability evaluation.

Shrawan Kumar, Ph.D., D.Sc., F.Erg.S.

Shrawan Kumar is a professor in Physical Therapy in the Faculty of Rehabilitation Medicine and in the Division of Neuroscience, Faculty of Medicine, at the University of Alberta. He joined the Faculty of Rehabilitation Medicine in 1977 and rose to the ranks of Associate and full Professor in 1979 and 1982, respectively. He holds B.Sc. (Biology and Chemistry) and M.Sc. (Zoology) degrees from the University of Allahabad, India, and a Ph.D. (Human Biology) degree from the University of Surrey, U.K. After earning his Ph.D., he did postdoctoral work in Engineering at Trinity College, Dublin, and worked as a Research Associate at the University of Toronto in the Department of Physical Medicine and Rehabilitation.

For his lifetime work, Dr. Kumar was recognized by the University of Surrey with the award of a peer-reviewed D.Sc. degree in 1994. He was invited as a Visiting Professor for the year 1983–1984 at the University of Michigan Center for Ergonomics in the Department of Industrial Engineering. He was a McCalla Professor in 1984–1985. He is a Fellow of the Human Factors Association of Canada, Human Factors and Ergonomics Society of the United States, and the Ergonomics Society of the United Kingdom. He was awarded the Sir Frederic Bartlett Medal for excellence in Ergonomics research by the Ergonomics Society of the U.K. in 1997. During the 48 years of existence of the society, Dr. Kumar is the seventeenth recipient of its highest honor. For his distinguished research, the University of Alberta awarded him one of the seven Killam Annual Professorship for the year 1997–1998. The Human Factors and Ergonomics Society of the U.S. also bestowed its top honor on him by awarding him the most prestigious award for 1997: Distinguished International Colleague.

Kumar has worked on more than 200 scientific peer-reviewed publications and works in the area of musculoskeletal injury causation and prevention with special emphasis on low-back pain. He has authored or edited seven books. He currently holds a grant from Natural Sciences and Engineering Research Council (NSERC). His work has been supported in the past, in addition to the above, by the Medical Research Council (MRC), Workers' Compensation Board, and National Research Council. He is Editor of the *International Journal of Industrial Ergonomics*, Consulting Editor of *Ergonomics*, Advisory Editor of *Spine*, and Assistant Editor of the *Transactions of Rehabilitation Engineering*. He also acts as a grant reviewer for NSERC, MRC, Alberta Occupational Health and Safety, and British Columbia Research.

Kumar has organized and chaired regional, national, and international conferences. Currently, he serves as Chair of the Rehabilitation Technical Committee of the International Ergonomics Association. As Chair of the Code of Ethics Committee of the International Ergonomics Association, he has additional valuable experience in larger and global issues.

Lieutenant Colonel Mary S. Lopez, Ph.D., C.P.E., OTR

Mary S. Lopez is the Manager of the Ergonomics Program at the U.S. Army Center for Health Promotion and Preventive Medicine. The program serves as the ergonomics consultant for the U.S. Army, responsible for ergonomic policies, program implementation and evaluation, field surveys, training courses, and educational materials.

She holds a doctorate in Industrial Engineering from Texas A&M University and a Master of Health Administration from Baylor University. She is an occupational therapist with more than 19 years of clinical experience and a Certified Professional Ergonomist. She is the chairperson of the Department of Defense Ergonomics Working Group and represents the Department of Defense on the Federal Agency Ergonomics Advisory Group.

Linda McQuistion, Ph.D., P.E., C.P.E.

Linda McQuistion is the Rehabilitation Engineer for the Ohio Rehabilitation Services Commission. As such she coordinates the provision of Assistive Technology services to vocational rehabilitation consumers and to agency employees receiving reasonable accommodations.

McQuistion holds a doctorate in Industrial Engineering from the University of Cincinnati, a Professional Engineer's License, and a Certification as a Professional Ergonomist. She serves on the editorial board of *Ergonomics in Design*, a publication of the Human Factors and Ergonomics Society, and has published in the fields of Rehabilitation Engineering and Reasonable Accommodation.

McQuistion has been named an EXEMPLAR Woman in Science and Engineering by the Ohio Academy of Science and was awarded the 1994 Meritorious Service Award by the Ohio Rehabilitation Technology Association. She is active in numerous professional organizations including the Human Factors and Ergonomics Society, the National Mobility Equipment Dealers Association, the National Rehabilitation Association, and the Rehabilitation Engineering and Assistive Technology Society of North America.

Victor Paquet, M.S.

Victor Paquet received a B.S. in Engineering Psychology from Tufts University (1991) and an M.S. in Industrial and Systems Engineering (Human Factors Engineering Concentration) from Virginia Polytechnic Institute and State University (1995). He is currently a doctoral student in the Department of Work Environment at the University of Massachusetts, Lowell. His research interests include ergonomic exposure assessment of nonrepetitive work and intervention evaluation methodologies. His dissertation will examine the validity of an observational work-sampling method for characterizing ergonomic hazards and address work-sampling strategies for quantifying ergonomic exposures in construction work.

Robert G. Radwin, Ph.D., C.P.E.

Robert G. Radwin is a professor at the University of Wisconsin, Madison, where he conducts research and teaches in the areas of ergonomics and human factors engineering. He holds academic appointments in Industrial Engineering and in the Biomedical Engineering Program, where he serves as Chair. He has an M.S. in Electrical Engineering and Bioengineering from the University of Michigan. His Ph.D. is from the University of Michigan, where he was a postdoctoral research fellow at the Center for Ergonomics. He is the recipient of a Presidential Young Investigator Award from the National Science Foundation and a Special Emphasis Research Career Award from the National Institute for Occupational Safety and Health. He is a fellow of the Human Factors and Ergonomics Society.

He serves as a reviewer for numerous scientific journals, conferences, and funding agencies; he sits on several international panels, editorial boards, and committees; and he chairs both the American National Standards Institute Z-365 Work Analysis and Design Subcommittee. He has consulted with numerous companies on ergonomic aspects of manufacturing processes and equipment design.

Radwin actively studies the recognition, causes, and controls of cumulative trauma disorders in manual work. His research is concerned with analytical methods for measuring and assessing exposure to physical stress in the workplace; ergonomics perspectives on the design; selection, installation, and use of manually operated equipment including hand tools; and functional deficits associated with musculoskeletal disorders and peripheral neuropathies.

Colonel Valerie J. Berg Rice, Ph.D., OTR/L, C.P.E., FAOTA

Valerie J. Berg Rice is an occupational therapist, an ergonomist, and an officer in the U.S. Army. She holds master's degrees in occupational therapy and health care administration and a Ph.D. in Industrial Engineering and Operations Research, with a specialization in Human Factors Engineering/Ergonomics. She is assigned to the U.S. Army Medical Department Center and School Center and School as Director of the Occupational Therapy Educational Program. Rice also organizes and directs a military short course for occupational therapists on combat fatigue, teaches ergonomics to Occupational and Physical Therapy students, and assists with military research, ergonomics, and executive management short courses.

Rice has conducted research on physically demanding military tasks and manual materials handling. Her research has included the design and evaluation of an ergonomic harness to carry stretchers and transport patients, manual materials handling (individual and team lifting, combined lifting/carrying performance, and determination of psychophysically determined lifting recommendations), the effects of pharmacologic agents on human performance, ergonomic evaluations of work settings such as dentistry, and psychosocial stressors. She is the author of more than 80 articles, reports, book chapters, and presentations on ergonomics/human factors, military performance, and occupational therapy. Her interests include human performance, industrial ergonomics, injury prevention, and special population needs.

Rice currently serves as President of the Board of Directors for the Board of Certification in Professional Ergonomics, Chair Elect of the Medical Systems and Rehabilitation Technical Group of the Human Factors and Ergonomics Society, and a member of the Continuing Competency Task Force for the American Occupational Therapy Association. She has served as a member of the Accreditation Council for Occupational Therapy Education and a faculty member for the American Occupational Therapy Association's (AOTA) continuing education series on implementation of the Americans with Disabilities Act. She is the official liaison between AOTA and the Human Factors and Ergonomics Society.

Ben Shirley, M.S.

Ben Shirley is a Senior Research and Design Engineer at Utah Medical Products Inc. This position involves steering committee decisions, project management, and design of medical devices for which he has received a number of patents. He received his B.S. degree in Mechanical Engineering from Brigham Young University in 1992, and received an M.S. degree from the University of Utah in Mechanical Engineering in 1994, majoring in human factors and ergonomics. His research emphasized the design and evaluation of wheelchairs to assist the elderly.

Ellen Rader Smith, M.A., OTR, C.P.E., C.V.E.

Ellen Rader Smith is an ergonomist and occupational therapist in private practice. As the owner of Ergo & Rehab Services, she provides ergonomic consultation services to industrial and office workplaces. She also provides hand and upper-extremity rehabilitation, performs work capacity and job-site assessments for industrial injured and disabled clients, and assesses persons for disability. Throughout Smith's ergonomic training programs, she emphasizes a practical and common sense approach to integrating ergonomics into the workplace and when modifying workplaces to meet specific users' needs.

Smith received her B.S. in Occupational Therapy from the University of Pennsylvania (1976) and her M.A. in Occupational Biomechanics and Ergonomics from New York University (1982). She is a Certified Professional Ergonomist and Certified Vocational Evaluator. She is a member of the Human Factors Society, American Occupational Therapy Association, American Society of Safety Engineers, and American Industrial Hygiene Association.

Karen Bruner Stroup, Ph.D.

Karen Bruner Stroup is Director of Riley Hospital for Children's Community Education Department. Previously, she served as Director of the hospital's Automotive Safety for Children Program, which continues today as a national resource for information and education on transportation of children with disabilities. Her research interests have broadened beyond transportation concerns for children with disabilities to include all areas of injury prevention education for children with special needs.

Carolyn A. Unsworth, Ph.D., OTR, B.App.Sci. (OccTher)

Carolyn A. Unsworth has taught courses over the past 6 years in cognitive and perceptual dysfunction at The Boston School of Occupational Therapy, Tufts University, and La Trobe University in Australia. Her research interests and publications include stroke rehabilitation, the clinical decision-making processes surrounding patient transfer from acute care to rehabilitation and discharge from rehabilitation, and the theory and assessment of function.

Paula C. Wilkoff

Paula C. Wilkoff attended the New York School of Interior Design and has been a practicing designer for the past 46 years. She is principal owner of a commercial design firm and devotes much of her time to the field of barrier-free design. Wilkoff's various projects have encompassed designs for corporate and professional offices and retail space, with an emphasis on accessibility. She was a principal contributor to the surveying of more than 13 million sq. ft of commercial space relative to compliance with Titles I and III of the Americans with Disabilities Act. She was a scenario development contributor to the textbook *Practicing Universal Design: An Interpretation of the ADA*, published by Van Nostrand Reinhold. Wilkoff has also written numerous articles relating to accessibility issues for trade magazines.

Wm. L. Wilkoff, FASID

Wm. L. Wilkoff, an Industrial Design graduate of Pratt Institute, has been practicing interior and industrial design for the past 46 years in the Washington, D.C., metropolitan area. He has been coprincipal and owner of a firm specializing in both residential and commercial design. For the past 25 years, since his appointment by American Society of Interior Designers (ASID) to the President's Committee on Employment of People with Disabilities, he has devoted much of his practice to the field of barrier-free design. He is a fellow of ASID and their representative to the American National Standards Institute, A117.1 Committee and the Americans with Disabilities Act *Accessibility Guidelines* Federal Advisory Committee which is developing new accessibility standards. He also serves on the District of Columbia Building Code Board, where he chairs the Committee on Accessibility. He coauthored the textbook *Practicing Universal Design: An Interpretation of the ADA*, published by Van Nostrand Reinhold, and has written numerous articles on this subject for various trade magazines. He has received many awards from both national and local chapters of ASID and the International Interior Design Association.

Preface

This text defines new specialty areas of practice bridging the fields of design and medicine, specifically those of human factors and ergonomics with health care and rehabilitation. The text is divided into six sections, an introductory section followed by five arenas of practice within the purview of health care and rehabilitation ergonomics.

The introductory section defines terms and the five areas of practice, provides a historical perspective, and describes a systems approach used in ergonomic practice. The systems approach includes techniques in analysis, design, and testing and evaluation. It provides a foundation for the rest of the text, as the systems approach is used in each of the consequent chapters.

The five areas of practice are ergonomics-for-one, ergonomics for special groups, industrial intervention—musculoskeletal ergonomics, user-centered equipment design, and the Americans with Disabilities Act. Each practice area section begins with an overview of ergonomic practice within that context, followed by chapters covering detailed case studies.

Several tenents of ergonomics are evident throughout this text: (1) Ergonomics applies to all human faculties, including but not limited to physical, mental, visual, and communication abilities, as well as subjective preferences and psychosocial issues. (2) Ergonomics applies to all settings in which humans function. (3) Ergonomics applies to all age and ability categories.

As ergonomics applies to all human faculties, the case studies presented in this text include physical, psychosocial, and cognitive examples. Equally, ergonomics does not only apply to vocational work; designing for the person also includes design of home, leisure, transportation, and public service environments, equipment, and processes. Therefore, the case studies include work, home, leisure, communication, industrial, health care, and public service settings. Because ergonomics applies to all age and ability categories, age ranges in the case studies include infants and children, adults, and the elderly.

Human factors and ergonomics is a profession unto itself, with its own professional societies, a process for accreditation of educational programs, and individual credentialing. However, ergonomic theories are used by practitioners with varied educational backgrounds. Therefore, although the majority of the contributing authors consider themselves ergonomists, others consider themselves professionals who use ergonomic techniques within their specialty areas. Their backgrounds include health care administration, industrial design, human factors and ergonomics, industrial engineering, law, medicine, occupational therapy, physical therapy, psychology, and rehabilitation engineering.

It is hoped that this text will be used by experienced clinicians and ergonomists alike to further their knowledge about this dual-edged practice arena, to hone their skills, and to acquaint themselves with the knowledge and capabilities brought by differing perspectives. It is also hoped that educational programs will use the text to educate students about possible specialization in health care or rehabilitation ergonomics. Using the case studies to pattern experiential learning programs or using the questions that arise from reading the text for the basis of masters theses and doctoral dissertations will do much to further development of the field. Truly, the future of our professional practice lies within our students. Finally, as one of the first texts focused on ergonomics in health care and rehabilitation, I trust it will only be one among many. As stated by Sue Bogner in the December 1996 special issue of *Human Factors*, this represents "a mere dusting of snowflakes on the tip of the iceberg. There is much work to be done."

Valerie J. Berg Rice

Acknowledgments

My deepest appreciation for all those who assisted with this text. Most important, I thank the authors who gave their expertise and knowledge and the time to put it together on paper. I especially thank Barbara Kornblau, who wrote two chapters for this text and coauthored another with me over the same time frame. My gratitude is extended to the editorial staff at Butterworth–Heinemann, especially Karen Oberheim, Medical Editor. I also thank those who offered encouragement: the members of the Board of Directors for the Board of Certification in Professional Ergonomics, especially Dieter Jahns, Jerry Duncan, and Hal Hendrik; the members of the Accreditation Council for Occupational Therapy Education, especially Florence Hannes and Paula Kraemer; my major advisor and mentor at Virginia Polytechnic Institute and State University, Harry Snyder; and Karen Jacobs, a comrade-in-arms for ergonomics in health care and rehabilitation. I also want to thank all of those members of the U.S. Army and Department of Defense who have worked with, supported, and mentored me during my military career, especially the following Assistant Chiefs of the Army Medical Specialist Corps: Colonel Lou Carmona, Colonel Roy Swift, Colonel Pete Bell, Colonel Wade Daigle, and Colonel Judy Riggan.

Section I

Introduction

Chapter 1
Defining the Terms

Valerie J. Berg Rice

Learning Objectives

On completion of this chapter, the reader should be able to define the following terms:

- Health care ergonomics
- Rehabilitation ergonomics
- Ergonomics-for-one
- Ergonomics-for–special groups
- Musculoskeletal ergonomics
- User-centered design
- Usability testing
- Work hardening

Key Words

Cumulative trauma
Design
Human factors
Human performance
Ergonomics
Health care

Abstract

Professionals in human factors/ergonomics have expanded their practice areas into health care and rehabilitation settings, applying ergonomic principles to the design of systems, environments, and products. Similarly, professionals in health care and rehabilitation have augmented their practice areas to include industrial applications and areas traditionally covered by other experts. The amplified interests of both groups and overlapping application of their skills has led to the development of two new fields of specialization: health care ergonomics and rehabilitation ergonomics. This chapter explains the areas of overlap, including ergonomics for one, ergonomics for special groups, musculoskeletal ergonomics, user-centered design, and application of the Americans with Disabilities Act (ADA). It also describes the educational background for health care/rehabilitation and human factors/ergonomics that do or do not apply to each area of overlap.

Introduction

In a special issue of the *Journal of the Human Factors and Ergonomics Society,* focused on health care, Bogner (1996a) stated that there is a "new frontier for contemporary human factors: health care." The reverse is also true. A new frontier exists for contemporary health care and rehabilitation: ergonomics.*

The extent of interests shared by medical and ergonomic professionals is reflected in the increase

---

*Numerous professions are becoming interested and involved in ergonomics, including physicians, occupational and physical therapists, nurses, and physicians assistants; engineers, human factors/ergonomics professionals, industrial and organizational psychologists, industrial designers, and biomechanists; and industrial hygienists, safety personnel, exercise physiologists, and athletic trainers.

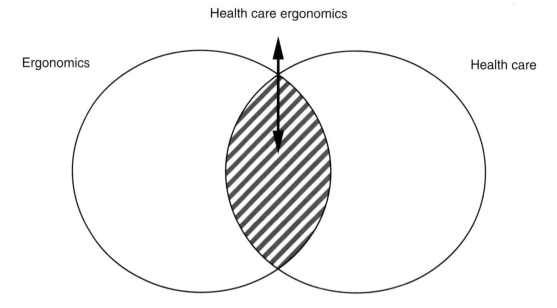

Figure 1-1. Health care ergonomics is the area of intersection between ergonomics and health care.

of (1) articles on these topics in professional journals, (2) new journals specifically focused on the application and research involved in the crossover between health care and ergonomics, and (3) special interest sections (i.e., technical groups) within their professional organizations. The application of ergonomics in health care has given rise to novel areas of specialty practice. Two of these areas are health care ergonomics and rehabilitation ergonomics.

Health Care Ergonomics

Health care ergonomics is a specialty in which design fields and patient-oriented fields combine skills to better serve patients and the general public. This specialty combines human factors engineering/ergonomics and health care and includes the domain formed at the intersection of the two disciplines (Figure 1-1). (Note that in this text, *human factors* and *ergonomics* are considered synonymous; for further clarification see Rice, 1995.)

> Human factors (ergonomics) is a body of knowledge about human abilities, human limitations, and other human characteristics that are relevant to design. Human factors engineering (ergonomics implementation) is the application of human factors information to the design of

tools, machines, systems, tasks, jobs, and environments for safe, comfortable, and effective human use (Chapanis, 1991, p. 2).

Therefore, health care ergonomics refers to the design of equipment, procedures, training, and environments within settings where health care is administered. Health care ergonomics includes such topics as the following (Gosbee, 1996; Rappaport, 1970, 1975):

- Design of emergency alarm and response systems within a health care setting
- Design of computerized record-keeping systems, along with software and hardware specifically for health care settings
- Design of a residential facility for the elderly, for adults with developmental delays, or for persons requiring an assisted living facility
- Development, design, and testing of equipment or procedures used in medicine
- Design issues in injury and illness prevention and patient outcome (efficacy) testing, including procedures and equipment designed to prevent injuries, diagnostic decision support, telemedicine, distance learning for medical topics, and shift work for health care providers

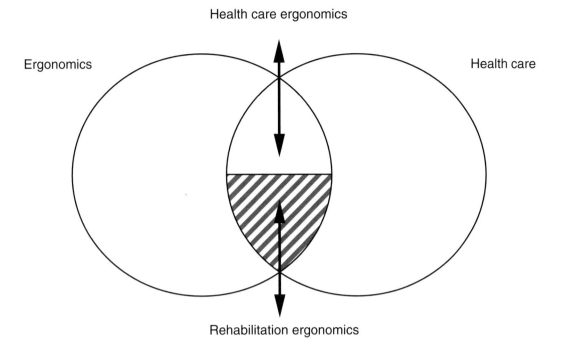

Figure 1-2. Rehabilitation ergonomics is a subset of health care ergonomics.

Rehabilitation Ergonomics

Just as rehabilitation is a subset of the broader category of health care, rehabilitation ergonomics is a subset of health care ergonomics. Rehabilitation ergonomics addresses the commonalties between the fields of human factors/ergonomics and rehabilitation (Figure 1-2). The sections of this text correspond to those common areas: ergonomics-for-one; ergonomics-for–special groups; ergonomics to prevent musculoskeletal injuries; user-centered design of environments, equipment, and procedures; and applications within the purview of the ADA.

Ergonomics-for-One

The term *ergonomics-for-one* was coined by McQuistion in 1993 and refers to designing to fit an individual, in this context, an individual with a disability. Instead of "fitting the task to the human" as in traditional ergonomics, the idea is to "fit the task to a particular individual," where fitting the task incorporates fitting the environment, equipment,

and process to the person. Although the use of the term is recent, the practice of ergonomics-for-one has been in existence since the origin of the fields of occupational and physical therapy. It is also an area in which the lay person has been known to create designs or home treatments for family members (Figure 1-3). It is, however, a relatively unusual application for many ergonomics practitioners.

In 1979, Cromwell wrote about the external influences impacting on occupational therapy. She stated:

> our original philosophy and focus when we were developing in the 20s: Human adaptive services to chronically ill people through the use of activities and settings for people who not only survive but also need to live! I believe our future function will be (remain) in this model, in the community, as generalists, acting in the role of the catalyst for helping patients/people solve increasingly complex problems of functioning in a highly technical society (Cromwell, 1979, p. 39).

The model of occupational therapy in the 1920s was to provide adaptive services for people who experienced an injury or illness, that is, to provide therapeutic activities to increase their abilities and

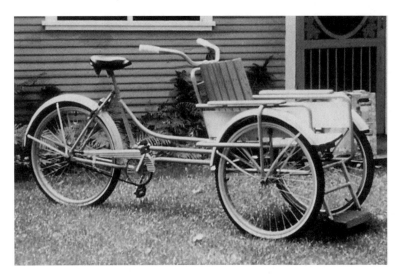

Figure 1-3. Homemade human factors: bicycle with front wheelchair attached. (Photograph courtesy of Susan Hallbeck, Ph.D., C.P.E.)

to provide environments in which they could continue to function as productive members of an evolving technological society. The vast majority of an occupational therapist's work took place in health care settings; however, once a patient had attained maximal functional capabilities, therapists did not say good-bye at the clinic door. They followed their patients into their homes and work sites. Typically, follow-up through planning for discharge, during follow-up consultation, or in making adaptations to work-oriented equipment in the clinic setting. Unfortunately, the direct relationship between therapeutic activity and occupation blurred during the push toward objective and scientific methodology following World War II. This occurred even though certain therapists were vigilant in reminding occupational therapists of their primary work-oriented knowledge base: occupation (Wiemer, 1979).

In the 1970s therapists were encouraged to practice in alternative sites such as housing, day care centers, schools, industry, workshops, prisons, and the community (Wiemer, 1979). Also during the 1970s, basic educational requirements for occupational therapists included the design of assistive equipment. Students were required to identify a patient's needs for adaptive equipment. The student then constructed the equipment, observed the patient's use of the equipment, and made adaptations to the equipment accordingly. Therapists provided consultation on assistive devices, redesign in the home or work environment, and reorganizing

tasks in order to ensure the highest possible functional capabilities for the individual patient.

Ergonomics-for-one, designing for the individual, is not new. However, technological advances have resulted in a level of dependence on specialists (designers and suppliers) for much of the assistive equipment used today, rather than therapists designing and constructing it themselves. In addition, persons with other backgrounds such as human factors/ergonomics, engineering, psychology, and computer technology realize they have much to offer in health care and rehabilitation. The field of rehabilitation engineering, for example, is made up of engineers who specialize in applying their technological skills to rehabilitation. No one field of study can claim exclusive rights to helping individuals. Thus, practitioners in many fields are contributing to designs for specific individuals who need assistance to achieve functional independence.

Ergonomics-for–Special Groups

As implied by its designation, *ergonomics-for–special groups* refers to designing for particular categories of people, rather than for a large range of people (as in traditional ergonomics) or designing for an individual (as in ergonomics-for-one).

Particular groups with special needs include children, the elderly, and those with permanent or semipermanent functional disabilities. Little research has been done to define the capabilities, limitations, and characteristics of the people in these diagnostic categories. Therefore, several approaches to defining the population in order to initiate the design process are suggested. Research and descriptive studies could be conducted on the groups as they are currently categorized, or they could be recategorized by diagnosis or functional abilities. A further possibility would be to group them first according to their diagnosis and then subdivide each diagnostic category into subcategories such as those with active, progressive diseases (multiple sclerosis, scleroderma, and arthritis) and those with nonprogressive injuries (spinal cord injury, quadra- or paraplegia, or traumatic brain injury). Only when descriptive information and performance information have been gathered on these special categories can ergonomic design be successfully implemented.

Descriptive information useful for ergonomic design includes anthropometry, reach, and range of motion. Useful performance information includes functional measures of grasp, strength, mobility, stamina (fatigue), vision, auditory perception, and cognitive function. The information necessary to describe each group would depend on the human capabilities affected by the disability or disease process. For example, the reach envelope of wheelchair users will differ according to their injury. The level of spinal cord injury will influence a wheelchair user's trunk stability and ability to lean forward or to the side. Traumatic bilateral amputation of the legs will also affect the trunk stability of a person in a wheelchair, but in a different manner than a spinal cord injury. If the patient has multiple sclerosis or has had a stroke, muscle weakness may be present in other areas of the body, and this can affect reach. Floyd's (1966) landmark research on the functional reach of wheelchair users diagrammed comfortable and maximal reach envelopes. Maximal reach required trunk stability and full trunk mobility. Although Pheasant's 1986 text presented anthropometric dimensions, these are not necessarily accurate for all diagnostic categories.

Some descriptive data and design for special groups have been reported, especially for the aging population. The elderly have received special attention in recent years, such as the compilation of anthropometric data shown in Table 1-1. This focus is partially due to the increased size of that population in our society and the consequent monetary support for such research. However, much remains to be done.

In terms of the disabled population, most research has been done with specific individuals, as case studies. The dearth of information in this is attributable, at least in part, to (1) a reluctance to collect information due to the unproven hypothesis that these groups have greater individual differences than the "normal" population, (2) lack of monetary support for the necessary research, and (3) the separation of clinical treatment from ergonomic design.

Industrial Intervention: Musculoskeletal Ergonomics

Musculoskeletal ergonomics involves the prevention of work-related musculoskeletal disorders (also known as *cumulative trauma disorders*), as described in the Occupational Safety and Health Administration's (OSHA) draft documents (1992, 1995), in the OSHA Guide for the Meatpacking Industry (OSHA, 1990), and by the National Institute for Occupational Safety and Health (1997). Musculoskeletal ergonomic programs include

- Analysis through techniques such as surveillance, work-site evaluation, task analysis, and sampling
- Problem identification, prioritization, and solution proposals
- Solution implementation through design of products and processes
- Work injury management, including early identification and treatment of persons with work-related injuries
- Education and training
- Testing for efficacy of the program

For many therapists, this area of application is the only area of ergonomics with which they are familiar. Part of the role of a rehabilitation practitioner is to provide patient education about his or her condition: what may have precipitated the condition; what may cause additional problems or an exacerbation of the symptoms; the course of treatment and possible course of the disease, illness, or injury; and home treatment programs they can administer for themselves. Therefore, it is obvious

Table 1-1. Available Anthropometric Data on the Elderly: Means and Standard Deviations

Age range (yrs) / Sample size	50–100[a] / 822	60–69[b] / 43	60–69[c] / 72	65–69[d] / 24	65–74[e] / 72	65–90[f] / 184	66–70[a] / 169	70+[b] / 12	70+[d] / 20	70+[c] / 28	72–91[e] / 130	75–84[e] / 40
Stature, against wall	—	172.8 (6.6)	—	171.9 (6.6)	—	—	—	171.5 (9.0)	170.4 (7.5)	—	—	—
Stature, free standing	157.1 (8.9)	—	172.6 (6.4)	171.2 (6.6)	—	169.0 (7.0)	—	—	169.6 (7.6)	171.9 (8.4)	168.4 (5.3)	—
Sitting height	79.9 (5.3)	90.8 (3.0)	90.8 (2.9)	90.0 (2.9)	—	—	—	89.5 (3.5)	89.0 (3.4)	89.8 (3.9)	88.3 (3.1)	—
Knee height	—	53.9 (2.5)	53.6 (2.5)	—	—	—	—	53.5 (3.4)	53.2 (2.9)	53.7 (3.2)	53.8 (2.1)	—
Trunk height	—	—	61.4 (2.6)	—	—	—	—	—	—	60.5 (2.8)	57.3 (3.2)	—
Popliteal height	42.1 (3.5)	—	42.1 (2.3)	—	—	—	—	—	—	42.1 (3.0)	44.0 (2.1)	—
Thigh height	—	—	19.7 (1.4)	—	—	—	—	—	—	14.8 (1.2)	—	—
Abdominal depth	—	—	25.7 (3.1)	—	—	—	—	—	—	26.5 (2.8)	27.5 (3.4)	—
Elbow breadth	—	—	7.2 (0.4)	7.2 (0.4)	—	—	—	—	7.2 (0.4)	7.2 (0.4)	—	—
Hip breadth	37.4 (3.9)	—	—	36.0 (2.3)	—	—	—	—	35.8 (1.7)	37.8 (2.4)	—	—
Bideltoid breadth	—	—	45.3 (2.4)	45.1 (2.1)	—	—	—	—	44.7 (1.6)	45.0 (1.7)	43.4 (2.3)	—
Bi-iliac breadth	—	—	29.7 (1.7)	29.7 (1.6)	—	—	—	—	30.0 (1.6)	30.2 (1.7)	31.2 (1.7)	—
Biacromial breadth	—	—	38.9 (1.7)	—	—	—	—	—	—	39.2 (1.8)	37.8 (1.6)	—
Upper chest breadth	—	—	23.9 (2.1)	24.0 (2.1)	—	—	—	—	24.4 (1.5)	24.3 (1.9)	24.3 (2.0)	—
Chest breadth	—	—	30.0 (2.2)	—	—	—	—	—	—	30.0 (1.6)	29.6 (2.1)	—
Face breadth	—	14.2 (0.5)	14.2 (0.5)	14.2 (0.5)	—	—	—	—	14.2 (0.5)	14.3 (0.5)	14.1 (1.9)	—
Hand breadth	7.7 (0.6)	—	8.5 (0.4)	8.5 (0.4)	—	—	—	—	8.5 (0.4)	8.6 (0.4)	8.4 (0.4)	—

Age range (yrs)	50–100[a]	60–69[b]	60–69[c]	65–69[d]	65–74[e]	65–90[f]	66–70[a]	70+[b]	70+[d]	70+[c]	72–91[e]	75–84[e]
Sample size	822	43	72	24	72	184	169	12	20	28	130	40
Head breadth	—	—	15.5 (0.5)	15.5 (0.5)	—	—	—	—	15.5 (0.5)	15.5 (0.4)	15.4 (0.5)	—
Nose breadth	—	—	3.7 (0.3)	3.7 (0.2)	—	—	—	—	3.8 (0.3)	3.8 (0.3)	—	—
Foot breadth	—	—	9.8 (0.6)	—	—	—	—	—	—	9.9 (0.5)	10.0 (0.5)	—
Seat breadth	—	—	36.0 (2.2)	—	—	—	—	—	—	36.4 (2.0)	—	—
Wrist breadth (R)	—	—	59.0 (3.0)	—	—	—	—	—	—	5.9 (0.2)	—	—
Head circumference	—	—	57.1 (1.4)	57.1 (1.3)	—	—	—	—	85.0 (1.4)	57.4 (1.6)	56.9 (1.8)	—
Calf circumference	—	—	35.9 (2.5)	36.0 (2.9)	—	—	—	—	34.7 (2.1)	35.3 (2.2)	34.3 (2.7)	—
Chest circumference, resting	—	—	99.6 (7.1)	99.9 (6.3)	—	—	—	—	99.6 (5.5)	99.7 (5.9)	96.2 (7.6)	—
Chest circumference, maximum	—	—	101.8 (6.9)	101.7 (6.1)	—	—	—	—	101.5 (5.4)	101.7 (5.7)	98.7 (7.4)	—
Chest circumference, minimum	—	—	97.6 (7.2)	97.5 (6.5)	—	—	—	—	97.8 (5.6)	97.9 (6.0)	94.5 (7.6)	—
Upper arm circumference	—	—	30.9 (2.7)	30.5 (2.6)	—	—	—	—	30.0 (2.4)	28.7 (2.8)	—	—
Waist circumference	—	—	95.5 (9.3)	97.4 (8.9)	—	—	—	—	7.1 (8.0)	97.0 (7.6)	—	—
Head length	—	—	19.6 (0.6)	19.6 (0.6)	—	—	—	—	19.5 (0.6)	19.7 (0.7)	19.7 (0.6)	—
Hand length	17.5 (1.2)	—	18.9 (0.9)	18.9 (0.9)	—	—	—	—	18.8 (0.9)	19.0 (1.0)	18.8 (0.8)	—
Ear length	—	—	7.2 (0.4)	7.2 (0.4)	—	—	—	—	7.3 (0.4)	7.3 (0.4)	7.5 (0.5)	—
Buttock-knee length	—	—	58.6 (3.0)	—	—	—	—	—	—	58.4 (3.2)	59.1 (2.4)	—
Buttock-popliteal length	46.3 (3.6)	—	48.2 (2.8)	—	—	—	—	—	—	48.1 (3.1)	47.2 (2.5)	—
Elbow to middle finger length	44.2 (2.8)	—	46.8 (2.0)	46.8 (1.9)	—	—	—	—	46.6 (2.5)	46.9 (2.8)	46.4 (1.8)	—

Table 1-1. *continued*

Age range (yrs)	50–100[a]	60–69[b]	60–69[c]	65–69[d]	65–74[e]	65–90[f]	66–70[a]	70+[b]	70+[d]	70+[c]	72–91[e]	75–84[e]
Sample size	822	43	72	24	72	184	169	12	20	28	130	40
Shoulder to elbow	—	—	37.3	37.4	—	—	—	—	37.0	37.4	36.9	—
			(1.8)	(1.7)					(2.1)	(2.2)	(1.7)	
Forward reach	—	—	84.2	—	—	—	—	—	—	85.9	86.9	—
			(3.7)							(5.4)	(3.8)	
Span	—	—	178.7	178.8	—	—	—	—	177.6	179.2	174.0	—
			(7.5)	(7.5)					(9.0)	(9.9)	(7.0)	
Span akimbo	—	—	93.5	93.5	—	—	—	—	92.7	93.4	90.6	—
			(3.9)	(3.8)					(4.5)	(4.8)	(3.9)	
Grip strength (left)	—	—	44 kg	—	—	—	32.9 kg	—	—	40 kg	26.7 kg	—
			(9.0)				(5.9)			(9.0)	(8.2)	
Grip strength (right)	—	—	47 kg	—	—	—	37.7 kg	—	—	42	28.8 kg	—
			(9.0)				(6.9)			(9.0)	(7.9)	
Skinfold (triceps) (R)	—	—	1.1	—	—	1.2	—	—	—	9.0	1.1	—
			(0.4)			(0.3)				(0.4)	(0.4)	
Skinfold (subscapular) (R)	—	—	1.7	—	—	—	—	—	—	1.5	1.6	—
			(0.8)							(0.7)	(0.7)	
Foot height	—	—	26.3	26.4	—	—	—	—	26.5	26.8	26.0	—
			(1.2)	(1.2)					(1.3)	(1.4)	(1.0)	
Weight (kg)	63.7	—	76.6	76.4	65.6	63.7	—	—	74.3	75.3	69.0	63.7
			(1.1)	(1.0)	(11.6)				(0.9)	(9.0)	(10.5)	(11.7)

Note: All measures in centimeters except weight measurements.
[a]Molenbroek, 1987 (average of males and females; data from the Netherlands).
[b]Borkan, Hults, & Glynn, 1983 (males only).
[c]Damon et al., 1972 (males only).
[d]Friedlander et al., 1977 (males only).
[e]Dwyer et al., 1987 (average of males and females).
[f]Pearson, Bassey, & Bendall, 1985 (average of males and females).
Source: Reprinted with permission from P.L. Kelly, & K.H.E. Kroemer. (1990). Anthropometry of the elderly: Status and recommendations. *Human Factors, 32,* 571–595.

that therapists and other rehabilitation personnel have been educating persons about work-related musculoskeletal disorders as long as such disorders have required rehabilitative intervention. For occupational therapists, task analysis is an integral portion of their basic education, because the breakdown of tasks into their component parts is essential to being able to use activity as part of the treatment process. Education, training, and rehabilitative treatment are within the traditional purview of rehabilitation practitioners. However, analysis of the work environment, surveillance, advanced design, and efficacy testing may have to be learned subsequent to most therapists' entry level education. Musculoskeletal ergonomics is considered an advanced specialty for therapists.

Musculoskeletal ergonomics is covered under the general topic of industrial ergonomics within most human factors/ergonomic curriculums. The depth and breadth of information provided may depend on the university program and the student's chosen specialty area; however, all students are exposed to the basic elements of industrial ergonomics and, therefore, musculoskeletal ergonomics. Students also receive considerable education in analysis, design, principles of training, and research. The area of knowledge they may be lacking is that of medical management, treatment, and the rehabilitation return-to-work processes.

The mental components of work are also considered in ergonomic application in a work site, which represents another area of overlap between ergonomists and health care professionals, both of whom work equally with the psychological and cognitive aspects of performance. Occupational therapists, nurses, psychologists, physicians, and physician assistants are some of the health care professionals who work with both physical and mental patient performance issues. Health care professionals are concerned with the effects of the stressors on the individual's work and their emphasis is the effect on the individual worker's health, family, and overall functioning. As health care providers, they typically provide treatment and suggest coping mechanisms for individuals working in high-stress environments. Ergonomists are primarily concerned with task demands, performance, and potential human error that can result in injury or decreased product quality. Examples of ergonomic research in this area have targeted groups working long hours under stress, such as medical residents, shift workers, aviators, military personnel, and air traffic controllers. The examples demonstrate that the ergonomist's approach to industrial intervention typically includes analysis and design issues that therapists may not include in their prevention of work-related musculoskeletal disorders.

User-Centered Equipment Design

The process of considering the end user in each phase of product development is the purpose of user-centered equipment design. Typically this means professional involvement in the analysis, planning, development, design, evaluation, implementation, and testing of new products. It involves usability testing of new or existing products and processes. Much of the evaluation of lower technology medical equipment is left to the discretion of the manufacturer. Little has been done to ensure ergonomic input into the design and evaluation of rehabilitation equipment, in terms of efficacy testing, ergonomic design principles, or user preference and acceptance. There is no federal program to support, nor are there specifications for, human factors/ergonomics in medical equipment design, such as exist for military systems (Bogner, 1996b).

An important aspect of user-centered design is the evaluation of equipment, processes, training, and instruction manuals for the purpose of preventing human error. According to a Harvard Medical Practice Study, roughly 100,000 preventable deaths occur to hospitalized patients per year (Leape, 1994). As Bogner (1996b) pointed out, this is twice the annual highway death rate, and the cost of preventable adverse events is approximately $25 billion (Bogner, 1994). The number of nonfatal injuries can be assumed to be far greater than the number of deaths, which makes this a far-reaching, serious issue.

Educational programs in ergonomics cover the design principles and research techniques necessary for user-centered evaluation to prevent human error. Experience in consumer product evaluation may be covered either in an experiential learning environment or by participation in sponsored research; however, the evaluation of medical or rehabilitation equipment within ergonomic curriculums is the exception rather than the rule. User-centered design and usability testing are not covered in rehabilitation curriculums. (In other contexts, *usability testing* traditionally refers to the evaluation of computer software.)

Americans with Disabilities Act

Implementation of the ADA (U.S. Department of Justice, 1991, 1992) should involve professionals from both design and health care fields. Existing transportation systems, housing, public buildings and parks, communication systems, work settings, and job interview procedures are some of the items that must be considered for redesign to accommodate individuals with disabilities. In turn, development of new systems and environments must include pertinent considerations in accordance with the ADA. Design professionals, such as engineers, ergonomists, industrial designers, and city planners are obviously necessary for this process. The involvement of health care personnel is also needed to help designers determine the potential capabilities and limitations of the user populations. Health care professionals also bring an awareness of assistive devices, disease progression, and emotional reactions to or symptoms of a disease. This knowledge allows them to contribute potential methods for designing environments and educating coworkers to minimize negative effects on the individual with a disability, as well as on the total work environment. Ergonomists are needed to ensure the newer improved design fits the individual or special groups in terms of ease of use and effectiveness.

Although many employers have indicated concern about the high cost of accommodating individuals with disabilities, 68% of accommodations are reported to cost $500 or less and 84% to cost $1,500 or less (Sanders, 1997). The roles that a health care or rehabilitation ergonomist might assume and the legal ramifications of consultation are covered in Section VI of this text. However, the reader is assumed to have a working knowledge of the ADA; for further information see the references listed in Section VI.

Work Hardening

Although work hardening is not considered to be a part of the field of ergonomics because of its thera-peutic nature, designing or identifying work tasks that will not exacerbate or contribute to work-related musculoskeletal disorders is accomplished by both ergonomists and health care professionals. (*Work-related musculoskeletal disorders* is considered synonymous with *cumulative trauma disorders* and injuries, but it is considered a more descriptive and all-encompassing term.) Identification of such tasks is part of comprehensive musculoskeletal ergonomics programs as described in OSHA's draft document (1992) and in the NIOSH (1997) publication on the elements of ergonomics programs. Task analysis may also be part of a work-hardening or return-to-work therapeutic process.

Work hardening is essentially the provision of clinically based work simulation, graded in levels of difficulty to help increase a patient's functional work-related abilities. The Commission on Accreditation of Rehabilitation Facilities (1989) defines work hardening as

> a highly structured, goal-oriented, individualized treatment program designed to maximize the individual's ability to return-to-work. The programs use the conditioning tasks that are graded progressively to improve the biomechanical, neuromuscular, cardiovascular, and psychosocial functions with real or simulated work activities.

Work hardening can also include increasingly difficult work assignments outside a clinical setting, with the ultimate goal of enabling patients to resume their original work tasks. Part of this process is to identify jobs and job tasks that are less demanding or have the fewest risk factors for work-related musculoskeletal disorders, related to the patient diagnosis. Should patients never reach their preinjury or illness status, the goal is to maximize their capabilities so they may return to some form of work and continue to earn a living. Work hardening has primarily been used in terms of vocational work, rather than home or leisure pursuits. Use of the term *work hardening* developed in the 1980s; however, its origins can be traced to the early 1900s.

Terminology

In this text, the terms *health care ergonomist* and *rehabilitation ergonomist* are proposed to describe specialties in which the knowledge and techniques of human factors/ergonomics are applied to areas of overlapping interest between human factors professionals/ergonomists and health care/rehabilitation practitioners. The terms suggest that the practitioner is an ergonomist who has specialized in health care or rehabilitation, just as *hand therapist* is a term applied to therapists who have specialized in the evaluation and treatment of hands and *pediatric neurologist* refers to a neurologist who has specialized in the treatment of pediatric patients. The first word (i.e., *hand, pediatric*) is a descriptor for the second word (i.e., *therapist, neurologist*). This connotation strongly advises health care practitioners who specialize in these areas to become well versed in ergonomic concepts, principles, and applications as they will likely be considered ergonomists. Likewise, ergonomists expanding their practice into medical and rehabilitation applications will need to increase their knowledge in those areas, as they are now adding a qualifier to their professional practice.

Conclusion

Health care ergonomics and rehabilitation ergonomics are specialties whose time has come. As Muto (1996) pointed out, human factors/ergonomics is well known in the aerospace, nuclear power, personal computing, and consumer products industries. Ergonomics is not as well known in health care and rehabilitation. However, Muto (1996) identified several factors that may help to change this situation and encourage the rapid development of the application of ergonomics in health care and rehabilitation:

1. Health care providers' desire to lower personnel and training costs by using equipment that is usable and maintainable by lower skilled workers
2. Manufacturers' desire to minimize exposure to litigation involving mishaps with medical equipment
3. Manufacturers striving to gain increased market share by developing state-of-the-art user interfaces
4. Increased attention given to human factors by regulatory agencies such as the U.S. Food and Drug Administration

In an attempt to define the field, several component areas within health care and rehabilitation ergonomics

were emphasized in this text: ergonomics-for-one, ergonomics-for–special groups, musculoskeletal ergonomics, and user-centered design. An application that incorporates the principles and procedures described in several of these component areas is the implementation of the ADA, also covered in this text.

The interests and expertise of ergonomists as well as health care and rehabilitation practitioners complement one another, as do their bodies of knowledge. The blending of the two fields of knowledge within areas of mutual interest will inevitably benefit consumers of all ages and abilities. As the specialties of health care ergonomics and rehabilitation ergonomics evolve and expand, new terminology, descriptions, and procedures will emerge and be disseminated by and among the professionals who share this exciting adventure.

References

Bogner, M.S. (1994). *Human error in medicine: A frontier for change*. Hillsdale, NJ: Lawrence Erlbaum.

Bogner, M.S. (1996a). Special section preface. *Human Factors, 38,* 551–555.

Bogner, M.S. (1996b). Medical human factors. In *Proceedings of the Human Factors and Ergonomics Society 40th Annual Meeting* (pp. 752–753). Santa Monica, CA: Human Factors and Ergonomics Society.

Borkan, G.A., Hults, D.E., & Glynn, R.J. (1983). Role of longitudinal change and secular trend in age differences in male body dimensions. *Human Biology, 55,* 629–641.

Chapanis, A. (1991). To communicate the human factors message, you have to know what the message is and how to communicate it. *Human Factors Society Bulletin, 34,* 1–4.

Clement, F.J. (1974). Longitudinal and cross-sectional assessment of age changes in physical strength as related to sex, social class, and mental ability. *Journal of Gerontology, 29,* 423–429.

Commission on Accreditation of Rehabilitation Facilities. (1989). *Standards manual for organizations serving people with disabilities*. Tucson, AZ: Commission on Accreditation of Rehabilitation Facilities.

Cromwell, F. (1979). External influences impacting occupational therapy. In *Occupational Therapy 2001*. Presented at the special session of the representative assembly, November 1978. Available from Rockville, MD: American Occupational Therapy Association.

Damon, A., Seltzer, C.C., Stoudt, H.W., & Bell, B. (1972). Age and physique in healthy white veterans at Boston. *Journal of Gerontology, 27,* 202–208.

Dwyer, J.T., Coleman, K.A., Drall, E., et al. (1987). Changes in relative weight among institutionalized elderly adults. *Journal of Gerontology, 42,* 246–257.

Floyd, W.F. (1966). A study of the space requirements of wheelchair users. *Paraplegia, 4(1),* 24–37.

Friedlander, J.S., Costa, P.T., Bosse, R., et al. (1977). Longitudinal physique changes among healthy white veterans at Boston. *Human Biology, 49,* 541–558.

Gosbee, J. (1996). What is the role and direction of human factors and medicine research? *Medical Systems and Rehabilitation Technical Group Newsletter, 8(3),* 1–2.

Leape, L.L. (1994). The preventability of medical injury. In M.S. Bogner (Ed.), *Human error in medicine* (pp. 13–25). Hillsdale, NJ: Lawrence Erlbaum.

McQuistion, L. (1993, January). Rehabilitation engineering: Ergonomics for one. *Ergonomics in Design,* pp. 9–10.

Molenbroek, J.F.M. (1987). Anthropometry of elderly people in the Netherlands: Research and applications. *Applied Ergonomics, 18,* 187–199.

Muto, W.H. (1996). Human factors in the medical laboratory: A practitioner's view. In the Medical Human Factors Panel Review chaired by M.S. Bogner, *Proceedings of the Human Factors and Ergonomics Society, 40th Annual Meeting* (p. 755). Santa Monica, CA: Human Factors and Ergonomics Society.

National Institute for Occupational Safety and Health. (1997). *Elements of ergonomics programs.* Atlanta: Centers for Disease Control and Prevention, U.S. Department of Health and Human Services.

Occupational Safety and Health Administration. (1991). *Ergonomics program management guidelines recommendations for meatpacking plants.* OSHA 3123.

Occupational Safety and Health Administration. (1992). OSHA advance notice of proposed rule-making for ergonomic safety and health management. *Federal Register, 57(149),* 34192–34200.

Occupational Safety and Health Administration. (1995, March 13). *Draft ergonomics protection standard.* (First issued in *Federal Register, 57[149],* 34192–34200.)

Pearson, M.B., Bassey, E.J., & Bendall, M.J. (1985). Muscle strength and anthropometric indices in elderly men and women. *Age and Aging, 14,* 49–54.

Pheasant, S. (1986). *Bodyspace—anthropometry, ergonomics, and design.* London: Taylor & Francis.

Rappaport, M. (1970). Human factors applications in medicine. *Human Factors, 12,* 25–35.

Rappaport, M. (1975). Preface. R.M. Pickett, & T.J. Triggs (Eds.), *Human factors in health care* (pp. xvi–xxii). (A collection of papers presented at an international symposium held in Lisbon, Portugal, June 1974.) New York: Heath.

Rice, V. (1995). Ergonomics: An introduction. In K. Jacobs, & C. Bettencourt (Eds.), *Musculoskeletal ergonomics for therapists* (pp. 3–12). Boston: Butterworth–Heinemann.

Sanders, M.J. (1997). The individual worker perspective. In M.J. Sanders (Ed.), *Management of Cumulative Trauma Disorders* (pp. 11–20). Boston: Butterworth–Heinemann.

U.S. Department of Justice, Civil Rights Division, & Office of the Americans with Disabilities Act. (1991). *ADA highlights Title II state and local government services.* Washington, DC: Government Printing Office.

U.S. Department of Justice. (1992). *The Americans with Disabilities Act Title III technical assistance manual.* Washington, DC: Government Printing Office.

Weimer, R. (1979). Traditional and nontraditional practice arenas. In *Occupational Therapy 2001.* Presented at the special session of the representative assembly, November 1978. Rockville, MD: American Occupational Therapy Association.

Chapter 2

Evolution of Health Care and Rehabilitation Ergonomics

Ellen Rader Smith

Learning Objectives

On completion of this chapter, the reader should be able to

- Describe the professional, societal, and regulatory factors that contributed to growth and diversification of practice areas for ergonomic and health care practitioners.
- Explain how the growth and diversification of ergonomics and health care have precipitated new specialty applications: health care and rehabilitation ergonomics.

Key Words

Aging
Disabled
Ergonomics
Human capabilities
Injury prevention
Rehabilitation equipment
Workplace adaptation

Abstract

This chapter traces the development and growth of the health care, rehabilitation, and ergonomic professions and their areas of overlapping interest. Fostering maximal functional independence of patients and enabling patients to return to their work environment are basic goals of rehabilitation. However, historical development of the rehabilitation professions saw a shift of focus from a work-based to a medical model after World War II. Beginning in the 1970s, allied health professionals increasingly applied ergonomic principles in their daily clinical practice; they also began moving their practices from the clinic into community and industrial settings. The resultant practice of matching the work environment and tasks with the capabilities of the returning worker is consistent with the ergonomic goal of providing the best human-system, product, or environment interface.

Human factors/ergonomics evolved from a primarily military and industrial base of practice into areas such as consumer products, computer science, and health care. Ergonomists have identified health care as an area of interest for applied research and implementation of ergonomic principles. In addition to professional growth, external events such as the issuing of federal guidelines, changes in work practices, and monetary constraints have influenced the health care and rehabilitation professions and the field of ergonomics. The consequent specialty areas of health care ergonomics and rehabilitation ergonomics can benefit individuals and specific populations by combining medical and ergonomic knowledge bases and by applying that knowledge to overlapping areas.

Introduction

The practice of ergonomics has seen steady growth and widespread application since World

War II. As ergonomics has expanded beyond its early roots in the military into other industries and workplaces, specialty areas have developed. These specialty areas evolved through the need to apply basic ergonomic tenets, of human-job, human-product, or human-environmental fits, to many circumstances:

- In places such as schools, planned communities, hospitals, and workplaces
- To products such as specialized medical, rehabilitation or technical equipment, and consumer products
- To people with special needs, including the aging, the disabled, musicians and other performing artists, mothers with babies and young children, shift workers, and medical personnel who physically handle patients

Health care ergonomics and rehabilitation ergonomics are areas of growing interest for professionals in both health care and ergonomics. As part of the health care continuum and rehabilitation process, a common goal and desire for all individuals is maximal functional independence in personal care, homemaking, avocational, and work activities. The areas of health care and rehabilitation ergonomics can help facilitate this goal, as they build on a fundamental ergonomic goal of best fitting and accommodating job demands or product design to abilities of the intended users.

Health care and rehabilitation ergonomics are natural extensions of the therapist's role in further facilitating the injured person's return to work, helping accommodate disabled persons in the workplace, and applying medical/rehabilitation expertise to the design of equipment and products for special populations. In the long run, the same principles can facilitate the daily performance and well-being of able-bodied and well populations.

Health care and rehabilitation ergonomics are also natural extensions of human factors/ergonomics; the health care industry too can benefit from the application of ergonomic design principles. The importance of designing systems, physical plants and facilities, medical and rehabilitation equipment, procedures, and training for maximum comfort, ease-of-use, acceptability, and productivity, while decreasing human error and injury applies to all settings.

Evolution of Rehabilitation

Occupational, physical and speech therapists, rehabilitation nurses, and vocational specialists play critical roles in the rehabilitation of persons with acute or chronic injuries and illnesses. During patient care, medical personnel address all facets of daily living activities: personal care, homemaking, and avocational and vocational tasks. Traditionally, occupational and physical therapy has been directed toward rehabilitation: maximizing the abilities of an injured person to perform home or work activities. (Therapists in this field may be referred to as *rehabilitation therapists.*)

A fundamental occupational therapy goal is to "enhance the capacity [of the client or patient] throughout the life span, to perform with satisfaction to self and others those tasks and roles essential to productive living and to the mastery of self and the environment" (Hopkins, 1978, p. 27); and "to maximize independence, prevent disability and maintain health" (American Occupational Therapy Association, 1994). Basic physical therapy goals are to enhance movement and function, as well as prevent reinjury.

More recent goals for both occupational and physical therapy include the determination of fitness requirements for specific jobs and performance abilities based on specific job demands. Vocational rehabilitation goals vary with the client. Options, in descending preference, are returning the client to the same job, returning to the same job with modification, finding an alternate job using the client's skill base, or retraining the client for a new occupation.

In the early 1900s, occupational therapists were vocationally focused and performed industrial therapy, primarily for the mentally ill. Passage of the Vocational Rehabilitation Act or Smith-Fess Act of 1920 (Public Law 66-236) directed occupational therapists into the vocational arena, particularly to prevocational programs provided in sheltered and curative workshops that offered physical and psychological restoration (Kornblau, 1996). Passage of this act laid the foundation for vocational rehabilitation by vocational specialists and evaluators as it is known today, and rehabilitation was defined as "the return to remunerative employment" (Jacobs, 1985, p. 2).

After the World Wars, in particular World War II, therapists responded to the needs of injured military personnel for increased medical service to maximize function and minimize disability (Cromwell, 1985). Thus began the transition of therapists from a vocational to medical model of care. Additional federal legislation in the late 1940s and 1950s fostered the ongoing development and proliferation of vocational and prevocational programs, most of which had a psychiatric base (Kornblau, 1996). While interest was waning among clinicians in the 1960s and early 1970s (Cromwell, 1985), the important role of therapists in vocational rehabilitation was emphasized as an integral tenet of occupational therapy by Florence Cromwell's writings on work-related programming and Mary Reilly's (1962) references on occupational behavior. The Federal Rehabilitation Act of 1973 and its amendments, sections 503 and 504 of Title V, further emphasized the role of vocational rehabilitation. It is felt that the Act became a driving force in preventing employment discrimination against persons with physical and mental handicaps (Rahimi & Malzahn, 1988).

Ogden (1985) noted a renaissance in occupational therapy and a return to its roots in the 1970s and 1980s with the development of work tolerance screening, work capacity evaluation, and work hardening programs in occupational medicine and return-to-work programs. Occupational rehabilitation programs, such as the Workers' Evaluation and Rehabilitation Center at Loma Linda University, began to develop in the early 1980s, particularly in California. In 1980, the American Occupational Therapy Association (AOTA) issued its position paper in the Role of Occupational Therapy in the Vocational Rehabilitation Process (AOTA, 1980).

Ishernhagen (1991) described a parallel development in the role of the physical therapist in "work injury management" during the 1970s and the expanded role of many occupational and physical therapists in the patient's total rehabilitation since the 1980s. In her discussion of the therapist's work injury management role, Ishernhagen (1988, p. 332) contrasts the "rehabilitation therapist's role in *working with a patient until return home is possible* with the occupational medicine therapist's role in *patient care continuing until the return to work process is complete*." The latter treatment approach moves beyond treatment of a specific musculoskeletal problem or diagnosis, to the complete rehabilitation process that culminates with the injured worker attaining the required functional levels for return to work.

Reconstruction therapists were the forerunners of occupational and physical therapists. The reconstruction program was established to "accelerate the return to duty of convalescent patients in the highest state of physical and mental efficiency consistent with the capabilities and the type of duty to which they are being returned" (Occupational Therapy, 1944, p. 1). Physical therapists primarily provided physical reconditioning while occupational therapists used fine, applied, or industrial arts to help individuals in their rehabilitation from acute illness/injury to vocational training (Hopkins, 1978).

Early pioneers in the development of work evaluation, work conditioning, and work hardening programs included Leonard Matheson, Keith Blankenship, Dennis Hart, Susan Ishernhagen, Melanie Ellexson, and Glenda Key. Their industrial programs included interdisciplinary rehabilitation teams of occupational and physical therapists, vocational evaluators, rehabilitation counselors and psychologists. These programs enabled therapists to provide accurate information about whether patients were fit to safely return to work, based on their current functional status. The information gained from various functional-capacity and work assessments plus on-site job evaluations helped the patient, physician, supervisor, employer, and other involved persons obtain relevant job-related and physical capacities information to assist the transition from "injured person within a medical care system" to a "person returning to work with an injury or disability in a competitive workforce."

Role in Education and Injury Prevention

In dealing with the patient or client injured in an industrial setting, rehabilitation specialists realized that the occupational rehabilitation process needed to address work-related or job-specific factors that could contribute to injury or reinjury. In the late 1980s, therapists moved into a preventive role when they began providing industrial consultation as they noted work-related injury trends among several patients (similar work and similar injuries, for example). The goal of these interventions has been to eliminate or reduce injury-related causality factors, and to develop educational and preventive strategies for both the injured worker and key work-site personnel (Rice, 1995a). Practical ergonomic concepts became integrated into occupational rehabilitation intervention and education programs. Many of these concepts were not new to therapists, who found that they represented natural extensions of joint protection, energy conservation, preferred lifting techniques, and home modification techniques.

In traditional medical settings and industry, a therapist's role includes education as part of treatment and prevention programs. In the 1970s, physical therapists became active educators in back schools; many of their first students had sustained a previous injury. The goal was to provide self-empowering methods to prevent new or further back injury. The methods used to train workers in safe lifting techniques vary, even as the successes of these schools as a primary method of back injury prevention varied (Snook, 1988). The initial focus of training workers in proper material handling techniques and conditioning expanded to address workplace and musculoskeletal ergonomic concepts critical to injury prevention and safety. On-site analysis by therapists also increased in an effort to better understand the physical demands of the work being performed. By the 1990s, the role of therapists in education and prevention was well recognized, especially in prevention of upper extremity cumulative trauma and back injuries. The term *industrial therapists* has been used to specify therapists in occupational medicine whose practice is located at the work site.

While industrial rehabilitation programs were proliferating, wellness programs also began to grow, providing increased teaching opportunities for allied health professionals. These programs are directed at well persons who want to maintain physical, emotional, and total well-being, as well as preventing disease and associated dysfunction. Therapists have become involved in corporate on-site physical fitness programs and other behavior-oriented approaches to achieving and maintaining positive health, including cardiac fitness, smoking cessation, treatment of substance abuse, stress management, and self-responsibility for health (Mungai, 1985).

The role of therapists in occupational medicine has expanded, with the biggest growth seen in the prevention of work-related musculoskeletal injuries. As occupational and physical therapists, occupational health and rehabilitation nurses, rehabilitation engineers, and vocational specialists have increased their active industrial roles, and augmented their knowledge and application of ergonomic principles, the specialty practice area of health care ergonomics has begun to emerge.

Many therapists specializing in industrial or occupational medicine have referred to the complete industrial rehabilitation process as *rehabilitation ergonomics,* although their view was more limited than that defined by Rice in Chapter 1. Matheson et al. (1997, p. 223) defined this practice area as "the relationship between the functional limitations and abilities of a person with a disability and the demands of a valued job within the context of a work environment for the purpose of matching that person to that job." Reflective of this growing area of interest is the formation of the Ergonomic Research Society and the National Interdisciplinary Committee on Health Rehabilitation Ergonomics by health care practitioners in 1993 (Jacobs & Bettencourt, 1995). Many of these groups' founding members were also involved in helping to establish the Occupational Injury Prevention Rehabilitation Society in 1996. There is also now a forum on rehabilitation ergonomics that began in the November 1996 issue of *Work*.

As noted in the previous chapter, rehabilitation ergonomics is considered an application area within the broader field of health care ergonomics. Health care ergonomics can be applied to the design of all medically related consumer products and nearly all aspects of daily living, as evidenced in a recent book: *Ergonomic Living* (Inkeles & Schencke, 1994). The therapist's role in facilitating self-independence for the performance of self-care, homemaking, work, or avocational activities affords many opportunities to apply ergonomic principles. For example, therapists teach joint protection and energy conservation techniques for arthritic patients. These methods have a strong biomechanical foundation that is fundamental to basic ergonomic principles. When therapists build up handle grips to facilitate grip, this could also be viewed as modifying the handle to meet specific ergonomic tool design specifications, such as recommended circumference or length. These therapeutic interventions or ergonomic modifications can reduce the required grip effort, increase user comfort and endurance, and enhance overall productivity. Ergonomics-for-one, applying ergonomic concepts to a single user or worker, can be viewed as re-engineering a daily activity or job task, to best meet the needs of the user.

Similarly, occupational therapists, with their emphasis on functionality, have been educated to provide treatment by making long or built-up handles to increase reach distances for individuals with limited shoulder motion or hand strength or control. Such an intervention could be considered a low technology ergonomic improvement. However, when similar modifications are made on a larger scale, usability tested, and sold to consumer markets, this modified tool might be described as an *ergonomic reacher*. Several rehabilitation supply companies are now marketing their products to health care providers and the industrial marketplace at the same time by creating a second catalog that emphasizes different applications of the same product.

Evolution of Human Factors/Ergonomics

Although ergonomics has only recently become commonplace to many health and safety professionals and consumers, the concepts of ergonomics have been recognized for more than 200 years. In the 1700s, the physician Ramazzini described the negative health effects of work as follows:

> the cause I assign [to] certain violent and irregular motions and unnatural postures . . . by which . . . the natural structure of the living machine is so impaired that serious diseases generally develop (Tichauer, 1978, p. 1).

We can go back even further and consider how cave dwellers and tradesmen before the Industrial Revolution made their own tools that contoured to their hands, felt comfortable, and enabled them to perform optimally. Although not called *ergonomics* at the time, the design of objects and equipment to serve basic human survival needs in "natural" environments can be considered an application of ergonomics design principles (McCormick & Sanders, 1982). This differs from the one-size-fits-all tools found on store shelves today. These examples clearly illustrate that the ergonomic principle of adapting equipment to meet users' needs predates the twentieth century.

Phases in the Development of Ergonomics

Christensen (1987) classifies the history of ergonomics into two major periods. The first period, the Age of Tools, goes back to prehistoric humans who made their own simple shelters, tools, and utensils. The next major period, the Industrial Revolution, was discussed in three distinct phases: the Age of Machines, 1750–1870, the Age of Power, 1870–1945, and a New Age: Machines for Minds, 1945–?. The Age of Machines marked the initial transition from the use of tools to machines. Human factors specialists (ergonomists) at this time, were active in the textile industry and in developing the use of steam power.

The Age of Power was characterized by applications in transportation, agriculture, and industry with an emphasis on adapting people to their work through selection, classification, training, and adjustment of work schedules (Christensen, 1987). The time and motion studies performed in the early twentieth century by early industrial engineers (sometimes called *efficiency experts*), such as Frederick Taylor and the Gilbreths, were aimed at improving work efficiency through task analysis and design (Chaffin & Andersson, 1984). Jobs were broken into their smallest task elements (called "therblings," based on Gilbreth spelled backwards). These elements were then either redesigned, simplified, or rearranged using only necessary movements for more efficient task completion. The principles that resulted from these studies represent an important developmental aspect of human factors/ergonomics and are still taught and used today.

The time of greatest growth in human factors/ergonomics occurred during and immediately after World War II. At this time, technology and the human sciences were applied to the problems that arose from the use of complex military equipment (Dul & Weerdmeester, 1993). Complex aircraft, radar, and other equipment created difficulties for operator performance and maintenance (Chapanis, 1951, as cited by Rodgers, 1983), as "man became the weak link in the system" (Damon & Randall, 1944, as cited by Rice, 1995a, p. 7). The need was recognized for design improvements for aircraft control panels (which required rapid information processing, sequencing, memory, and recall) and for other military equipment to increase ease and efficiency of use and maintenance. The ongoing third phase of ergonomic development, a New Age: Machines for Minds, is characterized by continued efforts to use people when critical decision making is required, and to use machines when the required functions could be considered automatic mental processing (McCormick & Sanders, 1982). This led to an ergonomic premise of allowing humans to perform where their unique abilities are required for cognition, information processing, reasoning, and decision making, or when responses depend on the processing of sensory and perceptual information; whereas machines are used to perform repetitive, rote, and automated tasks.

The U.S. Department of Defense recognized that conventional techniques of selection, classification, and training were not always sufficient for the operation and maintenance of complex systems. In new product and process design, the capabilities and limitations of people had to be considered early in the design and throughout each phase of development, acquisition, and use. This demanded attention to human dimensions and varying capability levels. Multidisciplinary teams of psychologists, engineers, anthropologists, and physiologists were formed to address these equipment design and training issues. In Great Britain, scientists on these teams believed that the scientific study of working efficiency could also be important under peacetime conditions (Pheasant, 1991). The early work of these multidisciplinary teams was referred to as *human engineering* and *engineering psychology* (Rodgers, 1983).

Contemporary Ergonomics

Since World War II, human factors ergonomic applications have proliferated in nonmilitary areas such as manufacturing, communication, and transportation. From the 1970s on, there has been widespread recognition of the importance of considering human factors in the design of nearly all products used by humans. This includes buildings and communities, consumer products, health services, high- and low-technology medical equipment, computer software and design, recreation equipment and facilities, and production processes.

Ergonomics has its roots in the human and behavioral sciences and engineering fields, including anthropology, anatomy, physiology, kinesiology, psychology, toxicology, engineering, industrial design, information technology, and industrial management (Dul & Weerdmeester, 1993). Traditional definitions address the person-machine system and

matching the person-machine system, or the job, to the worker or the product to the user. This match is felt to optimize working efficiency, health and safety, comfort and ease of use (Pheasant, 1991). Grandjean (1985) considers ergonomics to be the study of human behavior in relation to work. In addressing equipment design intended for human use, Murrell (1965) addresses factors beyond the physical product dimensions that must be considered: the intended user population, how information is received and processed to enable task completion, the physical and mental demands of the task and equipment to be operated, and the amount of time needed to make decisions and initiate appropriate action. Similarly, Dainoff (1986) views ergonomics as an applied science that addresses the design of the total environment with humans in mind and the ergonomic design goal of optimizing the person-thing relationship or the *fit*.

Meister (1971) describes human factors ergonomics as the application of behavioral principles and data to engineering design to maximize the human contribution and effectiveness of the system in which the person participates. Common to these definitions is the premise of adapting and designing workplaces, job tasks, and duties based on human capabilities. We can see the evolution of a systems approach to ergonomics, which has moved beyond a dual-faceted approach (person-job, person-product) to a multifaceted approach, such as the human-system interface technology (Hendrick, 1996) that has also helped pave the way for health care applications.

The Human Factors and Ergonomics Society has several technical groups whose interests reflect an overlap between ergonomics and health care. The interest of its Medical Systems and Rehabilitation Technical Group is "to maximize the contribution of human factors to the quality of life for people who are functionally impaired and to the effectiveness of medical systems (e.g., devices, computers, and managers)" (Human Factors and Ergonomics Society, 1997, p. 30). The Technical Group on Aging is concerned with "meeting the emerging needs of older people and special populations in a wide variety of life settings" (Human Factors and Ergonomics Society, 1997, p. 25). The International Ergonomics Association formed its Rehabilitation Ergonomics Committee in 1993, and offered its first international symposium in 1994 (Kumar, 1996). Thus, as the evolution of health care and rehabilitation has given rise to interest in human factors/ergonomics, so the evolution of human factors/ergonomics has encouraged application of ergonomic principles in the health care arena.

External Influences on Rehabilitation and Ergonomics

Many events have occurred in the past 20 years that have influenced the role of health care professionals working in industry, as well as influencing the growth of particular aspects of ergonomics. These include Occupational Safety and Health Administration (OSHA) regulations and guidelines, National Institute of Occupational Safety and Health (NIOSH) and American National Standards Institute (ANSI) guidelines, increased workers' compensation costs and pressure from insurers, an increased aging population, passage of the Americans with Disability Act (ADA), the growth of disability management programs, directives from world health organizations, and increased general consumer and manufacturer knowledge about ergonomics. The treatment or intervention that has resulted from these influences includes medical, health, and ergonomic practice areas that often overlap.

The federal 1973 Vocational Rehabilitation Act prompted employment opportunities for disabled individuals. Passage of the 1990 ADA was cornerstone legislation in expanding employment opportunities for the disabled. The reasonable accommodation process required by employers under Title I of the ADA can include adaptations of workplaces for the disabled. Provision of such reasonable accommodations seeks to bridge gaps between current job requirements and the worker's capabilities (McQuistion, 1993). Applying ergonomics in the design of work environments has helped to remove potential or existing incompatibilities in the human-machine work environment or person-job fit. This has resulted in more accessible workplaces for both disabled and able-bodied populations. In the past, health professionals may not have realized they were integrating ergonomic concepts in their rehabilitation role. It is now possible to say that many clinicians are consciously applying ergonomics as part of the total rehabilitation process.

At the same time the ADA was passed, the United Nations addressed the role of ergonomics in meeting the current and future needs of a growing number of aging, impaired, disabled, and disabled senior citizens, consumers, and workers (Kumar, 1992a). The World Health Organization established its World Program of Action to identify the issues faced by an aging population. These issues include the primary prevention of mental, physical, and sensory impairments; the rehabilitation of impaired persons; and equalization of opportunities for handicapped persons. In Mital and Karwowski's (1988) discussion of the role of ergonomics in rehabilitation, they view rehabilitation as a process of recognizing functional limitations of people with disabilities and designing the external environment around these limitations to benefit a given individual and society as a whole. In restoring disabled workers to productive and rewarding employment, ergonomic interventions help expand the employment opportunities for special populations by considering their specific needs.

Since 1980, NIOSH and OSHA have increased their attention to the development and prevention of musculoskeletal injuries in the workplace. NIOSH published its *Work Practices Guide for Manual Lifting* (1981) and revised it in 1994 to reflect more current information related to the prevention of back injuries. OSHA has issued citations under the General Duty Clause, Section 5 (a)(1) of the Occupational Health and Safety Act of 1970 to employers in the meatpacking, poultry, automotive, and manufacturing sectors who maintain unsafe workplaces that affect the health and safety of their employees. As a result of ergonomic issues uncovered during these citations, OSHA began an ergonomic rule-making process that continues to the present. These guidelines are intended to assist employers, as well as safety and health professionals, in providing safer workplaces that integrate ergonomic principles directed at injury prevention, worker comfort, and worker health.

In 1990, OSHA issued *Ergonomic Program Management Guidelines for Meatpacking Plants*, its first guidelines to address the identification and control of escalating rates of cumulative trauma disorders in the red meat industry. This document reviewed the elements that an ergonomic program might include: work-site analysis, hazard prevention and control, medical management, and training and education. This document became a stepping-stone for the development of OSHA's draft *Ergonomic Protection Standard* (1995, March), which would apply to all industries and the passage of California OSHA's *Repetitive Motion Injuries Standard* (1996, November).

In the late 1980s and early 1990s, several states introduced ergonomic legislation related to the use of video display terminals and their effect on the health and performance of their users. Some states issued guidelines (NJ Department of Health, 1989). On the local level, the *San Francisco Video Display Terminal Ordinance* (1990, December) was passed, as were VDT laws in Suffolk County, NY (1988), but both were overturned shortly after being enacted. The European community has also been actively involved in developing ergonomic standards, such as the International Standards Organization's current writing of its 17-part *ISO 9241, Ergonomic Requirements for Office Work with VDTs* (Williams, 1997).

American National Standards Institute (ANSI) has a subcommittee of ergonomic and health professionals, representatives from industry and labor, that have been working together since 1991 to develop their Z-365 standard, *Control of Work-Related Cumulative Trauma Disorders, Part I: Upper Extremities*. Both OSHA's ergonomic guidelines and ANSI's Cumulative Trauma Disorders (CTD) standard address the identification and control of injury-related work factors, job and workstation analysis and design, surveillance, training, and medical management. The medical management of work-related musculoskeletal disorders is a natural link where health care ergonomics can be applied to individuals or groups of individuals. Effective medical management requires a joint effort between health professionals in traditional and work-site settings, along with industrial safety, human resource, labor, and management personnel. Medical management also includes addressing ergonomic issues at home and work throughout the treatment continuum. Although the primary goals of ergonomic guidelines are to promote safety and health, another important goal is to reduce the direct medical and associated indirect financial costs associated with work-related injures. The cost-containment issue is often a driving force to help the total ergonomics team work together.

ANSI has been involved in other ergonomic-related standards, such as ANSI/HFS 100-1988, *Human Factors Engineering of Video Display Terminal Workstations*. This 1988 standard is being revised to reflect new findings and will include reference postures—rather than one recommended posture (the familiar series of 90 degree links)—and a section entitled *Working Environment and Systems Integration* (CTD News, 1997). In 1980, ANSI issued ANSI 117.1-1980, *Specifications of Making Buildings and Facilities Accessible to and Usable by Physically Handicapped People*. This issue is also addressed under Title II and III of the ADA, along with the accessibility of public transportation systems. These guidelines and legislation are additional examples of regulations that enable health care, vocational, and ergonomic specialists to work together in increasing building and transportation access for disabled populations.

OSHA, NIOSH, and ANSI guidelines; proposed and passed national and local legislation; passage of the ADA; and rising workers' compensation costs are among the factors influencing the rapid growth of ergonomics and subspecialty areas of health care and rehabilitation ergonomics. Disabled populations and able-bodied persons have benefited from the application of fundamental ergonomic principles to nearly all aspects of daily living.

Complementary Efforts

Ergonomics professionals and industrial rehabilitation specialists clearly share many complementary goals and processes. Achieving optimal worker performance by maximizing the fit between workers and their jobs is one such shared goal. In contrast to the primary rehabilitation goal of *helping individuals adapt* to given environments or situations, the primary goal of ergonomics is to modify the job, process, tool, or environment to meet or *adapt to the worker's needs* (Rader Smith, 1989). Both rehabilitation and ergonomics professionals advocate education, training, and worker participation in ergonomics programs, to help individuals to adapt. Ergonomics emphasizes design issues such as modifying activities or job tasks to accommodate human abilities (and limitations), and the process of tool, equipment, or environmental modification can be applied to meet specific needs of a population or an individual. In

Table 2-1. Rehabilitation and Ergonomics Compared

Rehabilitation	Ergonomics
Promote health	Ensure comfort
Prevent disability	Maintain well-being
Prevent dysfunction	Reduce/eliminate hazards
Relieve pain	Avoid pain
Restore function	Achieve effectiveness
Enable skill development	Arrange training
Adapt environment	Suggest job modification
Compensate for deficits using augmentative devices	Identify enabling devices and adjustments
Counsel social adjustment	Foster industrial relations

Source: S. Kumar. (1992a). Rehabilitation: An ergonomic dimension. *International Journal of Industrial Ergonomics, 9,* 101.

comparing several practice issues between ergonomics and rehabilitation, Kumar (1992b) found similar building blocks and goals for each area, as identified in Table 2-1.

The nature of work has significantly changed in the past 20 years. It has become more technical and specialized. Automation and the use of material handling equipment have eliminated much of the human effort from industrial workplaces. Computers are an integral part of many people's work. These changes, while enhancing overall productivity in the workplace, have been associated with some negative health effects, such as work-related musculoskeletal disorders (WRMDs), also known as *cumulative trauma disorders*, and psychological stress. Corporate downsizing can further increase the workload on employees who are generally already working to capacity. The U.S. Bureau of Labor Statistics reported approximately 332,000 cases of WRMDs in 1994. WRMDs were associated with an $11 billion price tag when direct medical and indirect costs of overtime, employee retraining, and production losses were considered (CTD News, 1996). Cost-conscious executive and risk managers realize that paying average WRMD injury costs of $3,000–$5,000 per incident is not a wise business practice. Workers' compensation insurance carriers are also motivated to curb these escalating costs. Spending money to positively affect change has led to the growth of work-injury management programs, occupational

health, industrial medicine, and proactive ergonomic programs.

Neglecting fundamental ergonomic principles increases the chances of incompatibility among various links in the total work production system and cycle, and results in system failures. Consistent with a safety and engineering approach, proactive ergonomic programs are being implemented, as part of the development and continuous improvement process, rather than as a quick fix to an identified problem. Whereas "ergonomics was once thought of as something nice to do, . . . now it's more often seen as something necessary to do" (Pulat & Alexander, 1991, p. 4). More data are becoming available supporting the theory that development of a constructive corporate attitude and awareness of ergonomics can help reduce workers' compensation costs, and that making ergonomic changes can positively affect worker behavior, health, and productivity, and an organization's profitability (Oxenburgh, 1991). Examples of collaborative and overlapping practice areas for ergonomics and rehabilitation are discussed in this section.

Health Promotion Programs

Health promotion programs have gained increased popularity in corporate America. In Pelletier's review of the health and cost benefits of 24 health promotion and industrial injury prevention programs surveyed between 1980 and 1991 (Kenny, Powell, & Reynolds-Lynch, 1995), he concluded that all the programs showed positive health and cost benefits. He also found reduced rates of employee absenteeism and turnover, productivity enhancements, and increased company allegiance. In today's results-oriented and managed health care delivery society, proactive programs are critical to reduce costs to employers, insurers, and injured workers.

Injury Prevention and Work Injury Management

Work injury management programs that facilitate the return to work of injured workers have proliferated since the 1980s. These programs include early identification and treatment, regular surveillance of the work site, and accurate record keeping, all of which require knowledge of symptomatology and a methodical system to identify personnel who are either at risk for developing symptoms or have initial symptoms commensurate with a WRMD. A combined effort between persons experienced in health care and ergonomics is needed.

"The application of ergonomics to preventive medicine" with the goal of preventing injuries through the application of ergonomic principles has been addressed by Pheasant in *Ergonomics, Work and Health* (1991, p. 5). WRMD injury prevention would include programs using education, training, and work-site evaluation. Surveillance conducted as part of the work injury management process could identify high-risk work areas, and thus help target injury prevention programs. A combined effort between persons experienced in health care and ergonomics can best implement these programs, which directly follow guidelines provided by OSHA's draft *Ergonomic Protection Standard* (1995, March 13) and ANSI's Z-365 standard, *Control of Work-Related Cumulative Trauma Disorders, Part I: Upper Extremities* (1996).

Health care personnel experienced in the evaluation and treatment of persons with occupational injuries are essential in returning these clients to work. Historically, the focus of rehabilitation efforts has been functional restoration and deficit compensation for persons who have suffered impairment. Today, rehabilitation efforts have broadened: Once functional restoration has been achieved, external factors at home or work are considered as part of the return to maximal function.

Industrial rehabilitation includes a natural progression from acute care treatment to restoring work capabilities to their maximum (using work capacity testing, work hardening, work conditioning, and counseling), followed by on-site intervention to complete the return-to-work process. Work-site adaptations must be considered when using graded activities to accomplish the return, or when a returning worker's capabilities are less than those required in a particular job. Work-site evaluation and intervention for an individual (also known as *ergonomics-for-one* or *reasonable accommodations*) can include modifying the workstation, tools, equipment, work load, work methods or pace, or environment to enable the best possible worker-job match and to minimize differences between a worker's current capacities and job demands. This process helps ensure a return to work with minimal

or no symptom exacerbation, which is an extremely important consideration because many injured or disabled persons may still have an impairment after even the best rehabilitation efforts. The skills and roles of health care providers and ergonomists complement each other in this process.

In the areas of evaluation and treatment, many therapists already integrate ergonomic principles into their clinical practice. Therapists are trained to understand the internal factors affecting human behavior and performance for healthy and disabled populations. To enable the successful application of ergonomics, therapists must become more familiar with factors beyond the individual client's control, such as total environment, the workplace and its organizational structure, and external motivating factors. To begin or further apply ergonomics, therapists need to become more cognizant of the work their patients perform, the postures and motions required of them, and any causal relationships between workplace risk factors and their medical conditions (Pheasant, 1991). The goal of this process is to provide therapists with a better understanding of the dynamic work environment and how it may have contributed to the patient's current condition, or how it could be affected on return to work. The therapist needs to work with trained ergonomists or engineers, who can then design and implement needed changes in the workplace, or obtain further knowledge and skills themselves on the way to becoming health care ergonomists. However, a therapist's understanding of the worker's functional limitations or those created by specific conditions is a skill set that ergonomists may not have, as their education is not within the medical or rehabilitation arena. Thus, the ergonomist looks to the therapist or health care practitioner for guidance. The collaborative work relationship established in this effort allows for the design or modification of workplaces and processes to facilitate the performance of injured or disabled workers. Often this benefits the abilities of nondisabled workers as well. The multidisciplinary team approach for return-to-work programs has been successful in reducing overall health care costs, as demonstrated in occupational rehabilitation models that include physical and occupational therapists, rehabilitation and vocational specialists, exercise physiologists, psychologists, and ergonomists (Mayne & Sawyer, 1994). This approach enables therapists, ergonomists, and other team members to address factors internal and external to a case for optimal results. Incompatibility between internal and external factors can lead to breakdowns in the worker-workplace interface, which may then result in physical-workplace system failures or worker injuries.

Disability Management Programs

Disability management programs have also proliferated in the past decade, in an attempt to control costs to industry of injury and disability. Interdisciplinary teams, usually headed by a rehabilitation specialist or nurse, consist of rehabilitation service providers, allied health professionals, psychologists, and ergonomists. The total care and treatment of the disabled person is monitored from the onset, so that all necessary services can be delivered promptly. Disability case management can be considered an alternate support system to control injury and disability problems by resolving barriers to safe and productive work performance (Shrey & Breslin, 1992). These authors further see the role of ergonomists in this process as critical to establishing successful accommodation strategies, when optimizing the worker-job fit, as it considers both the worker's capabilities and the job's requirements.

Design for Special Populations

Advances in medicine and increased life expectancies add to the continuous challenges to health care providers, rehabilitation technologists, product designers, and engineers to design and provide equipment for persons with special needs. Fostering the interface between equipment and each user's need can minimize functional limitations and perhaps even affect the disability process. This effort can include the ergonomic design of personal care items, clothing, mobility items, and child care aides.

The design of equipment requires attention to special anthropometric or body size measurements for the intended consumer. Population-specific anthropometric and strength data are needed to best design accessible living environments (Wright, Kumar, & Mital, 1994). An apparel research company recently sought the advice of occupational therapists to document the special clothing needs of adults with disabilities, so that their apparel could most appropriately be designed to reflect the special needs of this group (Stancliff, 1997). Applying ergonomics to the design of equipment for persons with various disabilities or medical impairments is an open area for therapists who understand their clients' functional capabilities (Rice, 1995a). A final step in the design/development process of medical rehabilitation (and other consumer) products is usability testing. According to Rice (1995b, p. 77), "this helps ensure that the final product does what it was designed to do, is acceptable to the people who use it, and is easy to use."

Zacharkow (1988) addresses posture, seating, and chair design issues for specific populations including school children, the elderly, disabled, wheelchair users, office workers, and drivers. In designing for wheelchair users, attention must be given to chair comfort, ease of operation, and accessibility to items that would be within the reach of a standing person. Similarly, upward reach distances can vary for the elderly as they age and possibly lose their erect stature. Other factors that must be considered for functionally impaired groups include hand control, dexterity, and strength; overall balance, coordination, and strength; head control; visual and hearing capabilities; and mental capacities.

Design issues clearly overlap with the rehabilitation practitioner's goals of maintaining an individual's functional independence throughout the life span. Israelski (1981) noted that it will take a great deal of creativity for human factors/ergonomic specialists to economically incorporate emerging technologies, such as speech synthesis and recognition devices, into designs for both disabled and nondisabled users. Special populations will be better served in years to come as health care ergonomics influences product design for all facets of human function that may be adversely affected by physical limitations, reduced auditory or visual capacities, slowed cognitive and information processing, reduced memory and reaction times, or dwindling social supports.

Adapting computers for the severely disabled using alternate input and recognition systems has already greatly enhanced the communication abilities of this population. A useful by-product of designing for the disabled is often more comfortable, efficient, safer, and more compatible designs for use by able-bodied persons. Health care professionals need to continue working with designers of all equipment they recommend for their clients. This could include the type of seating equipment and adaptations needed for the disabled at the computer, the most appropriate type of input device, and hardware and software issues related to the presentation and retrieval of information. Therapists are already active in this area, and they may also be integrating ergonomics into their treatment of clients.

Conclusion

The rapid advances in ergonomics that have occurred since World War II will, no doubt, continue into the twenty-first century. Similarly, the expanded role of health care professions in industry can be expected to continue, as long as WRMDs or "techno-injuries" occur in our highly specialized world, prolonged life spans persist, and medical and rehabilitation equipment is in demand. There has been a natural evolution combining particular aspects of health care and rehabilitation with ergonomics. These teams or persons that have specialized in health care and rehabilitation ergonomics will continue to be in demand. Interdisciplinary teams will include health care providers, vocational specialists, ergonomists, and engineers to deliver the necessary services that promote optimal human performance for individuals and groups of special populations in diverse environments.

The application of health care and rehabilitation ergonomics can and will increase functional performance in the home or workplace, for able-bodied or disabled individuals as well as for children and the elderly. As we enter the twenty-first century, the evolving role of health care and rehabilitation ergonomics will surely continue to develop and play a part in making the world more user-friendly for all of the world's populations.

References

American Occupational Therapy Association. (1980, April). *Role of occupational therapy in the vocational process.* A position paper. Rockville, MD: AOTA.

American Occupational Therapy Association. (1994). *Model occupational therapy practice act.* Rockville, MD: AOTA.

Americans with Disabilities Act of 1990. (Public Law 101–336). 42 USC #12101. Washington, DC: Government Printing Office.

American National Standards Institute. (1996). ANSI Z-365: Control of work-related cumulative trauma disorders, part I: Upper extremities. Unpublished draft. Available from National Safety Council, Itasca, IL.

California Occupational Safety and Health Standards Board. (1996, November). *Repetitive motion injuries standard.* Sacramento, CA: California Occupational Safety and Health Standards Board.

Chaffin, D., & Andersson, G. (1984). *Occupational biomechanics.* New York: Wiley & Sons.

Chapanis, A. (1991). To communicate the human factors message, you have to know what the message is and how to communicate it. *Human Factors Society Bulletin, 34,* 1–4.

Christensen, J.M. (1987). The human factors profession. In G. Salvendy (Ed.), *Handbook of human factors* (pp. 4–15). New York: Wiley & Sons.

Cromwell, F. (1985). Work-related programming in occupational therapy: Its roots, cause and prognosis. *Occupational Therapy in Health Care, 2(4),* 9–25.

CTD News. (1996). Average CTD comp case nears $4,000. *CTD News, 5(6),* 1.

CTD News. (1997). First look at ANSI/HFES 100 update. *CTD News, 6(2),* 7.

Dainoff, M., & Dainoff, M. (1986). *People and productivity: A manager's guide to productivity in the electronic office.* Toronto: Holt, Reinhart & Winston of Canada.

Dul, J., & Weerdmeester, B. (1993). *Ergonomics for beginners: A quick reference guide.* Washington, DC: Taylor & Francis.

Grandjean, E. (1985). Fitting the task to the man: An ergonomic approach (3rd ed.). Philadelphia: Taylor & Francis.

Hendrick, H. (1996, January). A vision for our future. *Human Factors and Ergonomics Society Bulletin, 39(1),* 1.

Hopkins, H. (1978). A historical perspective on occupational therapy. In H.L. Hopkins, & H.D. Smith (Eds.), *Willard and Spackman's occupational therapy* (5th ed.). Philadelphia: Lippincott.

Human Factors and Ergonomics Society. (1997). *Directory and yearbook, 1997–1998.* Santa Monica, CA: Human Factors and Ergonomics Society.

Inkeles, G., & Schencke, I. (1994). *Ergonomic living: How to create a user-friendly home and office.* New York: Simon & Schuster.

Ishernhagen, S. (1988). *Work injury: Management and prevention.* Rockville, MD: Aspen Publishers.

Ishernhagen, S. (1991). Physical therapy and occupational rehabilitation. *Journal of Occupational Rehabilitation, 1(1),* 71–82.

Israelski, E. (1981, September 18). Opening Remarks. Human Factors Applications for Disabled Persons. Proceedings of a Symposium, Metropolitan Chapter of the Human Factors Society (pp. 2–6). New York.

Jacobs, K. (1985). *Occupational therapy: Work-related programs and assessments.* Boston: Little, Brown.

Jacobs, K., & Bettencourt, C. (Eds.). (1995). *Ergonomics for therapists.* Boston: Butterworth–Heinemann.

Kenny, D., Powell, N., & Reynolds-Lynch, K. (1995). Trends in industrial rehabilitation: Ergonomics and cumulative trauma disorders. *Work: A Journal of Prevention, Assessment and Rehabilitation, 5(2),* 133–142.

Kornblau, B. (1996). The occupational therapist and vocational evaluation. *AOTA Work Programs Special Interest Section Newsletter, 10(1),* 1–4.

Kumar, S. (1992a). Rehabilitation: An ergonomic dimension. *International Journal of Industrial Ergonomics, 9,* 97–108.

Kumar, S. (1992b). Preface. *International Journal of Industrial Ergonomics, 9,* 93–95.

Kumar, S. (1996). Preface. *International Journal of Industrial Ergonomics, 17,* 77–79.

Matheson, L., Ishernhagen, S., & Hart, D. (1997). Rehabilitation ergonomics. A client-center ecological approach. *Work: A Journal of Prevention, Assessment and Rehabilitation, 8(2),* 223–225.

Mayne, E., & Sawyer, J. (1994, October). Integrating ergonomics into the rehabilitation process: A multidisciplinary approach for successful return to work. Proceedings of the Human Factors and Ergonomics Society 38th Annual Meeting (pp. 715–718).

McCormick, E., & Sanders, M. (1982). *Human factors in engineering and design,* 5th ed. New York: McGraw Hill.

McQuistion, L. (1993, January). Ergonomics for one. *Ergonomics in Design,* pp. 9–10.

Meister, D. (1971). *Human factors: Theory and practice.* New York: Wiley & Sons.

Mital, A., & Karwowski, W. (1988). *Ergonomics in rehabilitation.* Philadelphia: Taylor & Francis.

Mungai, A. (1985). The occupational therapist's role in employee health promotion programs. *Occupational Therapy in Health Care, 2(4),* 67–78.

Murrell, K.F.H. (1965). *Ergonomics: Man in his working environment.* London: Chapman & Hall.

New Jersey Department of Health, Public Employees Occupational Safety and Health. (1989). *New Jersey guidelines for use and functioning of VDTs.*

Occupational Safety and Health Administration. (1995, March 13). *Draft ergonomics protection standard.* (First issued in Federal Register, 57, No. 149, 1992, August 3.)

Occupational Safety and Health Administration. (1990, August). *Ergonomics program management guidelines recommendations for meatpacking plants* (OSHA 3121). Washington, DC: Government Printing Office.

Occupational Safety and Health Administration. (1990, September). *Ergonomics program management guidelines recommendations for general industry.* Washington, DC: Government Printing Office.

Occupational therapy. (1944). *War Department training manual* (pp. 8–291). Washington, DC: Government Printing Office.

Ogden, L.D., & Wright, M.C. (1985). Work related programs in occupational therapy: A renaissance. *Occupational Therapy in Health Care, 2(1),* 109–126.

Oxenburgh, M. (1991). *Increasing productivity and profit through health and safety.* Chicago: CCH International.

Pheasant, S. (1991). *Ergonomics, work and health.* Gaithersburg, MD: Aspen Publishers.

Pulat, B.M., & Alexander, D. (Eds.). (1991). *Industrial ergonomics: Case studies.* Norcross, GA: Industrial Engineering and Management Press.

Rader Smith, E. (1989). Ergonomics and the occupational therapist. In *Work in progress: Occupational therapy in work programs* (pp. 127–155). Rockville, MD: AOTA.

Rahimi, M., & Malzahn, D.E. (1988). A physical ability evaluation system used in rehabilitation engineering. In E. Mital, & W. Karwowski (Eds.), *Ergonomics in rehabilitation* (pp. 115–128). Philadelphia: Taylor & Francis.

Reilly, M. (1962). Occupational therapy can be one of the great ideas of 20th century medicine. *American Journal of Occupational Therapy, 16(1),* 1–9.

Rice, V.J. (1995a). Ergonomics: An introduction. In K. Jacobs, & C. Bettencourt (Eds.), *Ergonomics for therapists* (pp. 3–12). Boston: Butterworth–Heinemann.

Rice, V.J. (1995b). Human factors in medical rehabilitation equipment: Product development and usability testing. In K. Jacobs, & C. Bettencourt (Eds.), *Ergonomics for therapists* (pp. 77–93). Boston: Butterworth–Heinemann.

Rodgers, S. (Ed.). (1983). *Ergonomic design for people at work, 1.* Belmont, CA: Lifetime Learning Publications.

San Francisco Video Display Terminal Worker Safety Ordinance. (1990, December 27). File #118-90-5.

Shrey, D.E., & Breslin, R. (1992). Disability management in industry: A multidisciplinary model for the accommodation of workers with disabilities. *International Journal of Industrial Ergonomics, 9,* 183–190.

Snook, S. (1988). Approaches to the control of back pain in industry: Job design, job placement and education/training. *Occupational Medicine: State of the Art Reviews, 3(1),* 45–59.

Stancliff, B. (1997). Apparel research company needs OT input. *OT Practice, 2(2),* 11.

Suffolk County, NY. (1988). Video Display Terminal Law. Local Law No. 21.

Tichauer, E. (1978). *The biomechanical basis of ergonomics: Anatomy applied to the design of work situations.* New York: Wiley & Sons.

U.S. Department of Health and Human Services. (1981). *NIOSH work practices guide for manual materials lifting.* Washington, DC: Government Printing Office.

U.S. Department of Health and Human Services. (1994, January). *Applications manual for the revised NIOSH lifting equation* (PB94–176930). Washington, DC: Government Printing Office.

Vocational Rehabilitation Act of 1973. Public Law 93-1112. Washington, DC: Department of Health, Education, and Welfare.

Williams, J. (1997, April). Ergonomics standards update. *Human Factors and Ergonomics Society Bulletin 40(4),* 3–5.

Wright, U., Kumar, G.M., & Mital, A. (1994, October). Research design data for the elderly. *Proceedings of the Human Factors and Ergonomics Society 38th Annual Meeting* (pp. 137–41).

Zacharkow, D. (1988). *Posture, sitting, and standing, chair design and exercise.* Springfield, IL: Thomas.

Chapter 3

Ergonomics: A Systems Approach

Valerie J. Berg Rice

Learning Objectives

On completion of this chapter, the reader should be able to

- Explain the systems perspective as used in ergonomics/human factors and compare and contrast it with the health care/rehabilitation approach.
- Define and give examples of analysis, design, and testing and evaluation as used in ergonomics/human factors.

Key Words

Analysis
Design
Systems
Human capabilities
Human limitations

Abstract

This chapter introduces and explains human factors/ergonomics from a systems perspective and discusses the typical approach by the practitioner from a macro to a microlevel during application of ergonomics. It also defines and provides examples of the three-step process of analysis, design, and test and evaluation used in human factors/ergonomics and applied throughout this text. This three-step process is compared and contrasted with the three-step process used in health care and rehabilitation, which consists of evaluation, intervention and treatment, and re-evaluation (or in a research context, the third step is referred to as *efficacy* or *outcome testing*).

Introduction

Impediments in linking two fields, such as human factors/ergonomics and health care, include the difficulties introduced by lack of knowledge of one another's fields of practice and their specific goals, processes, and vocabularies. The previous chapter introduced the fields of practice of health care/rehabilitation, and human factors/ergonomics, as well as identifying differences and similarities in the two disciplines. This chapter reiterates some of the main goals of each field and addresses the processes and vocabularies. Although health care and rehabilitation are not synonymous terms, often what applies to one applies equally well to the other, especially in this context. In other words, within this chapter, most of the information presented will apply to both health care and rehabilitation, unless otherwise stated.

Goals

Rehabilitation is focused on the individual patient and the "social, economic, vocational, and cultural implications of a patient's disorder; the stress is on the personal impact of disability and chronic pain and their effects on family, friends, and community" (Corso, 1984). That is, rehabilitation of the patient involves helping the patient regain the physical and mental capabilities necessary to accomplish life roles. These include work, leisure, rest and sleep, as well as family roles. (Although this terminology is typically used in occupational therapy, the resumption of life roles is integral to all disciplines involved in rehabilitation.) Looking at a broad view, health care practitioners focus on the physical and emotional health and wellness of individuals, who are part of a larger society.

Human factors/ergonomics is focused on designing the environment so that it matches the capabilities and limitations of humans, as well as ensuring comfort, ease of use, and preference. This includes the design of machines, equipment, processes, and home or work-site layouts with the final goals of maintaining health and enhancing productivity. Although the traditional focus has been on the work environment, it now includes leisure and domestic pursuits as well. As stated by Dryden and Kemmerling (1990), "On one hand we have the patient-centered disability-oriented approach of the medical specialist; on the other, we have the behavior-centered, ability oriented, path taken by the industrial engineers."

Interestingly, these two fields can complement each other. In working with patients, the health care or rehabilitation practitioner may assist patients in gaining (or regaining) a state of wellness and an optimal (for them) level of functioning. Because the optimal level of functioning differs for each person, the patient may need assistive devices or alternative designs of the environments in which work, play, rest, or sleep occurs. In these situations, the therapist can perform a medically based functional examination and view the results in conjunction with the prognosis and possible side effects of the illness or injury. This information is essential for the human factors engineer/ergonomist in designing an environment to fit an individual or a particular patient population. Human factors engineers/ergonomists use knowledge and design skills to formulate questions pertinent to the design of equipment or settings. Without additional training beyond the basic professional education, the health care/rehabilitation practitioner lacks design skills; the human factors/ergonomics practitioner lacks medical knowledge such as functional deficits, prognosis, and side effects associated with illness and injury. A combined effort between the two disciplines can eliminate disparities and better meet system and patient needs.

Process

A health care practitioner or therapist first considers the patients' health issues, then his or her functional status, the people the patient need to interact with, and his or her environment. Thus, the therapist (or health care practitioner) thinks first of the patient, and the process radiates out from there. This can be seen as beginning at a micro (patient) perspective and moving toward a macro view. Although health care and rehabilitation use a systems approach, the perspective is different from the human factors/ergonomics professional.

Human factors engineers/ergonomists take a macroergonomic systems approach. Surrounding the element of interest are a myriad of system components comprising an entire system. The system components influence the element of interest. The macroergonomic systems approach considers the entire system. All of the components that may impact on the portion of the environment being analyzed are considered. In other words, the first inclination is to focus on the larger, macro level and move to the micro perspective.

The human factors engineer/ergonomist and health care professional must be aware of each other's thought processes, when conversing and working with one another. For example, when investigating cumulative trauma injuries, the therapist may start with the individual workers by conducting interviews and reviewing medical records. The human factors practitioner/ergonomist may begin by defining the system and its mission and requirements, followed by examining plant records, workplace layout, and work processes. Ideally, if they are there to perform an ergonomic evaluation for the prevention of cumulative trauma injuries, eventually they will each cover the same ground. An ergonomic evaluation should be inclusive; the quality and comprehensiveness of the evaluation should not dependent on the individual evaluator. If the human factors engineer/ergonomist and health care professional understand each other's field of practice, they will cover the pertinent information and consult with persons who have the expertise they lack. Unfortunately, if they do not understand each other's field of practice, the therapist may perform an incomplete ergonomic analysis; the consequence can be incomplete resolution of problems or incomplete provision of preventive measures, possibly leading the employer into a false sense of security regarding the safety of workers. If unaware of the health care perspective, the ergonomist may not adequately set up a medical prevention program, referral process, or baseline medical evaluation for early intervention, or provide a sufficiently detailed explanation of cumulative trauma (and potential preventive treatments). An ergonomist may also fail to accommodate an individual's unique needs by neglecting to prepare a design that can be adjusted as the patient's condition changes (either improving or declining).

Three-Step Process

Both fields of practice use a three-step process, but with different terminology, professional practices, and expectations occurring at each step. The health care/rehabilitative three-step process includes evaluation, treatment/intervention, and re-evaluation. The human factors/ergonomic professional uses a three-step process of analysis, design, and test and evaluation. An abbreviated view of the rehabilitative/health care process is presented, followed by a detailed description of the human factors/ergonomic process.

Rehabilitation: Evaluation

During this first step, the patient is evaluated, typically in accordance with standard operating procedures for the injury or illness. Immediate health needs are addressed and the patient is stabilized. If the illness or injury is judged to have residual effects that could impact on the patient's life, then further evaluation is conducted (possibly through referral to another practitioner). The patient's physical and mental abilities may be assessed using standardized testing, along with identification of limitations and potential to improve (as necessary and in accordance with the illness or injury). The patient's abilities are defined primarily in terms of deficits that can be rectified through patient treatment (for example, muscle weakness treated with strength training, or cognitive problem solving treated through retraining or substitution).

A medically based functional capacity evaluation may be conducted to determine the patient's ability to conduct activities of daily living, work tasks, and leisure pursuits. The resulting information can be compared with norms or with specific requirements of their work, leisure, or home environments. If the rehabilitation process will be long

term or certain limitations are expected to be permanent, then further evaluation of the patient's home or work environment may be warranted. For example, if home health care is provided, it often includes an evaluation of the patients' home—to determine the need for ramps, assistive devices, and alterations to rooms, shelves, or other areas—as well as evaluation and treatment of the patient in the home.

The main focus of the rehabilitative evaluation is the patient. The environment of the patient is only evaluated if the consequences of the illness or injury justify such an evaluation. For example, an occupational therapist will ask the patient about life roles and activities (i.e., occupations) to ascertain the level of functioning, whether treatment goals are needed in these areas, and whether assistive devices are necessary.

Rehabilitation: Treatment/Intervention

The treatment/intervention process includes specific patient treatment based on the injury or illness, subsequent disability, and functional capabilities. The majority of patient treatment is medical in nature, using techniques such as graded, focused physical exercise, splinting, cognitive retraining, and physical modalities such as ultrasound and heat. However, occupational therapy and work hardening involve the use of specific work, home, or leisure activities to achieve their objectives. Both use treatment techniques of graded activity (physical and mental), gradually increasing the demands on the patient in accordance with the requirements of the roles that particular patient would like to eventually resume. Treatment/intervention may include alterations to the home or work environment for those with long-term or chronic disabilities. These alterations may include gradual changes in the environment to coincide with the patient's improved status, or the changes may become permanent, if the highest functional level for that patient has been reached.

Rehabilitation: Re-Evaluation

Throughout the course of treatment, re-evaluation occurs on a periodic basis, generally using the same measures used during the initial, baseline evaluation. The measures used are based on goals set during the initial evaluation and subsequent re-evaluations. They may include physical measures of strength and coordination or task performance measures such as level of independence during activities of daily living. The functional information derived from these evaluations and re-evaluations of a patient are absolutely essential during ergonomics-for-one or return-to-duty applications. The efficacy of patient treatment and the basis for discontinuation of treatment are determined by the results of the patient re-evaluation. Research in this area is referred to as *outcome research.*

Human Factors/Ergonomics: Analysis

The macroergonomic viewpoint and a systems perspective are evident during the initial phase of the process, that is, during analysis. In a work setting, the tasks performed by an individual contribute to the system and to the accomplishment of the missions and goals of that system. All elements pertaining to the situation at hand are evaluated during analysis, typically in a top-down approach. Problems are identified and questions regarding the adequacy of the designs involved are developed. During the analysis, the problems to be prevented or rectified through design are identified. The solutions (designs) can only be as good as the questions asked, meaning that the analysis process guides the design process. If an incomplete analysis is done, it is possible that the identified problems will only be a portion of those problems which need to be corrected. Thus any design solution would probably address only part of the problems. According to the Board of Certification in Professional Ergonomics (1996), analysis can include mission analysis, function analysis, and task/job analysis and synthesis (note the movement from the total system to specific tasks, from macro to micro).

Mission analysis involves defining missions and objectives as well as the resource allocations needed to achieve the mission and objectives. For example, usability testing of rehabilitation equipment (such as a walker) might involve defining the mission (to provide assistive devices to individuals with mobilization difficulties), as well as the objectives: primary (walking and negotiating obstacles in the home,

yard, grocery store, and parking lots), secondary (carrying assistance), and perhaps tertiary objectives (allowing for seated resting on the walker itself) to be achieved through the use of the equipment (Rice, 1995). During the evaluation of a manufacturing work site, the analysis might involve defining company, plant, and division missions and objectives. In so doing, the human factors/ergonomic professional would identify the personnel, finances, and other resources necessary to achieve the objectives. All of this information is important to meet the goals of human factors/ergonomics: enhancing performance, promoting comfort and safety, and implementing user information such as preferences and educational and cultural background to make the process as user-friendly as possible.

Function analysis involves identification, classification, and evaluation of the functions accomplished by human and machine that have implications for staffing, training, and design. For example, some functions are achieved by a piece of machinery, such as the Baltimore Therapeutic Equipment (BTE), providing physical resistance to the patient's actions and recording the amount of resistance the patient was able to willingly overcome, while the humans (therapist and patient) provide the input for the amount of resistance, the parameters to be measured, subjective evaluation of patient fatigue, and interpretation of the results. In this case, the ergonomist identifies the functions most appropriately allocated to the machine versus the human when designing the BTE.

During task analysis, the psychological and physical abilities necessary for task performance are identified, along with the procedures and equipment used in achieving the task (Stammers, Carey, & Astley, 1990). For example, during usability testing of medical equipment the knowledge, skills, and abilities required of those who will be operating equipment would be identified. This testing can include the mental processes and distinctions required during a task (such as reasoning and decision making), as well as the physical motions used and their frequency, the resistance encountered (strength needed), and the body positions assumed. The task is broken into its component parts, yet still considered within the context of the system in which it is used. Although task requirements may be similar, the operators of the medical equipment may differ in their ability to complete the task due to educational, cultural, and language differences. All operators (users) should be considered.

Meister (1985, p. 1) refers to mission/function/task analysis, along with operational sequence diagramming, error analysis, and various computerized models as *analytic techniques*, which he asserts are often used in engineering design, test facilities, and simulated systems. He uses the term *measurement methods* to apply to those methods used in functioning systems (systems that already exist and are functional), such as observation, interviews, questionnaires, ratings, and objective measures.

> The purpose of the analytic techniques is to aid in the design of the human subsystem so that the performance of the superordinate system will be maximized. The purpose of the measurement methods is to gather information about personnel function to assess the adequacy of human subsystem performance with reference to the terminal outputs of the overall system; and/or to understand the relationship between the human subsystem and the overall system (Meister, 1985, p. 2).

During the analysis and development of a *new* system, analytic techniques are used in a laboratory setting to begin to identify important items of design, whereas measurement methods are used to assess the operation in an applied setting (Meister, 1985, pp. 9–10). In actuality, many of the techniques are overlapping and can be used in either setting. Practicing rehabilitation or health care ergonomists will probably be assessing existing systems, and they will use both analytic techniques and measurement methods to describe an applied setting. For a review of analytic techniques and measurement methods, see Meister (1985) and Wilson and Corlett (1990).

Information gained during mission, function, and task analyses is used to assess the adequacy of an existing design or to provide input for a new design. One method of accomplishing this is for the human factors professional/ergonomist to interpret the information and compare and contrast it with previous findings in research and literature. Thus begins the transformation in which the information can be used in the design phase of the process. For example, the problem may be worker injuries and lost work time resulting from cases of cumulative trauma to upper extremities, such as carpal tunnel syndrome. At the same time the problem is being defined, questions are developed regarding the design of the work—physical, psychosocial, and organizational aspects of the job that may contribute to a cumulative trauma injury. Perhaps the design of the workplace or tools appears to have resulted in direct pressure over the carpal tunnel. In this case, the human factors/ergonomics professional would cite specific studies that defined the increase in carpal pressure resulting from direct pressure using a similar tool, along with any epidemiological studies that associated direct pressure over the carpal tunnel with a significant increase in risk of reported injury. If the information does not exist in the literature, the human factors professional/ergonomist would obtain the best available information, or might choose to conduct the research of interest. Human factors/ergonomics is a field based in research (Table 3-1), which is continually updated. Citation of the rationale of why a particular design is considered problematic increases the practitioner's credibility and the willingness of employers to expend funds for corrections.

Human Factors/Ergonomics: Design

Design for People

Information gained through analysis is used to create alternative design concepts that will satisfy known requirements and constraints while achieving the specified objectives. It is the job of the human factors/ergonomic professional to ensure that behavioral aspects (human capabilities, limitations, comfort, and preferences) are considered in a design. Health care professionals commonly misinterpret this to mean that human factors professionals/ergonomists are more concerned with the effectiveness and efficiency of the mechanical aspects of the system than they are with the health and welfare of the human operator. This is not the case. The difference is one of perspective.

For example, the purpose of a furniture manufacturing plant is to manufacture quality furniture that customers will purchase, and ergonomic design input must address that purpose. Human workers form one component of the system, and their health and welfare have definite and significant impact on system performance and output (the system includes all elements, such as manufacturing, marketing, and administration). How-

Table 3-1. Research Requirements

Human Factors and Ergonomics Society[a]	American Physical Therapy Association[b]	American Occupational Therapy Association[c]
Introductory master's level program Appendix A. Curriculum. Core Research methodologies: Students must be trained to execute projects including data collection, data analysis, preparation of technical reports, statistical procedures, experimental design Research experience: Master's thesis Doctoral entry level; the following must also be included: Ability to formulate research questions Doctoral dissertation with an emphasis on theory or conceptual development	Introductory master's level program Section 3.8.3.(10–12) Research learning experiences: Evaluate published studies related to physical therapy practice, research, and education Secure and critically evaluate information related to new and established techniques and technology, legislation, policy, and environments related to patient or client care Participate in scholarly activities to contribute to the body of physical therapy knowledge (e.g., case reports, collaborative research)	Introductory bachelor's level program Section II.B.5 Program content shall include: Research: The necessity and value of research The essential components of a protocol Interpretation of studies related to occupational therapy and the application of results to practice

[a]*Human Factors and Ergonomics Society Accreditation Self-Study Report Guide.* (Revised May 1995). Available from the Human Factors and Ergonomics Society, P.O. Box 1369, Santa Monica, CA 90406-1369.
[b]American Physical Therapy Association. (Effective January 1, 1998). *Evaluative criteria for accreditation of education programs for the preparation of physical therapists.* Available from the Commission on Accreditation in Physical Therapy Education, American Physical Therapy Association, 111 North Fairfax Street, Alexandria, VA 22314.
[c]American Occupational Therapy Association. (1991, updated in 1995). *Essentials and Guidelines for an Accredited Educational Program for the Occupational Therapist.* Available from the Accreditation Council for Occupational Therapy Education, P.O. Box 31220, Bethesda, MD 20824-1220.

ever, the primary mission of the plant is not to prevent cumulative trauma injuries; instead the prevention of injuries is an objective necessary to achieving the primary mission of making furniture and competing successfully with other furniture manufacturers. Therefore, when a human factors/ergonomic practitioner introduces the human element into the design, it is stated in terms of the system's mission and performance. For example, recommended ergonomic changes to a manufacturing process should be submitted with a cost-benefit analysis. The costs of implementing a change might include initial financing and an increase of 3 seconds in product assembly time, resulting in fewer products produced per month. This potential financial loss might be offset by benefits such as financial and productivity gains achieved by decreasing injury claims, lost work days, and retraining requirements, while increasing morale.

The very definition of human factors/ergonomics is to design for human use, thus concentrating on including the person in what otherwise might be a pure engineering approach. People are a focus of the human factors engineer/ergonomist, just as they are of a health care practitioner. One profession medically treats people, the other designs for people. Neither professional definition or practice is complete without the human element.

During analysis, the mission, goals, and objectives of the system and pertinent subsystems were identified. In developing a new design or re-evaluating an existing design, various alternatives are considered from the standpoint of human performance. The intent is for the operator to perform their functions and tasks effectively, without excessive workload, and without error (or with minimal error). Thus, tasks the worker must perform are evaluated in terms of known human capabilities and limitations, taking into consideration cultural expectations and probability of error; the design concepts that pass through this filter are selected and tested.

Ask Defining Questions

Several authors suggest that the step between analysis and design be bridged by a listing of germane questions that have arisen from the analysis, and which the design should answer (Meister, 1985, pp. 4–5, 9; Sanders & McCormick, 1987, pp. 541–542). Table 3-2 suggests questions and concerns that might be considered when designing a control panel.

The questions identified during analysis should center around a specific set of problems, such as cumulative trauma injuries, or a global assessment of the workplace, such as when performing a plant-wide ergonomic functional analysis. Responsible practitioners must clarify with their client their own capabilities as ergonomists, and whether they are performing a specific service (microergonomic) or using an extensive approach (macroergonomic). For example, health care professionals may choose only to perform consultant activities regarding cumulative trauma, rather than assess and design to prevent human error.

In usability testing, the actual design (or redesign) of a product occurs after discussions between a user group (subject matter experts) and investigators; establishment of design objectives; and analyses of tasks and functions (Rice, 1995). At this time, performance criteria are developed and incorporated into product design. Guiding questions during preliminary design might include items such as the following (Meister, 1985):

- Of the various design alternatives available, which is the most effective from the standpoint of behavioral performance?
- Given a system configuration, will system personnel be able to perform all required functions effectively?
- Will personnel encounter excessive workload?
- What factors are responsible for potential error and can these be eliminated?

These generic questions can be applied to designing a wheelchair, a kitchen for a disabled individual, or a manufacturing assembly line. Often the answers to the questions will lead to the design of several alternative solutions. Depending on the expense of developing these alternatives, some may be created in the form of an adjustable mock-up with the critical dimensions of the product adjusted through a range of values. To ascertain the user's

Table 3-2. Examples of Concerns to Be Addressed in the Design of a Complex Control Panel

1. Reach and accessibility (anthropometrics)
2. Resistance of the controls (strength, force)
3. Ability to distinguish controls (tactile and visual recognition of shapes)
4. Principles of design layout (criticality, sequence, and frequency)
5. Feedback that the control has been activated
6. Sensory modality most appropriate for use
7. Whether the information displayed for the operator is within human information-receiving capabilities (to include limitations imposed by dual tasking)
8. Whether human judgment is required for proper operation
9. Whether speed or precision mandates are reasonable for the situation
10. Identification of hazards
11. Whether extenuating circumstances (heat, cold, noise) might interrupt the process and result in a safety concern
12. Whether fail-safe measures should be designed into the system
13. The training that is required of operators (length of time, training aids, training updates, costs)
14. Whether there are psychosocial concerns (e.g., work fulfillment, social interaction, team building, responsibility for their own work)

comfort, ease of use, preference, and other psychophysical elements, a "fitting trial" (also known as *initial usability testing*) or a "walk-through" (Pheasant, 1986) will yield information that can be included to help refine the design. Other methods of evaluation include mathematical and computerized modeling techniques.

To reiterate, the design process entails taking the information gained during the analysis, reformatting it into questions or objectives that could be answered through a more human-centered design, creating a design to respond to those questions, and implementing the design either in the form of a trial (mock-up) or actual item. Designs can take many forms, and the term need not refer only to a product or physical object. A process can be redesigned, such as a training program, health reporting system, wellness program, or communication flow within a company. The design should alleviate or correct as many of the problems or questions identified by the analysis as possible. Each question or problem area should be prioritized, and constraints (finances, physical space, time, etc.) should be considered in selecting the final design. Trade-offs are inevitable and the ideal design may not be the design selected.

Accessing Design Information

Some health care or rehabilitation professionals have voiced their desire to take a few design courses to improve their skills in human factors/ergonomics. However, relatively few courses titled "design" in human factors/ergonomic curricula are offered, just as there are few, if any, courses titled "patient treatment" in health care/rehabilitation curricula. Instead, design is embedded in the professional courses and texts. Introductory texts on workplace design discuss principles such as designing for the intended population and for a range of the expected population of users. The typical design range includes the smaller 5% female population to the larger 95% male population. Other design principles include consideration of costs, service, maintenance of equipment, and locating items in terms of importance, frequency, and sequence of use.

Some courses and texts on human factors/ergonomics might describe and define human limitations and capabilities, whereas others expect this knowledge before a student's beginning course work. When human limitations and capabilities are included in a text, they are covered in terms of the physical body—anthropometric dimensions, strength, vision, hearing, speech, tactile discrimination, and olfactory discrimination (work physiology and biomechanics are often covered in separate courses)—and mental aspects: cognitive information processing, response to stimuli, mental workload, and stress. Generally, such texts also identify environmental issues that influence performance (such as the effects of workspace clearance dimensions and reaches, clothing, temperature, vibration, acceleration, scheduling and biorhythms, alcohol, as well as the results of research on performance measures and user preferences). Systems, controls, and human control of systems are also introduced. The reader, with assistance from instructors, uses his or her professional judgment to integrate, translate, and apply this information to the design of equipment, space, or organizational structure.

Professional judgment, based on comprehensive knowledge of the area of practice, will have a great deal of impact on users. This same professional judgment must be applied in the decision whether to use known information (such as normative data, probability data, relevant principles) or whether to conduct specific studies to answer the questions that have arisen from analysis, before beginning the design process.

Other information on design may be found in subsections of professional texts with titles such as *engineering solutions, administrative solutions,* or *guidelines* within a section or chapter describing particular design problems seen by ergonomists. Some examples of the inclusion of design ideas in subtopics include descriptions of physically demanding work such as manual materials handling, repetitive work, shift work, and the office environment (Alexander, 1986; Chaffin & Andersson, 1991; Konz, 1995; Rodgers, 1986). The best resources for an armchair review of the design process are texts that present both problems and solutions, such as Rodgers (1986), Pulat and Alexander (1991), and for universal designs that can be used to comply with the Americans with Disabilities Act, Wilkoff and Abed (1994). Reviewing the proceedings from conferences that concentrate on an applied approach, or journals that emphasize the application of ergonomic principles, can also give a reader an idea of the design process. Learning through another's mistakes can also be informative, and Casey (1993) presents fascinating and often horrifying descriptions of incidents when human factors principles were either not used in the original design or were not adhered to.

Obviously, practitioners cannot simply take a few courses on design to substantially increase their level of practice and understanding in human factors/ergonomics. A comparison may help to illustrate the point. For health care practitioners, Standard Operating Procedures (SOPs) may guide the majority of their practice. However, for an occupational therapist (OT) in a traditional practice, the SOP can only be a guide. The OT treatment plan, possible assistive devices, and workplace design alterations will be based on the occupations practiced by the patient. An *occupation* is defined as the activities that occupy that patient's time. A patient with an upper extremity amputation who previously worked as an automotive mechanic, played billiards during his leisure time, has a small son, and has a home that he does repairs on will have a very different treatment plan than a patient of the same age, with the same injury, who is a homemaker, mother, and who cares for her elderly parents. In essence, treatment and design are based on particular knowledge foundations, and then are learned through guided reading and practice with an instructor, mentor, or coworker. This is also true in the field of human factors/ergonomics. Patient treatment and design for the human vary notably, depending on the context and circumstances.

Human Factors/Ergonomics: Test and Evaluation

Once a design or alternative concept is selected and implemented, there must be an evaluation to determine whether it is achieving the objectives it was designed to achieve. Were the identified questions answered or problems solved? Whereas a therapist may regard any improvement in the functional ability of a single patient as "proof" that their intervention has "worked" (a 10-lb gain in grip strength or an increased ability to dress oneself), the ergonomist looks for a statistically significant finding, typically with an alpha level of 0.05. It is generally not considered sufficient that "most people like the new design" or even "60% of the workers like the new design"; instead statistical analysis of multifaceted measures is suggested. Once again, the human factors/ergonomics professional typically is interested in each facet, such as functional (performance), injuries/illnesses, and subjective preferences, as well as the impact on the system as a whole. The rationale for using statistics is the desire to know how unequivocal the data are (whether they could be due to chance) and whether alternative solutions may be plausible (Meister, 1985). Also of interest is whether the findings have practical value and can be generalized to situations other than the one studied.

Not all designs receive final testing and evaluation. For example, a walk-through can be used with an existing product to identify problem areas and remedies. If the product is prohibitively expensive to produce, then a series of evaluations, using walk-throughs and mock-ups may serve to refine the product until a final design is selected. For example, the military requires "development tests" be conducted for each development phase of major system design in acquisition programs. The final design may or may not be evaluated further in an operational setting using performance objectives. The ideal situation is to perform a series of evaluations during the development of a product and prior to production, and to perform operational tests once the product is complete. Operational tests should be performed in the environment in which the product or process will be used, and with the population who will be involved with the item. Designs that are not tested with the appropriate user population are noticeably deficient in their execution, as noted in the contemporary text *The Design of Everyday Things* (Norman, 1990). For example, a redesign of city road and traffic signs can be implemented and make perfect sense to the designer when viewing the city road maps on a system of charts, but may be terribly confusing to the tourist from out of town. Dashboard controls in a vehicle may be appropriately spaced with adequate feedback and tactile information for a bare hand, but may cause errors when the operator wears gloves in the winter.

During testing and evaluation, the system, product, or process is evaluated to ensure that human characteristics have been adequately considered during the design, and that they serve their purpose effectively and safely (Sanders & McCormick, 1987). In most situations, testing and evaluation should be systematic and completed in scientific fashion. In many cases, testing and evaluation may be considered synonymous with a field experiment, and the stipulations that accompany the experimental method should be followed (Drury, 1990). The dependent measures should be related to the use of the item or process and can include "work performance, physiological effects, accidents, effects on health, learning time, job satisfaction, attitudes and opinions, and economic considerations, to mention a few" (Sanders & McCormick, 1987, p. 540). Objective as well as subjective measures should be included. Seldom can the answers be provided by using a single measure. Meister provides a list of generic performance measures. Recognizing the complexity of selecting performance measures for operational testing, he also provides guidance on how to select among measures:

> The evaluator should select measures that are 1. highly related to the output or product of the performance being measured, 2. objective, 3. quantitative, 4. unobtrusive, 5. easy to collect, 6. require no specialized data collection techniques, 7. are not excessively molecular and therefore

require no specialized instrumentation, and 8. cost as little as possible monetarily and in terms of evaluator effort (Meister, 1985, p. 263).

Of course, the dependent measures of interest will drive the instrumentation and collection techniques selected.

It is also possible to repeat the measures used during the analysis to demonstrate the changes that have occurred as a result of the design changes. This might be done with implementation of design changes geared to decreasing the incidence of cumulative trauma injuries. The number of reported injuries before and after implementation may be compared, taking into account a possible Hawthorne effect; that is, having any attention paid to the worker result in a positive effect (Roethlisberger & Dickson, 1939). Observation times should be stipulated, and a longer observation time may yield more credible results.

Testing and evaluation is the portion of the process that is most often neglected. Results of testing and evaluation are often used by employers, potential employers, politicians, and the general public to determine the value of human factors/ergonomic design implementation. As stated by Hendrick (1996, p. 1),

> Managers have to be able to justify an investment in terms of its concrete benefits to the organization—to the organization's ability to be competitive and survive . . . we must better document the costs and benefits of our efforts and share these data with our colleagues, business decision makers, and government policymakers.

The results do not always have to be in monetary terms; however, it is important to demonstrate that inclusion of ergonomics/human factors makes a difference. The difference may be increased productivity, sales, morale, or consumer satisfaction, as well as decreased injuries and medical claims. Similar statements to that made by Hendrick have been made in health care professions, calling for outcome research to demonstrate the effectiveness of specific interventions. Effectiveness can be measured in terms of functional ability of the patient, time to return to work, and patient satisfaction. Whether you refer to them as *efficacy* studies or *outcome studies* and whether practitioners think the evaluation is adequate or not, the results are often used to indicate the financial, practical, and social value of our professions.

Research

This text is directed at field application of human factors/ergonomics and more specifically at those areas of overlap between human factors/ergonomics and health care/rehabilitation. However, because human factors/ergonomics is a research field, it is important to mention research in regard to the three activities covered in the previous section: analysis, design, and test and evaluation. Research efforts may also use three phases, although in a different sequence. They may analyze the situation, conduct testing and evaluation of the current situation, and use the results to develop design concepts and suggest design guidelines, or they may analyze, develop a design prototype or alternatives, and perform testing and evaluation on the prototypes. For example, Petzall (1996) analyzed the situation for public access for wheelchair users in Sweden. Petzall determined the heights of typical curbs, pedestrian crossings, and transportation system step obstacles. As a result of the analysis, Petzall developed a research question regarding the heights of step obstacles that could be traversed with a manual wheelchair maneuvered by an assistant. He then selected two wheelchair designs commonly used in Sweden, and conducted testing and evaluation of the perceived exertion of an assistant, forces generated, task completion time, and comfort ratings of wheelchair patients using independent measures of five right-angled step heights. At the conclusion of the testing and evaluation, step-height design guidelines were provided for public transport systems when the wheelchair-bound individual could get assistance. Thus, his sequence was analysis, test and evaluation, and design.

Conclusion

The three phases of analysis, design, and test and evaluation can be used in a variety of professions. It is not the process that makes this human factors/ergonomics, it is the content. Again, this can be an area of confusion. Evaluating a flexor tendon injury, fashioning a splint, and evaluating the effectiveness of that splint is not human factors/ergonomics, even though the steps of evaluation (analysis), design, implementation, and re-evaluation were used. However, evaluating the needs of upper extremity amputees, designing an artificial limb that meets the capabilities and limitations of potential users, as well as the requirements of the environment (levels of precision and prehensile force, as well as climatic restraints), and testing the new limb with a user population may benefit from the expertise of an ergonomist.

A three-step process has been presented in this text for those individuals who are less familiar with the field of ergonomics/human factors. Use of a three-step process, applying ergonomic knowledge and principles in each, should result in a thorough ergonomic investigation. The crux of human factors/ergonomics is ensuring that the environment, tool, or process is as closely matched with human capabilities (physical and mental) as possible, while considering the restraints resulting from their internal environments (personal preferences, cultural expectations, educational level, ingested food or chemicals, and sleep deprivation) and external environments (heat, cold, altitude, noise, and physically constrained spaces).

References

Alexander, D.C. (1986). *The practice and management of industrial ergonomics*. Englewood Cliffs, NJ: Prentice Hall.

Board of certification in Professional Ergonomics Directory. (1996). (Available from BCPE Corporate Office, P.O. Box 2811, Bellingham, WA 98227.)

Casey, S. (1993). *Set phasers on stun*. Santa Barbara, CA: Aegean Publishing Company.

Chaffin, D.B., & Andersson, G.B. (1991). *Occupational biomechanics*. New York: Wiley & Sons.

Corso, J.F. (1984). Human factors in medical rehabilitation: Some major problem areas. *Proceedings of the Human Factors Society, 28th Annual Meeting*, San Antonio, TX (p. 649). Santa Monica, CA: Ergonomics Society.

Drury, C.G. (1990). Designing ergonomics studies and experiments. In J.R. Wilson, & E.N. Corlett (Eds.), *Evaluation of human work* (pp. 101–129). New York: Taylor & Francis.

Dryden, R.D., & Kemmerling, P.T. (1990). Engineering assessment. In S.P. Sheer (Ed.), *Vocational assessment of impaired workers* (pp. 107–129). Gaithersburg, MD: Aspen Publishers.

Hendrick, H.W. (1996). Sharing human factors success stories. *Human Factors and Ergonomics Society Bulletin, 39(9)*, 1, 5.

Hill, S.G. & Kroemer, K.H.E. (1986). Preferred dedination and the line of sight. *Human Factors, 28*, 127–134.

Konz, S. (1995). *Work design: Industrial ergonomics*. Scottsdale, AZ: Publishing Horizons.

Meister, D. (1985). *Behavioral analysis and measurement methods*. New York: Wiley & Sons.

National Institute for Occupational Safety and Health. (1997). *Elements of ergonomic programs*. Centers for Disease Control and Prevention, U.S. Department of Health and Human Services.

Norman, D. (1990). *The design of everyday things*. New York: Doubleday.

Petzall, J. (1996). Traversing step obstacles with manual wheelchairs. *Applied Ergonomics, 27(5)*, 327–341.

Pheasant, S. (1986). *Bodyspace—anthropometry, ergonomics and design*. London: Taylor & Francis.

Pulat, B.M., & Alexander, D.C. (1991). *Industrial ergonomics: Case studies*. Norcross, GA: Industrial Engineering and Management Press.

Rice, V.J. (1995). Human factors in medical rehabilitation equipment: Product development and usability testing. In K. Jacobs, & C. Bettencourt (Eds.), *Ergonomics for therapists*. Boston: Butterworth–Heinemann.

Rodgers, S.H. (1986). *Ergonomic design for people at work* (Vol. 2). New York: Van Nostrand Reinhold.

Roethlisberger, F.J., & Dickson, W.J. (1939). *Management and the worker*. Cambridge, MA: Harvard University Press.

Sanders, M.S., & McCormick, E.J. (1987). *Human factors in engineering and design*. New York: McGraw-Hill.

Stammers, R.B., Carey, M.S., & Astley, J.A. (1990). Task analysis. In J.R. Wilson, & E.N. Corlett (Eds.), *Evaluation of human work* (pp. 134–160). New York: Taylor & Francis.

Wilkoff, W.L., & Abed, L.W. (1994). *Practicing universal design: An interpretation of the ADA*. New York: Van Nostrand Reinhold.

Wilson, J.R., & Corlett, E.N. (Eds.) (1990). *Evaluation of human work*. New York: Taylor & Francis.

Section II

Ergonomics-for-One

Chapter 4

Ergonomics-for-One: An Introduction

Linda McQuistion

Learning Objectives

On completion of this chapter, the reader should be able to

- Define ergonomics-for-one, rehabilitation engineering, assistive technology, rehabilitation technology, and adaptive aids.
- Understand the systems approach to accommodation.
- Complete a task analysis of essential job functions.
- Effect accommodations.

Key Words

Rehabilitation engineering
Accommodation
Assistive technology
Rehabilitation technology
Task analysis

Abstract

The concept of ergonomics-for-one uses highly individualized assessment to accommodate an individual with limitations. A systems approach to achieving such an accommodation is demonstrated, including a technique and forms for task analysis.

Introduction

Ergonomics-for-one is the application of ergonomic principles and techniques to match the specific demands of a given pursuit (such as work, education, leisure, home activities) to an individual's functional capabilities. The emphasis is on fitting the task to a specific individual, not to a population as when working in more traditional ergonomic applications.

Ergonomists usually apply their specialized skills to groups of current or potential users for broad implementation, such as designing automobile interiors for the general population, reconfiguring control panels in a nuclear power plant, or recommending the purchase of adjustable office furniture for all clerical staff in an insurance agency. In this role, the ergonomist designs the most effective product or environment for a given population. However, when the intended user is a person with special needs, such as an injury or a disability, the ergonomist must design specifically for that individual; thus the designation *ergonomics-for-one*.

The practice of ergonomics-for-one is not new, nor is it new to the practice of occupational therapy: For decades, therapists have developed assistive devices to provide a better fit between a client and a work or home environment.

Significance of Ergonomics-for-One

Successful application of ergonomics-for-one results in a life change for the individual to whom it is applied. When this concept is applied to a person with a disability, the outcome can be quite significant. In addition, the ripple effect can be quite impressive. For example, when an injured worker cannot be completely rehabilitated to prior capability, but can be returned to productivity, the job is saved, the worker is productive and earning income, and the employer's workers' compensation costs are reduced.

Ergonomics-for-one can be used to help an individual born with a severe disability join the workforce for the first time, resulting in greater financial independence, an enhanced contribution to society by becoming a taxpayer, and possibly the elimination of the need for public assistance. A student with a disabling condition may now be able to attend classes with other students, participate in extracurricular activities, and complete work assignments. This may, in turn, open the door to a college education. Even seemingly small changes, such as improving a person's ability to more fully participate in activities of daily living and homemaking can be significant: It can increase independence, reduce the need for personal attendant care, and may even eliminate the need for nursing home residence.

Practicing Ergonomics-for-One

Individuals who apply the concepts of ergonomics-for-one may be referred to as *rehabilitation engineers*, *rehabilitation technologists*, or *assistive technologists*. These terms are often used interchangeably to refer to the vast array of professionals who perform these types of services. Such professionals include ergonomists, occupational therapists, physical therapists, industrial designers, computer specialists, speech-language pathologists, industrial nurses and physicians, engineers from traditional engineering disciplines (industrial, mechanical, electrical, human factors, computer, biomedical) and rehabilitation engineers (trained in rehabilitation engineering curricula).

Rehabilitation engineering refers to the application of technological, scientific, and engineering principles to the rehabilitation process by degreed or licensed engineers. Individuals performing similar activities—but not including engineering design—are considered rehabilitation technologists or assistive technologists. All are performing ergonomics-for-one. Thus, for the sake of simplicity and consistency *all* will be referred to throughout the chapter as *ergonomists*.

It is also important to realize that each of the professional groups mentioned above brings a unique perspective and set of skills to the application of ergonomics-for-one. Often the best solutions are developed via interdisciplinary teams. This is especially true for a person with a severe disability involving multiple impairments and requiring intervention in multiple environments (such as work, school, and home).

Federal Legislation

Federal legislation assigns specific definitions to the terms *rehabilitation engineering*, *rehabilitation technology,* and *assistive technology*. The Technology-Related Assistance for Individuals with Disabilities Act of 1988 (as amended) (Public Law 100-407, Section 3[1][2]), provides definitions for assistive technology as follows:

1. Assistive technology device. The term a*ssistive technology device* means any item, piece of equipment, or product system, whether acquired commercially off the shelf, modified, or customized, that is used to increase, maintain, or improve functional capabilities of individuals with disabilities.
2. Assistive technology service. The term *assistive technology service* means any service that directly assists an individual with a disability in the selection, acquisition, or use of an assistive technology device. This term includes
   a. the evaluation of the needs of an individual with a disability, including a functional evaluation of the individual in the individual's customary environment;
   b. purchasing, leasing, or otherwise providing for the acquisition of assistive technology devices by individuals with disabilities;
   c. selecting, designing, fitting, customizing, adapting, applying, maintaining, repairing, or replacing of assistive technology devices;
   d. coordinating and using other therapies, interventions, or services with assistive technology devices, such as those associated with existing education and rehabilitation plans and programs;

e. training or technical assistance for an individual with disabilities, or, where appropriate, the family of an individual with disabilities; and

f. training or technical assistance for professionals (including individuals providing education and rehabilitation services), employers, or other individuals who provide services to, employ, or are otherwise substantially involved in the major life functions of individuals with disabilities.

The Rehabilitation Act of 1973 (as amended) (Public Law 100-407, Section 361.5[39]) defines rehabilitation technology as

> the systematic application of technologies, engineering methodologies, or scientific principles to meet the needs of and address the barriers confronted by individuals with disabilities in areas which include education, rehabilitation, employment, transportation, independent living, and recreation. The term includes rehabilitation engineering, assistive technology devices, and assistive technology services.

Both pieces of legislation emphasize the fact that services or devices are being provided to "individuals" with disabilities not "populations" of persons with disabilities. This same emphasis is found in Title I of the Americans with Disabilities Act of 1990 (Public Law 101-336, Section 101) with respect to the provision of reasonable accommodations by employers:

> The term *reasonable accommodation* means:
> (i) Modification or adjustments to a job application process that enable a qualified applicant with a disability to be considered for the position such qualified applicant desires; or
> (ii) Modifications or adjustments to the work environment, or to the manner or circumstances under which the position held or desired is customarily performed, that enable a qualified individual with a disability to perform the essential functions of that position; or
> (iii) Modifications or adjustments that enable a covered entity's employee with a disability to enjoy equal benefits and privileges of employment as are enjoyed by its other similarly situated employees without disabilities.

In general, the three aforementioned pieces of federal legislation are aimed at removing barriers and increasing independence for individuals with disabilities. Achieving these goals can involve changes to the method, tools, equipment, workstation, or environment that are customarily in place to enable a person with a disability to accomplish a given task or function in an alternative manner. This involves an assessment of the individual's capabilities and limitations and an analysis of the tasks or functions to be accomplished. A comparison of the two exposes any gaps between the capabilities of the individual and the requirements of the task. The ergonomist's skills must then be used to effectively bridge this gap to provide an effective accommodation, which is the heart of ergonomics-for-one.

Accommodation Process: Systems Approach

Systems Analysis

An ergonomist may be called on to accommodate an individual with a disability in a wide variety of circumstances: employment, education, functional daily living, or leisure. This chapter primarily emphasizes the employment setting; however, the concepts and methodology presented may be generalized to the other situations. The accommodation process is most effectively achieved through a systems approach (Figure 4-1).

Systems Model

The system is composed of the following elements:

1. Essential task functions
2. Tools, equipment, information, and workstation traditionally used to complete the task
3. Inputs and outputs to the system
4. Environment within which the task is accomplished
5. Individual with a disability who desires to complete the task

The ergonomist must assess all elements of the system to make the most appropriate accommodation. It is important to note that ergonomists must develop their own, personalized, process of assessment. The order and manner in which the elements within the system are studied defines the individual ergonomist's process. An assessment of the accommodation system can begin with any of the five elements, provided all elements are eventually studied. Note that the

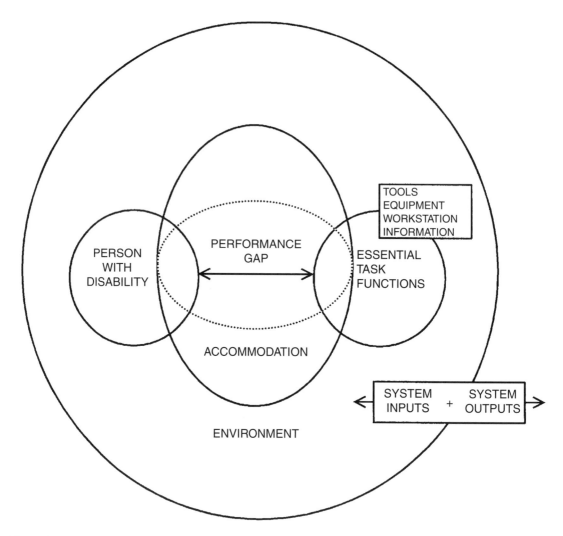

Figure 4-1. Diagrammatic representation of the accommodation process using a systems approach.

process can be iterative in nature: As the ergonomist progresses through the assessment, the discovery of additional constraints or the need for more information regarding a previously studied element may prompt the ergonomist to revisit the element, or to run through the entire process again. This is most likely to happen when the ergonomist is attempting to save costly time by not overanalyzing a situation or when the ergonomist is inexperienced with the process.

System Elements

Defining Essential Task Functions. The definition of essential task functions will vary with respect to

circumstances. Consequently, the setting (e.g., employment, education, functional daily living, or leisure) will dictate the definition.

Within the realm of employment, the essential functions of a job are defined by Title I of the Americans with Disabilities Act of 1990 (ADA) (Public Law 101-336) as follows:

> (n) Essential Functions
> (1) In general. The term "essential functions" means the fundamental job duties of the employment position the individual with a disability holds or desires. The term "essential functions" does not include the marginal functions of the position.
> (2) A job function may be considered essential for

any of several reasons, including but not limited to the following:

(i) The function may be essential because the reason the position exists is to perform that function;

(ii) The function may be essential because of the limited number of employees available among whom the performance of that job function can be distributed; and/or

(iii) The function may be highly specialized so that the incumbent in the position is hired for his or her expertise or ability to perform the particular function.

According to the ADA provisions, functions pertaining to a job are considered essential under three circumstances. In the first circumstance, "the reason the position exists is to perform that function." Clearly, the job of cab driver exists to drive the cab and pick up and deliver customers. Thus, driving, with or without an accommodation would be considered an essential function. In another example, the job of butcher exists to cut meat. The ability to perform this task would, therefore, be considered an essential function.

The second circumstance that renders a job function essential is that there are a "limited number of employees available among whom the performance of that job function can be distributed." For instance, in a small restaurant, the people who wait on tables might be required to perform several tasks if the number of employees is limited. They would have to be able to seat customers, take orders, serve food, bus tables, and collect money.

Another familiar example is that of a unionized plant where the terms of a collective bargaining agreement may limit or prohibit the reassignment of certain job functions to workers in other job classifications. A task may be considered essential even when it is only performed for a short time each day: The only time an employee may be required to perform data entry may be during peak times (e.g., in a federal tax processing center). However, because all employees are needed to perform this function at that time, it is essential to the job.

According to the ADA, the final circumstance in which a function is considered essential is when the function is "highly specialized" and the individual is "hired for his or her expertise or ability to perform the particular function." The function of designing certain tools must be done by a licensed engineer; similarly, welding operations performed in the construction of an oil refinery must be done by personnel trained in this specialized task.

Assessing Job Function. The ergonomist should first assess the job the way it would be performed by an employee without a disability. Next the ergonomist may need to work with the employer, the supervisor, and the employee to determine which functions are essential to that job, consulting the written job description if one exists. Each function should be viewed from the perspective of what outcome or result it is intended to achieve.

Consider the job of telephone receptionist. Traditionally, the receptionist takes phone messages by hand and physically places the handwritten slips into the appropriate slot in a vertical organizer. The essential functions of the job are to receive and record information from phone calls and convey that information to the appropriate individuals, regardless of how it is recorded or delivered. Consider the job of palletizing 50-lb sacks of sand: The existing job description states that the worker lifts the 50-lb sack from the conveyor and places it appropriately on a pallet. The essential function is not manually lifting the sack but rather moving the sack from the conveyor to the pallet. This outcome-based mindset ultimately simplifies the design of the accommodation because only the true function requirements are being studied.

Tools, Equipment, Workstation, Information. The ergonomist must determine what resources are traditionally used to accomplish the job. These resources may be as obvious as a large farm implement or a paint brush, or as familiar as writing instruments or kitchen aids. Equipment used to assist in achieving the job functions may include motorized vehicles, such as fork lifts or trucks; industrial machinery, such as drill presses or band saws; medical equipment, such as electron microscopes or electrocardiography monitors; telephone systems; and office equipment, such as copiers and folding machines. The workstation may be a simple desk and chair, an adjustable computer table, a workbench, a station on an assembly line, a mechanic's pit, a checkout counter, or a cutting table. Finally, informational resources may include telephone calls, electronic mail, reference manuals, computer disks, work orders, or verbal instructions.

In examining these resources, the outcome or result that is being achieved through their use should again be the focus. This will simplify the ultimate definition of the accommodation.

System Inputs and Outputs. The ergonomist must identify the things that enter and leave the system with which the individual must interact. This may include customers, patients, parts on an assembly line, packages, mail, or electronic mail. The ergonomist must determine the required outcomes as a result of these interactions. For example, customers must be greeted and seated, parts must be added to a subassembly on the line, and packages must be placed on a pallet for shipping. Once again, the outcome-based approach will simplify the definition of the final accommodation.

Environment. The environment in which the job will be accomplished must also be assessed. Factors that may be pertinent such as noise, lighting, fumes, dirt, and ventilation should be noted. The ergonomist should also ascertain whether the job could be performed in an alternative location, and if so, this should be examined. Finally, if pertinent, the architectural accessibility of the environment should be assessed.

Person with the Disability. The ergonomist must make a determination of the capabilities and limitations of the individual with the disability, who may be able to provide some or all of the information, but consulting other sources may be necessary. Please note that it is impossible to accurately predict a person's abilities solely on the basis of a medical diagnosis. However, consultation with someone knowledgeable in the diagnosis may clarify whether further changes in the client's status should be anticipated:

- Many disabilities go through stages—disabilities can wax and wane.
- Disabilities can change due to environmental conditions.
- Disabilities may change due to stress or fatigue.
- An individual may be deemed by his or her physician to be completely rehabilitated but still regain some residual function.

A particular disability may manifest itself differently in different individuals or at different stages. In addition, multiple impairments can result from a single disability. Preparing foundational information regarding the disability will help the ergonomist formulate specific questions to determine the individual's functional capabilities.

Functional analyses provides another means by which to assess capabilities and limitations, including range of motion, lifting capacity, strength, endurance, fine motor control, visual deficits, learning disabilities, hearing impairment, and memory loss. One way to minimize the time and cost associated with traditional functional analysis is to first assess the essential functions. Once the essential functions and their requirements are clear, the ergonomist can move to targeted analyses aimed at gleaning only necessary information. These assessments address the germane questions only, as opposed to the comprehensive obtained through functional capacity testing done as part of a medical examination or when returning an injured worker to work. For example, if one only needs to know the level of magnification required by an individual with a visual impairment to read 10-point type, why order an entire low-vision evaluation?

Again, knowledge of the disability is important. What is measured as a functional capacity today may not be accurate next week in some situations. The ergonomist must be aware of this.

Existing medical documentation may also be a valuable source of information. A functional assessment that is not job related might be valuable. In addition to finding out about specific impairments and medical and surgical interventions, for example, such an assessment might reveal that the client has physician imposed limitations on lifting, stooping, bending, or walking.

If the situation is job related and the individual has requested a reasonable accommodation, then the employer may already have this type of information on file. The employee or applicant may have had to submit this information to show evidence of the disability and justify the accommodation.

Performance Gap

By comparing the requirements of the essential task functions to the capabilities of the individual with the disability, a performance gap, if any exists,

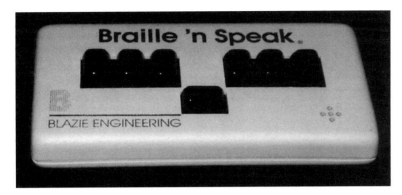

Figure 4-2. The Braille 'n Speak (Blazie Engineering, Forest Hill, MD) is a commercially available portable computer. Blazie Engineering's device is equipped with braille keys for use by an individual who is blind and proficient in braille utilization.

should be exposed. This gap may occur because the individual is unable to perform an essential function using the current method or existing tools or equipment, cannot access the present workstation, or is not capable of negotiating the existing environment. The performance gap defines the specific areas in need of accommodation.

Accommodation Design

The ergonomist's skills can be used to bridge the performance gap by identifying an accommodation, which allows the individual to perform the essential tasks in an alternative manner.

Types of Accommodations

The accommodation defined by the ergonomist may involve any or all of a variety of components: job restructuring, provision of assistive devices or adaptive aids, alternative tools and equipment, workstation modification, and environmental changes.

Job Restructuring. The ergonomist may design an alternative method for task completion. Consider the example of the receptionist's job that involves taking phone messages and placing them in the appropriate slot in a vertical phone message organizer. On inquiry, the tasks are determined to be essential, and traditionally, the messages are handwritten. The individual for whom the job is being considered cannot write the messages by hand or physically place them in the message organizer. However, everyone in the office has e-mail capabil-

ities. As an accommodation, the receptionist will record the phone messages in a computer file and send them to the appropriate employees via e-mail.

Provision of Assistive Devices or Adaptive Aids. Items that have been designed specifically to overcome limitations caused by various types of disabilities are known as assistive devices and adaptive aids (Figure 4-2). Common examples are telecommunication devices for the deaf or hearing impaired, braille printers, alternative keyboards, and three-wheeled scooters. Extensive databases of such devices exist, such as AbleData (Trace Research and Development Center, University of Wisconsin, Madison). To avoid "reinventing the wheel," the ergonomist should be familiar with these products.

Alternative Tools and Equipment. The ergonomist may recommend an alternative tool or piece of equipment, all of which are commercially available. Electric cutting shears may replace manual scissors for an individual with carpal tunnel syndrome (Figure 4-3). Existing tools or equipment may also be modified to fit the individual being accommodated. For example, to accommodate a grasping impairment, the ergonomist may build up the grip diameter of a soldering pencil or recommend a modification of the hand controls on an industrial punch press. It should be noted that such alterations may result in a violation of the Occupational Safety and Health Administration (OSHA) code and should only be undertaken by an appropriately licensed engineer. Another adaptation might be the addition of jigs or fixtures to hold materials or parts in place during a task (Figure 4-4). These devices are particularly useful in accommodating

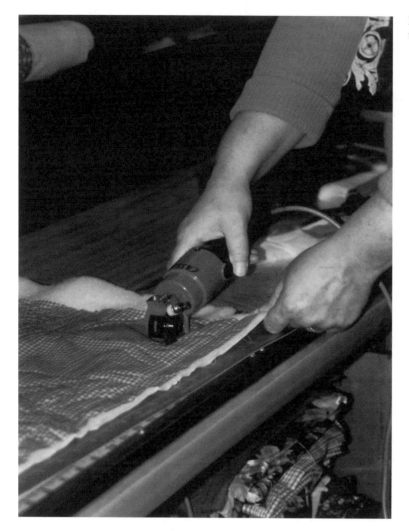

Figure 4-3. Individual using electric shears to cut quilting material.

individuals with visual impairments or the use of only one hand due to amputation, stroke, or head injury.

Workstation Modification. The ergonomist may use traditional skills to alter workstation heights and depths, define appropriate reach envelopes, provide an improved layout, or customize a workstation with motorized height adjustment or low-friction turntables.

Environmental Changes. Environmental changes may involve altering the physical environment to make it architecturally accessible for an individual using a wheelchair. Issues of temperature may need to be addressed when disabilities, such as multiple sclerosis, are involved because individuals possessing this disability often have difficulty regulating body temperature. Lighting may need to be altered for individuals with visual impairments. For example, an individual with retinitis pigmentosa may need to work in diminished light to avoid further deterioration of vision. Controlling excessive noise can be of benefit to individuals with hearing impairments as well as those with attention deficit disorders.

Accommodation Hierarchy

When recommending an accommodation there is a hierarchy that should be followed whenever possible. This hierarchy begins with the least radical change. The first level of modification that the ergonomist should consider is that involving simple changes such as rearranging the workstation or alter-

Figure 4-4. Employee with a visual impairment uses a custom designed jig that holds a file folder stationary while he crimps a small metal tab onto the corner.

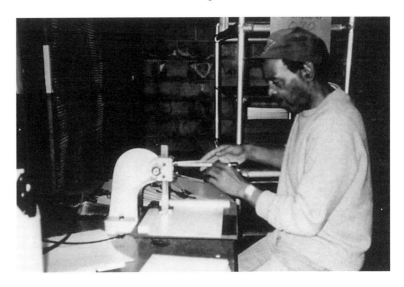

ing the methods used. Second, the ergonomist may consider the recommendation of a commercially available off-the-shelf item. Such products should carry warranties, have proven track records regarding reliability and maintainability, and are usually less costly and less time-consuming to procure than modified or custom designed products.

At the third level of the hierarchy lie the modified off-the-shelf products. In this situation, the ergonomist identifies the off-the-shelf product that most closely satisfies the defined need and modifies it to obtain a more exact fit. Keep in mind that modifying a commercially available product may void a manufacturer's warranty, result in OSHA violations, or pose a safety hazard to the designer or end user. It should, therefore, be approached with caution. The final stage in the hierarchy is the provision of a custom-designed solution (Figures 4-5 through 4-7). Custom fabrication has the distinct advantage of providing an exact fit—the ultimate application of ergonomics-for-one.

The hierarchy should be viewed as a guide and should not drive the selection of the most appropriate accommodation. The ergonomist must choose the accommodation that best fits the individual.

Consumer Choice

When working through the assessment and accommodation process, the ergonomist must always work closely with the person being accommodated. The ideas, recommendations, and personal preferences of the individual should be taken into account. If the ergonomist fails in this area, it could result in failure of the accommodation—the individual with the disability must be willing to use the recommended accommodation to make it a success.

Other Considerations

In defining an accommodation, the ergonomist must also consider the following constraints: cost, portability and durability, environmental conditions, and reliability and maintainability.

Cost. In many cases, cost will be the bottom line. Anything that the ergonomist can do to minimize costs will help ensure that the recommended accommodation will be implemented and that such services will be requested in the future. Some methods for containing costs are as follows:

- Obtain pertinent materials in advance of site visits or face-to-face evaluations; these include job descriptions, medical background, workstation layouts, and photos or videotape of the job and the site.
- Be familiar with the vast array of existing assistive devices and commercial products—

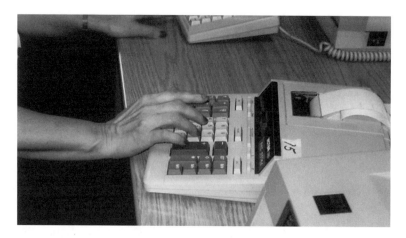

Figure 4-5. Employee with carpal tunnel syndrome exhibits excessive wrist extension while using computer keyboard and adding machine.

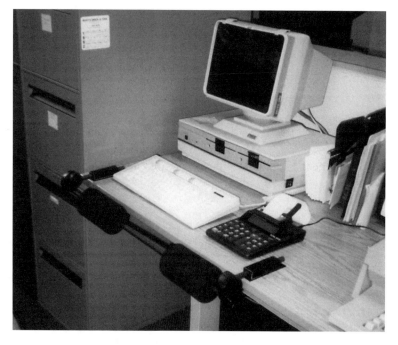

Figure 4-6. Custom wrist support, the Roll-N-Slide (designed by rehabilitation engineer Keith Johnston in conjunction with the Ability Center of Toledo, OH) was supplied to employee with carpal tunnel syndrome.

such as lifting devices, pallet levelers (Figure 4-8), and ergonomically designed hand tools—so that off-the-shelf items can be recommended where possible.

- Perform the task analysis before functional assessment to minimize the cost and extensiveness of the latter.
- Develop a systematic approach using standardized forms for recording information, which will increase the likelihood of obtaining essential or clarifying information on the initial site visit. Failure to obtain sufficient information might require a second site visit or lead to an inappropriate accommodation.
- Refrain from jumping directly to a solution before systematically analyzing the situation. Putting an incorrect solution in place can be very costly. You must define the problem correctly before you can solve it!

Figure 4-7. Employee exhibits appropriate wrist posture while using the Role-N-Slide. The device also allows the employee to slide the wrists forward for key access or side-to-side to access the keyboard or the adding machine.

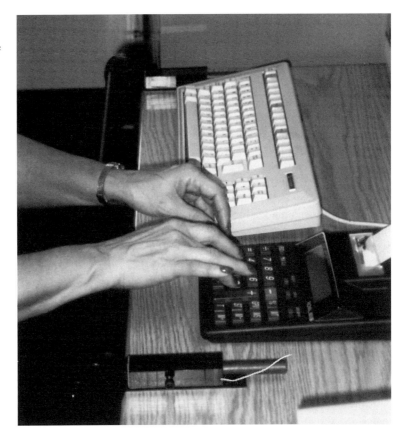

Figure 4-8. Commercially available Southworth Rotating Palette Leveler.

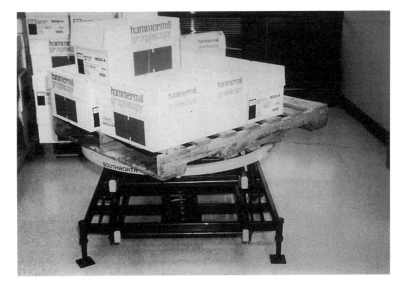

Portability and Durability. If the individual being accommodated must carry or otherwise transport a recommended device, then the issue of portability should also be considered. The ergonomist must consider the weight and dimensions of the object, the individual's lifting and carrying capabilities, and the method of transport. Is the client in a wheelchair? How durable is the device? Can it be jostled? Can it survive if dropped?

Environmental Conditions. The ergonomist may need to consider environmental factors when recommending an accommodation. For instance, is the individual or the device under consideration sensitive to moisture, temperature extremes, or dirt?

Reliability and Maintainability. The ergonomist should consider reliability and maintainability in the recommendation process. If a device is not highly reliable or requires a great deal of maintenance, it will soon be sitting on the shelf.

Consequences of the Design

The ultimate goal of any accommodation is to enable an individual with a disability to perform a task safely and efficiently. In so doing, the following principles should be kept in mind:

1. The design should take full advantage of a person's capabilities.
2. The design should not stress a person beyond his or her limitations.
3. The design should not aggravate the existing disability, nor should it cause a new disability (McQuistion, 1993).

Test and Evaluation

The ergonomist should follow up after the completion of an accommodation, to determine the success of the ergonomic intervention. Consider the following factors:

- Essential functions—Can the individual being accommodated now perform the essential functions?
- Productivity—Is the accommodated employee able to meet established production quotas or expectations? If new methods, equipment, tools, or adaptive devices have been provided, consider the learning curve effect when examining productivity. The ergonomist must provide all involved parties with a realistic picture.
- Personal satisfaction—Is the accommodated individual pleased with intervention? Inclusion of the individual, as appropriate, throughout the assessment and design phases promotes employee satisfaction.
- Ease-of-use—Are the components of the intervention relatively easy to use and maintain once the employee and any coworkers affected have been appropriately trained? Without ease-of-use, the accommodation will likely be abandoned.
- Universal design—Does the intervention benefit other employees? Employees without disabilities can sometimes benefit from the accommodation when it is discovered that a new method, tool, or piece of equipment will enable them to be more productive or work more safely.
- Cost savings—Does the introduction of the intervention allow discontinuation or reduced use of a more costly accommodation? For instance, introducing a document scanner and a voice output–screen reader package to a blind employee's computer setup would eliminate the need for someone to act as a reader. The benefits include cost savings, greater independence, and increased versatility and control over the scheduling of the work day (the employee can read documents at will instead of only when the reader is available). Another example of cost savings can be seen when someone with a worker's compensation claim returns to work as a result of the intervention. The employer can realize savings in workers' compensation premiums as well as savings in hiring and training a substitute employee.

Systems Approach Regardless of Setting

Most of the aforementioned information has been presented with an emphasis on the employment setting. However, the processes discussed above can be generalized for application to education, functional daily living, and leisure. Regardless of setting, the ergonomist should still apply the systems approach.

Education

The essential functions associated with education vary with the grade level of the student, the school, the teacher, and other factors. Essential functions may include taking notes in class, participating in class discussions, and completing homework assignments. The ergonomist's approach, nonetheless, is similar to that used in the employment situation: Determine the required outcomes for each essential function, and ascertain the individual's capabilities so as to define the accommodation. If note taking in class is essential, and the student is unable to accomplish this manually, the ergonomist must seek alternatives. An assessment of typing skills—with or without assistive devices—should determine whether taking notes using a laptop computer is an option. A team approach can be essential to success. In an educational setting, the team may consist of the student, teachers, parents (if the student is a minor), a school-based health care professional, and the ergonomist.

Functional Daily Living

The goal of the ergonomist within this realm is to increase independence with respect to self-care (activities of daily living), homemaking, and community access. Because this area can be vast and all encompassing, it is important to work with the individual to be accommodated, family members, and the funding agency (where applicable) to clearly define essential functions. This will assist the ergonomist in maximizing the level of accommodation within a given budget. If, for example, homemaking is a stated priority, the essential homemaking tasks should be defined. If food preparation is determined to be the most essential then efforts will concentrate on defining the essential functions of this task (e.g., cutting, cooking, baking, cleanup), assessing the layout of the kitchen, and examining kitchen implements and appliances. A wide variety of adaptive aids, often called *aids to daily living* (ADLs), are commercially available. Information regarding specific sources can be obtained from the Centers for Independent Living present in all states.

Leisure

Accommodating an individual for sport and recreational activities is an instance of complete consumer choice. Because many such activities normally emphasize physical activity, there may be an increased need for functional assessment in this realm. The area of adaptive leisure aids has exploded in the marketplace. Assistive aids exist for adaptive bowling, fishing, hunting, photography, skiing, cycling, horseback riding, playing cards and board games, needlepoint, and many other interests. This type of information is available from Independent Living Centers.

Task Analysis Methodology

Task Analysis

The topic of task analysis is presented here as it applies to an employment setting. However, the information and technique presented below can be readily generalized to include applications of education, functional daily living, and leisure.

Definition

Job analysis is a tool for examining job content. Such analyses can vary greatly with respect to the technique employed, the types of information gathered, and the level of detail desired. The most important feature of any such technique is its comprehensiveness. The technique must assist the ergonomist in achieving a complete and thorough analysis.

Technique

Each ergonomist must adopt his or her own technique for accomplishing task analysis. An example of one such technique is presented below. A set of forms is provided to assist you in the application of this technique. This technique is comprehensive in nature as well as being highly flexible. It can be easily customized to accommodate jobs that vary widely with respect to the level of repetitiveness, the number and nature of tasks, and the existence of multiple task environments.

Forms and Instructions

Figures 4-9 and 4-10 present a set of forms for use in job analysis. The term *environmental analysis* is used for the heading to remind the ergonomist that the job is composed of more than the actual functions performed by the worker. Recall from the previously presented systems model that one must also consider tools, equipment, workstation, information requirements, system inputs/outputs, and environmental conditions—all of the elements within the work environment.

Detailed instructions for completing the Environmental Analysis forms are presented below. The form in Figure 4-9 is used to collect general information:

1. Name. List employee name or identification number.
2. Job Title. List both the official job title or classification as well as a descriptive title that more accurately depicts the job if necessary.
3. Required Skills, Education, and Training. This information may appear on the job description or may be obtained from the employer.
4. General Task List. Break the job down into its component tasks and list each. If a job description is available it may be helpful to attempt this in advance. It can then be refined during the actual assessment.
5. General Environmental Conditions. List environmental factors that apply to all job tasks. Also list issues related to architectural accessibility of the workplace if applicable.

The form presented in Figure 4-10 is used to collect detailed information regarding the individual tasks listed in the General Task List in Figure 4-9. In other words, one copy of the Environmental Analysis Part B form in Figure 4-10 should be filled out for *each* task listed in the General Task List on the Environmental Analysis Part A form in Figure 4-9.

1. General Task Description. The ergonomist should list one task from the General Task List and provide a brief description.
2. Task Elements. Break the task down into its individual elements.
3. Essential Nature. These criteria can assist in determining whether or not a function is essential.
   a. Criticalness. Use some measure to indicate to what degree the element is essential. One such measure may be a numeric scale ranging from one (not critical) to five (extremely critical).
   b. % of Time/Day. In an average day, what percentage of time is spent performing this element?
   c. Task Frequency. State the number of times this element is performed within a given time increment. If the task element is highly repetitive it may be appropriate to state this information in times/minute. If the element is rarely performed times/hour or times/day may be better.
4. Task Element Requirements. These items define the methods used in the individual task elements.
   a. Body Position. List the body position used while performing the element (sitting, standing, bending)
   b. Motion. Give the specific motions involved to accomplish the element. The body parts involved should also be listed when appropriate and whether both hands or feet were used. If the job is not highly repetitive in nature, gross movements or tasks may be listed (such as typing, grasping a phone, moving a box). Highly repetitive functions may need to be reduced to elemental motion segments. Consider an assembly job; motions may include reach for part with left hand, place part on subassembly with left hand, hold part with left hand, apply pneumatic nut driver with right hand. These individual motions and hand designations can become important if, for example, one is accommodating an individual with a right arm amputation.
   c. Motion Distance. State the distance covered by the motion listed in (b) above.
   d. Movement Location. For the motion defined in (b) and (c) above list the location range relative to the body areas in which the motion occurs. Typical range indicators include floor to knee, knee to waist, and elbow to shoulder.
   e. Weight. Provide the weight of the objects being held, lifted, carried, or pushed.
5. Tools Utilized. List all tools currently used to perform the element.
6. Equipment Utilized. List all equipment currently in use, including the use of safety equipment.
7. Information Requirements. List all informa-

ENVIRONMENTAL ANALYSIS - PART A

NAME: _____

JOB TITLE: _____

REQUIRED SKILLS, EDUCATION OR TRAINING: _____

_____

_____

GENERAL TASK LIST:

_____

_____

_____

_____

_____

_____

_____

_____

_____

GENERAL ENVIRONMENTAL CONDITIONS: _____

_____

_____

_____

_____

_____

_____

Figure 4-9. Sample form for performing Part A of environmental analysis. (Form and technique were initially developed by Linda McQuistion and Mark Ficocelli for the Ohio Rehabilitation Services Commission and were published in *National short-term training program: Americans with Disabilities Act* [McQuistion, 1992]. They appear here in modified form.)

ENVIRONMENTAL ANALYSIS- PART B

GENERAL TASK DESCRIPTION: _____

TASK ELEMENTS

ANALYSIS CRITERIA				
CRITICALNESS				
% OF TIME/DAY				
TASK FREQUENCY				
BODY POSITION				
MOTION				
MOTION DISTANCE				
MOVEMENT LOCATION				
WEIGHT				
TOOLS UTILIZED				
EQUIPMENT UTILIZED				
INFORMATION REQUIREMENTS				
TASK SPECIFIC ENVIRONMENTAL CONDITIONS				
VISUAL CONSIDERATIONS				
SAFETY & HAZARD CONSIDERATIONS				
WORK STATION (ATTACH SKETCH)				
SYSTEM INPUTS/ OUTPUTS				

Figure 4-10. Sample form for performing Part B of environmental analysis. (Form and technique were initially developed by Linda McQuistion and Mark Ficocelli for the Ohio Rehabilitation Services Commission and were published in *National short-term training program: Americans with Disabilities Act* [McQuistion, 1992]. They appear here in modified form.)

tion needed to perform the task element and the purpose for the information. Also note the type of media being used to convey the information and to whom it is being given.

8. Task-Specific Environmental Conditions. List only those factors specific to the task element. For example, when performing a given element there may be a problem with fumes, glare, or noise.

9. Visual Considerations. When necessary, the human factors specialist should list the attributes that may affect visually intense elements (i.e., those requiring a great degree of visual concentration or focus). These include color, contrast, size, distance, and movement.

10. Safety and Hazard Considerations. List existing and potential safety issues. These might include unguarded machinery, open pits, pinch points, or chemical exposures.

11. Workstation. Briefly describe the current workstation by listing its components (adjustable computer desk, workbench, check-out stand). Attach a sketch if necessary.

12. System Inputs/Outputs. List the inputs/outputs associated with the task element. Indicate the nature and purpose of each.

Case Example

Analysis

To demonstrate the use of the task analysis technique and forms, the case of the shipping clerk is presented. The shipping clerk position being studied is responsible for filling orders for packs of order forms. This individual, Johnny Lee, obtains an order form request from the receptionist. He then gathers the packages of forms requested from two 3-tiered shelves and takes them to a packing table. Johnny completes a packing slip and places it in the box along with the forms. Holding a tape dispenser gun in one hand, he applies tape to the box while rolling the box over with the other hand. He then removes the shipping label from the order form and applies it to the box. Johnny places the box on a pallet for shipping. He then returns the order form and a copy of the packing slip to the receptionist and obtains a new order form.

Figures 4-11 and 4-12 present completed Environmental Analysis forms for the shipping clerk position. The general information is presented in Figure 4-11. Figure 4-12 demonstrates task 5 from the General Task List: Packs Forms. This task is broken down into four task elements. One column of information is then completed for each element.

The individual to be accommodated has cerebral palsy. He states that he has difficulty ambulating, lifting, and stooping. A physical assessment revealed the following:

1. Individual ambulates independently for short distances.
2. He is observed holding onto walls or other supports for balance much of the time.
3. Abnormal muscle tone is observed throughout his body affecting balance, ability to stoop and bend, and upper extremity coordination.
4. Upper extremities are functional in range of motion.
5. Tremors and deficits in coordination affect his fine motor skills.
6. Labored breathing was exhibited throughout the assessment while lifting boxes and pushing loaded cart.
7. Pelvic obliquity was observed looking at individual from behind (right hip higher than left).
8. No cognitive deficits were observed.

The therapist performing the physical assessment referred the employee to the state vocational rehabilitation program as a potential job-save situation. The ergonomist then worked with the employee, the employer, and a third-party payer representative (vocational rehabilitation counselor). Next, the completed Part A and Part B Environmental Analysis forms were studied and the requirements of the job were compared to the capabilities and limitations of the individual to be accommodated, thereby defining the performance gaps. These are the gaps to which the ergonomist must apply the concepts of ergonomics-for-one and then define the accommodation.

After observing the individual in the performance of his job, meeting with the employee and supervisor, and studying the information as above, the ergonomist was able to determine the following:

1. Essential Functions. Two other individuals also perform this job; but they work different

ENVIRONMENTAL ANALYSIS- PART A

NAME: Johnny Lee

JOB TITLE: Shipping Clerk (Form Packer/Shipper)

REQUIRED SKILLS, EDUCATION OR TRAINING: On-the-Job training

GENERAL TASK LIST:

1). Obtains order form from receptionist

2). Collects forms requested on order form

3). Takes forms to packing table

4). Completes packing slip

5). Packs forms

6). Places packed box on pallet for shipping

7). Returns copy of packing slip to receptionist along with order form

GENERAL ENVIRONMENTAL CONDITIONS: _____

1). Cool temperature - warehouse setting

Figure 4-11. Part A of Environmental Analysis form completed for shipping clerk position.

ENVIRONMENTAL ANALYSIS- PART B

GENERAL TASK DESCRIPTION: 5). Packs Forms

TASK ELEMENTS

ANALYSIS CRITERIA	Places Empty Box On Shipping Table	Places Forms & Packing Slip In Box	Seals Box	Labels Box
CRITICALNESS (range, 1–5)	5	5	5	5
% OF TIME/DAY	5%	30%	3%	2%
TASK FREQUENCY	5 Times/Hr.	5 Times/Hr.	5 Times/Hr.	5 Times/Hr.
BODY POSITION	Standing	Standing	Standing	Standing
MOTION	Reaching one hand	Reach/Grasp/ Move/Release Forms	Roll Box While Taping	Peel/Move/ Stick Label
MOTION DISTANCE	3 Ft.	1 Ft. into Box	Box Circumference	1Ft.
MOVEMENT LOCATION	Shoulder to Waist	At Waist	At Waist	At Waist
WEIGHT	1 Pound	5 Pounds/ Package of Forms	Up to 30 Pounds	-
TOOLS UTILIZED	-	-	Tape Gun	-
EQUIPMENT UTILIZED	-	-	-	-
INFORMATION REQUIREMENTS	-	Packing Slip	-	Order Form
TASK SPECIFIC ENVIRONMENTAL CONDITIONS	-	-	-	-
VISUAL CONSIDERATIONS	-	Reading Forms #'s & Packing Slip & Order Form	-	Reading Labels
SAFETY & HAZARD CONSIDERATIONS	Long Reach for Empty Box	-	Rolls Box to Tape	-
WORK STATION (ATTACH SKETCH)	Packing Table at Waist & Shelf at Shoulder	Same	Same	Same
SYSTEM INPUTS/ OUTPUTS	Empty Box	Order Form/ Forms & Packing Slip	-	Order Form

Figure 4-12. Part B of Environmental Analysis form completed for shipping clerk essential job function: packs forms.

shifts than the employee to be accommodated. Because all of the above-mentioned elements must be completed and no other employee is available to assist, it was determined that all of the listed elements should be considered essential.

2. Performance Gaps. Due to the physical limitations related to his disability (cerebral palsy), the employee displayed the following performance deficits:

    a. Difficulty walking to the receptionist's desk to obtain order forms and return completed order forms and packing slips.

    b. Difficulty gathering the requested forms:

        i. Trouble walking the shelving aisles to gather forms

        ii. Balance problems when retrieving forms from bottom shelf

        iii. Pain/difficulty reaching forms on top shelf

        iv. Difficulty carrying forms; pain and trouble carrying volume of forms necessitating multiple trips to fill each order

    c. Pain and difficulty reaching for empty box

    d. Difficulty holding and manipulating tape gun and filled box

    e. Extreme difficulty in lifting and transferring filled box from packing table to pallet

    f. Low production rate. The employee is very slow and deliberate in the performance of all job tasks. Consequently, he is unable to meet established production quotas.

Potential Design Solutions

The following potential solutions could bridge the above-mentioned performance gaps.

1. Job sharing across job classifications: Can the receptionist or a designee deliver the order forms to the shipping clerk and retrieve the filled order forms and packing slips?

2. Would the vocational rehabilitation agency provide a three-wheeled scooter to help overcome ambulation problems?

3. If a three-wheeled scooter were provided, would the employer fund a custom basket that could be used for gathering forms?

4. Would a scooter seat with swivel and height adjustment capabilities assist the employee in order picking of forms?

5. Could the shelves of forms be reorganized so that no forms would be stored on the top shelf? Could the most frequently requested forms be stored on the center shelf?

6. Consider the purchase of a pallet leveler—a hydraulic/pneumatic/spring-loaded platform that lowers as weight is added to the platform to keep the uppermost surface at a near constant height. Thus, as subsequent layers are added to the pallet, one is always placing the box at the same height. This makes it possible to position such a device next to a work surface and virtually slide a box from the work surface to the pallet.

7. Consider a rotating feature for the pallet leveler so that the employee can, via a low friction turntable, rotate the platform into position to receive the next box. This would eliminate the need for the employee to push a box to the opposite side of the pallet for positioning.

8. Consider reconfiguring the packing table: to avoid the long reach for empty boxes, to ensure appropriate work-surface heights for performing the packing elements, and for transferring boxes to the pallet.

9. Is there a better method for sealing the boxes? A better tool? A device to hold the box while it is being sealed?

In considering these and other potential interventions make sure that input is sought from the employee, the employer, and the counselor throughout the process. This helps ensure that all parties will be satisfied with the solution and also helps avoid embarrassing mistakes. You certainly would not want to spend a great deal of time and effort working up a wonderful proposal based on providing a rotating pallet leveler, only to discover *during* your big presentation that the company had already considered this idea and had to abandon it due to the inability of the floor to bear the additional weight! Take nothing for granted!

Test and Evaluation

In evaluating the success of the intervention, the ergonomist must determine whether the shipping clerk can now perform the essential duties. Second, is he able to meet the established production quotas for number of boxes packed, or is he likely to reach this goal in a reasonable amount of time? If the answer to these two questions is yes, the ergonomist knows that the intervention is a functional success and the individual's job will be saved.

To further evaluate the accommodation, the ergonomist should determine to what extent all parties are satisfied with the intervention. Additionally, find out whether other employees who will be using the intervention understand how to properly use and maintain the tools and equipment. If other employees will be using components of the intervention, it is likely that the productivity and safety of these employees will improve.

Conclusion

To appropriately and effectively provide an ergonomic intervention for a person with a disability, the ergonomist must apply ergonomics-for-one. This systems approach enables the ergonomist to perform a comprehensive analysis. The information obtained from the analysis phase allows the ergonomist to design and implement a best-fit accommodation. Follow-up procedures test the accuracy and effectiveness of the intervention, enabling fine-tuning and changes when necessary. A final evaluation will show the overall success.

Acknowledgments

The author acknowledges Barbara Babaryk, for her tremendous word-processing efforts in the creation of this chapter and her endless patience, and Mark Ficocelli, of Ficocelli Design, for his assistance in the development of the Environmental Analysis forms and technique.

References

Americans with Disabilities Act of 1990. Public Law 101-336. Title I, Section 101. Washington, DC: U.S. Government Printing Office.

McQuistion, L. (1993). Rehabilitation engineering: Ergonomics-for-one. *Ergonomics in Design, January,* 10.

McQuistion, L. (1992). *Job accommodation in national short-term training program: Americans with Disabilities Act.* Chicago: Region V Rehabilitation Continuing Education Program.

Rehabilitation Act of 1973 (as amended). Public Law 103-73. Section 361.5. Washington, DC: U.S. Government Printing Office.

Technology-Related Assistance Law for Individuals with Disabilities Act of 1988 (as amended). Public Law 101-407. Section 3. Washington, DC: U.S. Government Printing Office.

Suggested Reading

American Association of Retired Persons, & Stein Gerontological Institute. (1993). *Life-span design of residential environments for an aging population.* Washington, DC: American Academy of Retired Persons.

Cooper, R. (1995). *Rehabilitation engineering applied to mobility and manipulation.* London: IOP Publishing.

Jageman, L. (1984). *Adaptive fixtures for handicapped workers.* Menomonie, WI: University of Wisconsin-Stout.

Kumar, S. (Ed.). (1997). *Perspectives in rehabilitation ergonomics.* Bristol, PA: Taylor & Francis.

Mann, W.C., & Lane, J.P. (1991). *Assistive technology for persons with disabilities: The role of occupational therapy.* Rockville, MD: American Occupational Therapy Association.

Mueller, J. (1990). *The workplace workbook: An illustrated guide to job accommodation and assistive technology.* Washington, DC: Dole Foundation.

Chapter 5

Physical Disability Case Study: Work Accommodations for an Individual with Phocomelia

Linda McQuistion

Learning Objectives

On completion of this chapter, the reader should be able to

- Understand a team approach to accommodation.
- Apply the systems approach to accommodation.
- Complete a basic task analysis of essential job functions.
- Effect accommodations.
- Evaluate accommodations.

Key Words

Rehabilitation engineering
Accommodation
Assistive technology
Rehabilitation technology
Task analysis

Abstract

This chapter presents a case study of a job accommodation for an individual with phocomelia. A team approach is used to accomplish this accommodation for a program specialist position. The use of a task analysis technique and associated forms is demonstrated.

Case Study: Program Specialist

Background

The Job

The position being studied is a program specialist for a state agency. This program specialist serves as the executive secretary for a council that deals with disability-related issues. This job involves coordinating council activities and providing administrative support. The position requires the provision of technical assistance regarding disability-related issues to employers, government agencies, and the general public. The individual must generate written council materials, write reports, and compose testimony. The job also requires the incumbent to sit on committees and advisory boards.

The Employee

The individual to be accommodated is a female whose disability is phocomelia due to thalidomide. Phocomelia is a developmental anomaly characterized by the absence of the proximal portion of a limb or limbs. As a result, the hands or feet are attached to the trunk by a single, small, irregularly shaped bone. This condition may result when the drug thalidomide is taken early in the mother's pregnancy.

The employee has two hands attached to the trunk as described above, extremely limiting her

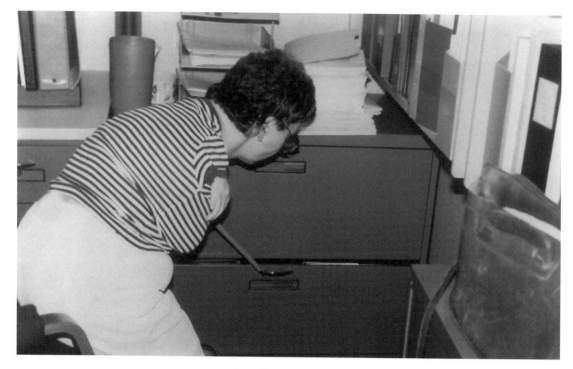

Figure 5-1. Employee with disability uses reacher to open drawer.

reach. She has one foot similarly attached, which limits her mobility and necessitates the use of a joystick-driven power wheelchair. She drives a modified van that incorporates a wheelchair lift and hand controls. For assistance, the employee has a dog and a reacher composed of a loop hook and dowel rod (Figure 5-1).

Preliminary Accommodation

When the employee was hired for this position, the employer instituted a temporary accommodation until a more formal accommodation could be undertaken:

- Bookshelves were lowered to provide some accessible storage.
- Secretarial assistance was arranged for retrieval of inaccessible materials.
- Handles were placed on desk and file drawers so employee could use the loop hook reacher to open drawers.
- A headset was provided for phone use.

Analysis

Essential Functions

The essential functions of the job were defined by consulting the written job description and meeting with the employee and supervisor. These functions are shown in the General Task List in Figure 5-2. Each essential function was listed on an individual Environmental Analysis–Part B form such as that shown in Figure 5-3.

Task Elements

The task elements of each function listed on Part B were then defined and listed across the top of the grid. As an example, consider the first essential function in the General Task List, "coordinates council activities," which involves making phone calls to secure a meeting site and typing meeting notices and agendas.

Figure 5-3 shows a breakdown of the requirements for each task element of this essential func-

ENVIRONMENTAL ANALYSIS- PART A

NAME: _____**K.L.**_____

JOB TITLE: **Program Specialist (Executive Secretary)**

REQUIRED SKILLS, EDUCATION OR TRAINING: _____

_____

_____

GENERAL TASK LIST:

1). _____Coordinates council activities (i.e., site arrangement, etc.)_____

2). _____Develops disability awareness programs_____

3). _____Provides administrative support to the council_____

4). _____Arranges/conducts meetings/seminars_____

5). _____Provides disability-related information to public (i.e., individuals,_____

_____employers, etc.)_____

6). _____Develops printed materials_____

7). _____Prepares written testimony regarding disability-related legislation_____

8). _____Assists government agencies with respect to disability-related issues___

9). _____Serves on committees/advisory boards, etc._____

GENERAL ENVIRONMENTAL CONDITIONS:_____

1). _____Cramped quarters in employee's office_____

2). _____Heavy paper clutter_____

3). _____Elevated office noise due to open office panel system_____

4). _____Entire building - ADA accessible_____

Figure 5-2. Environmental Analysis: Part A completed for program specialist position.

ENVIRONMENTAL ANALYSIS - PART B

GENERAL TASK DESCRIPTION: 1). Coordinating council activities

TASK ELEMENTS

ANALYSIS CRITERIA	Secure Meeting Site	Produce Meeting Notices and Agendas		
CRITICALNESS (range, 1–5)	5	5		
% OF TIME/DAY	10%	10%		
TASK FREQUENCY	1/day	1/day		
BODY POSITION	Sitting/Leaning	Sitting/Leaning		
MOTION	Grasp Phone Writing	Typing		
MOTION DISTANCE	2 ft.	—		
MOVEMENT LOCATION	At worksurface	Must go out to main office to use computer		
WEIGHT	Phone	—		
TOOLS UTILIZED	Pen	—		
EQUIPMENT UTILIZED	Telephone	Computer		
INFORMATION REQUIREMENTS	Telephone Directories Calendar	Notes Calendar		
TASK SPECIFIC ENVIRONMENTAL CONDITIONS	—	—		
VISUAL CONSIDERATIONS	Read fine print in directories	Read computer screen		
SAFETY & HAZARD CONSIDERATIONS	Leaning for phone	Old computer— keyboard attached*		
WORK STATION (ATTACH SKETCH)	Desk in office	Desk in office Table in Main Office		
SYSTEM INPUTS/ OUTPUTS		0: Meeting Notices		

Figure 5-3. Environmental Analysis: Part B completed for one essential function of the program specialist job. This function is "coordinating council activities." *The inability to position the keyboard and monitor separately can be associated with wrist problems (e.g., carpal tunnel syndrome), neck and shoulder pain, and eye strain.

tion. Once examined this way, the ergonomist can see that this function primarily involves telephone and computer use.

Figure 5-4 considers essential function number five from the General Task List—"provides disability-related information to the public." The function involves the following activities:

- Performing research regarding disability-related laws, policies, and pertinent matters
- Responding to telephone calls regarding information requests
- Providing written responses
- Meeting with individuals

Figure 5-4 gives the breakdown of the task elements for this essential function. Initial review shows that this function involves telephone and computer use, as did the first essential function but adds a dimension: Providing disability-related information to the public can also involve researching resource materials and meeting with individuals in the office.

After examining several of the essential functions it becomes apparent that all of these functions require some combination of five elements:

1. Research and accessing resource materials
2. Telephone use
3. Writing
4. Computer use
5. Meeting with one or two individuals

It is often the case when dealing with an informational type position, as opposed to a more physical job, that the worker uses a basic set of elements to accomplish a great many functions. The role of the ergonomist then becomes one of accommodating these elements.

Existing Workstation

The employee's current office (Figure 5-5) is 6 × 8 ft. The work surfaces vary from 24 to 30 in. deep and are located 8–9 in. above compressed seat height. The office cubicle is part of an overall open office architecture used throughout the building. As a result, the existing work surfaces are individual surfaces that attach to the cubicle walls.

The individual being accommodated transfers into a large office chair to work and parks her power wheelchair within her cubicle. She uses the assistance of a dog that also stays within her office. Shelving units surround the interior of the cubicle at a height of approximately 4 ft. and more are located above her desk. The task-lighting units and light switches are located under these shelves.

The ergonomist was informed at the start of the project that the employee's unit would be moving to another section of the building. A new, unoccupied space was available to configure as an office space for this individual, so time was not spent sketching the existing workstation.

Existing Equipment

A telephone and computer system were in use. As part of a preliminary accommodation, the employer had supplied a headset, but it was not in use by the employee at the time of the assessment. She indicated that the headset was awkward, heavy, and often shorted out. As a result, the employee used a standard phone and handset located on the work surface (Figure 5-6). She must place one foot on the floor and lean forward quite far to access the phone.

The computer system in use was a Wang one-piece terminal (keyboard and monitor in one unit), which was located on a table outside of her office in a common area. The Wang terminal was part of a network. As such, her secretary was able to access her documents to finish formatting, printing, and so forth. The Wang had its own word processor which was not compatible with other word-processing systems (such as Word-Perfect). The Wang system had no e-mail capabilities, and no floppy drives were available.

A second network, a DEC system, was also available within the building. E-mail capabilities did exist with this system allowing access to the organization's 70 offices statewide. The employee did not have access to this system.

Informational Resources

The employee has a large volume of informational resources including files, books, manuals, and legal documents. She has approximately 30 linear feet of materials, 16 linear feet of which are not accessible to the employee; and 12 linear feet are accessed with varying degrees of difficulty.

ENVIRONMENTAL ANALYSIS - PART B

GENERAL TASK DESCRIPTION: 5). Provides disability - related information to the public

TASK ELEMENTS

ANALYSIS CRITERIA	Perform Research	Telephone Responses	Written Responses	Small Meetings
CRITICALNESS (range, 1–5)	5	5	5	5
% OF TIME/DAY	40%	20%	10%	< 1%
TASK FREQUENCY	1/Hr.	4/Hr.	4/Day	1/3 Days
BODY POSITION	Sitting	Sitting/ Leaning	Sitting/ Leaning	Sitting
MOTION	Reaching Writing	Grasp Phone Writing	Typing	Writing Reaching for resources
MOTION DISTANCE	Varies - to 4 Ft.	2 Ft.	—	Varies - to 4 Ft.
MOVEMENT LOCATION	Varies - from floor - waist to overhead	At workstation	Must go to Main Office	Varies - floor-overhead
WEIGHT	Up to 15 lbs.	Phone Headset (8 oz)	—	Up to 15 lbs.
TOOLS UTILIZED	Pen	—	—	Pen
EQUIPMENT UTILIZED	—	Telephone	Computer	—
INFORMATION REQUIREMENTS	Resources: Directories, Legal Doc., Manuals, etc.	Telephone Directory Resource Material (Dir., etc.)	Resource Materials	Resource Materials
TASK SPECIFIC ENVIRONMENTAL CONDITIONS	—	—	—	No space in office to meet with 1-2 people-are sitting in her doorway
VISUAL CONSIDERATIONS	Locate/Read Directories, etc.	Read fine print in directories	Read computer screen	Read resources
SAFETY & HAZARD CONSIDERATIONS	Overhead reach/ filing	Leaning for phone headset	Carrying larger resource books One piece computer	Carrying resources
WORK STATION (ATTACH SKETCH)	Books, Desk & shelves	Desk	Desk in office table in main office	Office Desk
SYSTEM INPUTS/ OUTPUTS		0: Phone info.	0: Letter, memo, etc.	I: 1-2 people

Figure 5-4. Environmental Analysis: Part B completed for one essential function of the program specialist job. This function: "provides disability-related information to the public."

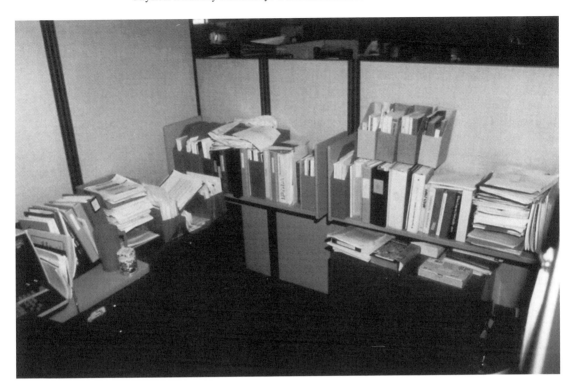

Figure 5-5. Employee's existing workstation.

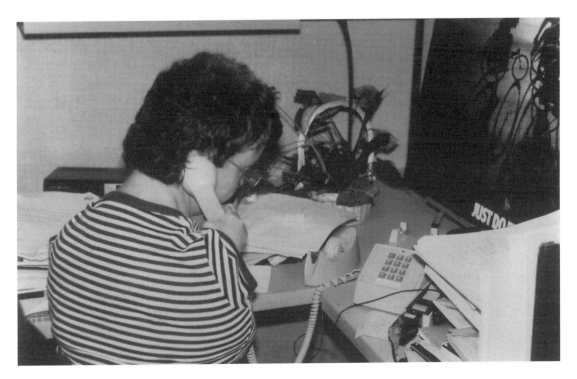

Figure 5-6. Employee using existing telephone.

This individual also keeps several piles of documents (totaling about 2 linear feet) on her desk because of insufficient accessible storage.

It was determined that approximately 20 linear feet of the resource materials are used frequently and, therefore, need to be made accessible. The remaining 10 linear feet of materials are used only occasionally and can be stored in overhead shelves, which would require assistance for retrieval. This is acceptable to the employee.

She currently retrieves materials stored overhead by using her loop hook reacher to pull the book off the shelf; she allows the book to fall to the work surface, from which it can be retrieved. This process presents a safety hazard to the worker.

Environmental Conditions

Architecturally, the building comprises 40,000 sq. ft of space in a single story. The entire building meets the accessibility guidelines of the Americans with Disabilities Act of 1990. It is laid out with an open office architecture using panels to create individual cubicles. As a result, there is often a great deal of noise from use of telephones, copiers, and employee conversations.

The employee's cubicle is crowded and cluttered: Books and documents are stacked on the desk, floor, and shelves. She transfers from her power wheelchair to an office chair to work. These two chairs, along with the employee's dog, take up most of the available floor space, thus no meeting space remains.

Job Specific Functional Assessment

Anthropometric measurements were taken and the following was determined:

- Static reach was approximately 6 in. for fingertips and 4 in. for grasp
- Functional reach was approximately 12.5 in. as employee leaned forward
- All other reaches required the employee to lean out of her chair and balance on one leg (employee uses a platform shoe on one foot)
- Optimal work surface height was determined to be 13 in. above compressed seat height. The

employee types one-handed, using only her right hand.

Design

Team Approach

A team approach was used in this case to define, design, and implement the accommodation. Such an approach is used to take advantage of the expertise of professionals from various disciplines and helps emphasize the fact that the employee should be involved in defining the accommodation.

The team on this case was composed of the employee, an ergonomist, an industrial designer, and a computer specialist. The ergonomist met with the employee's supervisor to procure information regarding the essential functions and any other pertinent information. It was at this meeting that the ergonomist learned of the office move. The ergonomist then held a preliminary meeting with the employee (the supervisor did not feel the need to be present) to determine the scope of the accommodation. A comprehensive analysis took place next, involving the employee, ergonomist, and industrial designer. Because the industrial designer would create the detailed layout and design drawings, work with fabricators, and supervise and assist the actual construction of the workplace, it was appropriate for this individual to be present for the assessment. The computer specialist was called in after the basic computer needs were defined.

Performance Gap

After assessing all parts of the accommodation system, the following items requiring accommodation were identified:

- Phone use. Use of the phone itself is cumbersome. Entering phone numbers is time-consuming. Accessing phone numbers from phone books, directories, or card files is difficult and slow.
- Resource material. It is difficult for the employee to access resource materials. Resources on floppy disks cannot be accessed with current computer setup.

- Meeting space. No space currently exists for employee to meet with individuals in her office.
- Computer use. Employee cannot effectively access her current computer. She has no access to e-mail. She has no means for reviewing information on floppy disks. Needs to maintain capability of passing documents to secretary.
- Work-surface dimensions. Employee cannot reach items at the back of her work surface. Employee must lean over excessively to write.
- Floor space. The floor is cluttered with stacks of resource materials. There is barely enough space for the power chair, office chair, and assistance dog.
- Light switches. Switches for task lighting are not accessible.
- Task interactions. Phone use often occurs while accessing resource information or using the computer, or both. Conferences with one or two individuals in her office often involve accessing resource information.

The Accommodation

After examining all of these issues, the accommodation was defined as follows.

Workstation Layout. Figure 5-7 shows the newly designed office space.

1. Work surfaces. All primary work surfaces will be 18 in. deep. This is the shortest depth possible that will maximize the reach envelope of the employee (functional reach = 12.5 in.) while still accommodating equipment (phone, computer, etc.).
2. Accessible storage. Turntables (Figure 5-8) will be used to house all materials that must be readily accessible. Each turntable will have approximately 8 linear feet of storage space. Lateral file cabinets will be located under one work surface. The file cabinet is accessible and provides 5 linear feet of file space split between two drawers. The bottom drawer is accessed with difficulty.
3. Nonaccessible storage. Six linear feet of space is available in two overhead bookshelves. Assistance is required to access this material.
4. Meeting space. A space of 4.0 × 5.5 ft will be provided at the front of the office to

accommodate meetings with one or two individuals. A free-standing conference extension will be provided for this purpose. When not used for meetings, the conference extension will double as an additional work surface (Figure 5-9).
5. Wheelchair parking. A space will be provided at the front of the cubicle in which the employee can park her power wheelchair.

Light Switches. Switches for task lighting will be located in an accessible location, just under the work surface.

Computer Issues. Several issues were resolved through these accommodations:

1. Provide PC, WordPerfect, printer. A personal computer will be provided to the employee along with WordPerfect software. In addition to document generation this will enable the employee to search diskettes for resource information, such as ADA regulations.

Specifications

386 SX Wang PC	0.28 dot pitch VGA monitor and card
25-MHZ processor	4 expansion slots (3 full slots for future use; half slot for modem)
80-MB hard drive	3½ in. floppy drive
4-MB RAM	5¼ in. floppy drive

2. Provide access to Wang network. This requires cabling of employee's office as well as purchase of a WLOC network card. This will continue to allow the employee's secretary to access her documents and vice versa.
3. Provide access to DEC network. This requires a modem, ProComm Plus software, cabling, and a cable connector. This will enable the employee to use the interoffice e-mail system. The modem and associated software will enable the employee to dial the phone through the computer.
4. Provide alternate keyboard. To minimize required movement distances while keying, a nonstandard keyboard will be provided. The smaller 81-key compact keyboard was found to be satisfactory (Figure 5-10).

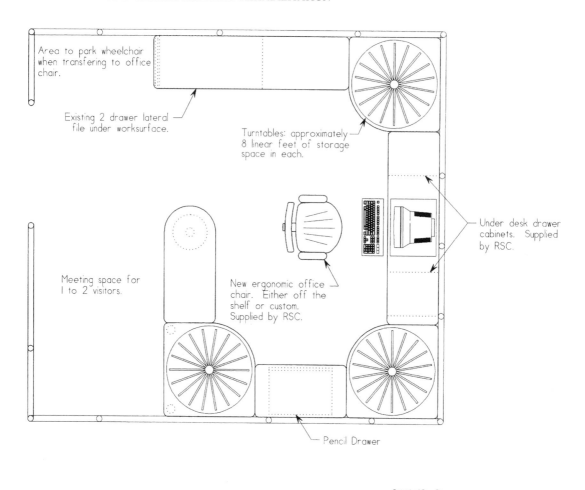

Area to park wheelchair when transfering to office chair.

Existing 2 drawer lateral file under worksurface.

Turntables: approximately 8 linear feet of storage space in each.

Under desk drawer cabinets. Supplied by RSC.

Meeting space for 1 to 2 visitors.

New ergonomic office chair. Either off the shelf or custom. Supplied by RSC.

Pencil Drawer

EQUIPMENT LAYOUT
Revision 1

Designed and Drawn By
FICOCELLI DESIGN
6454 HILLTOP AVENUE
REYNOLDSBURG, OHIO 43068
(614) 577-0695

Figure 5-7. Layout drawing of workstation for employee accommodation.

5. Keyboard mounting. The employee types with the right hand only. The keyboard must be precisely mounted for appropriate access. A Bogen Arm (a camera mounting device) was used to mount the keyboard. The keyboard can be moved into position during use or pushed away when not needed (Figure 5-11). The original design layout (see Figure 5-7) called for the computer to be in a traditional straight-on position directly in front of the employee. However, the employee preferred to have the computer angled for comfort and ease of use as shown in Figures 5-11 and 5-12.

6. Scanner. The secretary will be trained to use the document scanner (already at the organization) to scan documents for the employee so that she can access them via her PC.

Phone Issues

1. Headset. An appropriate, lightweight headset will be provided.
2. Computer phone directory. The employee can use the modem to dial phone numbers using a directory of frequently dialed numbers, which will be set up in a computer file.

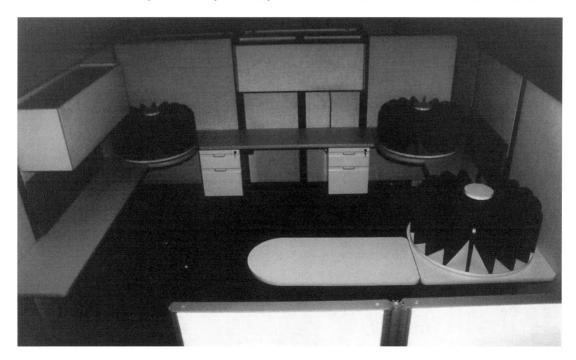

Figure 5-8. Workstation layout demonstrating specific accommodations: turntables for storage, narrow work surfaces, and file cabinets under work surface.

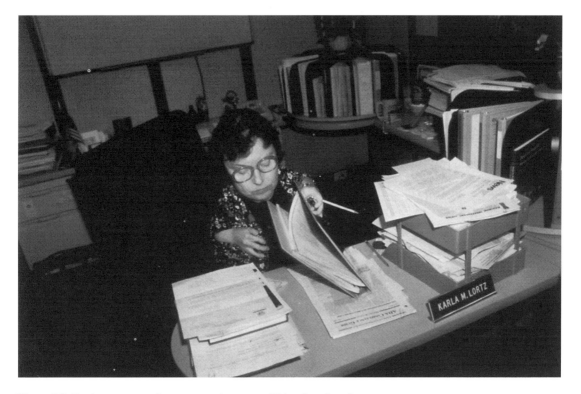

Figure 5-9. Employee uses conference extension as an additional work surface.

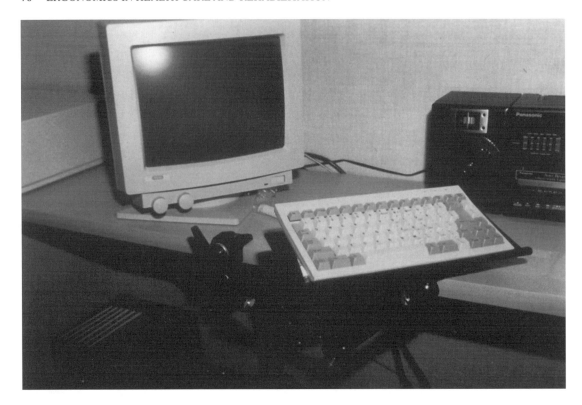

Figure 5-10. Computer setup showing compact keyboard.

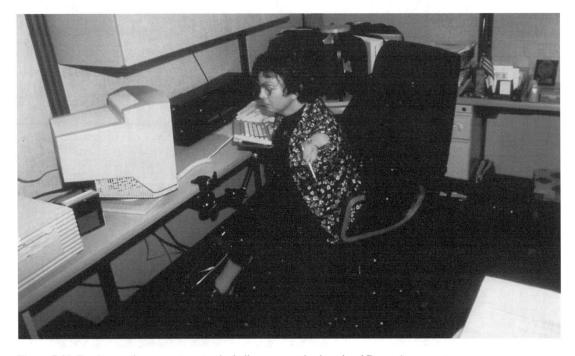

Figure 5-11. Employee using computer setup including compact keyboard and Bogen Arm mount.

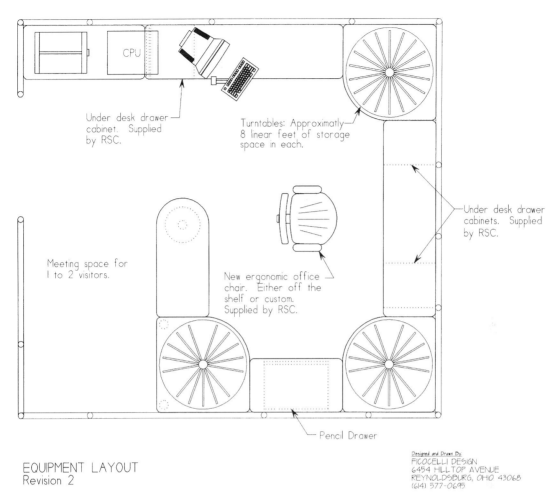

EQUIPMENT LAYOUT
Revision 2

Designed and Drawn By:
FICOCELLI DESIGN
6454 HILLTOP AVENUE
REYNOLDSBURG, OHIO 43068
(614) 577-0695

Figure 5-12. Revised layout drawing of workstation for employee accommodation.

Build New Office Cubicle. After considering the aforementioned items and dimensions it was determined that the new cubicle should be 10.5 × 10.5 ft. An unused space was secured and work on the accommodation proceeded in the new location while the employee continued to use her old office.

Training. Once all of the accommodations were put in place, the employee moved into the new work space, and she was given training in the use of the PC and printer, DOS, WordPerfect, the modem, the DEC, e-mail, and the phone directory.

Evaluation

Once the employee had the chance to use the new office space for several weeks, a follow-up meeting was arranged. Employee feedback resulted in the following changes (Figure 5-12 shows the revised layout).

Changes

- Move computer. The employee spends a great deal of time at the computer. This meant that her back was usually to the door, and she was

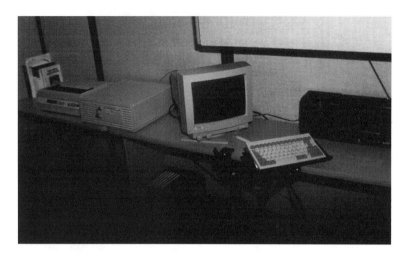

Figure 5-13. Additional work surface for printer.

unable to see anyone entering her office. She wanted the computer relocated to the side of her office;

- Add work surface. The employee found it impractical to park her wheelchair in the space provided at the front of the office. She found it more convenient to locate the chair off to one side within her main work area. Given that the area provided for the chair was not used, she asked for an additional work surface to better accommodate her printer (see Figures 5-12 and 5-13).
- Alter turntables. The employee had several oversized binders of resource information that would not fit into the slots on the turntables. Some slots needed to be enlarged.

Effectiveness

Subjective evaluation was used to determine the effectiveness of the final accommodation. As a result, it was determined that

- The employee was able to make more phone calls per day.
- Phone calls were easier to make.
- Small meetings were successfully accommodated in her office.
- She was able to generate more written responses.
- Resource retrieval was much easier.
- She was able to use information supplied on diskette.
- It was much easier to use resource materials while using the phone or the computer.
- Writing and note taking were made easier.
- The employee was able to perform all essential functions of her job efficiently, comfortably, and safely.

Acknowledgments

The author acknowledges the following individuals for their participation on the accommodation team: Mark Ficocelli, Industrial Designer; John Hassell, Computer Specialist; Karla Lortz, Employee to Be Accommodated. The author also thanks Barbara Babaryk for her patience and hard work in the word processing and construction of this document.

Chapter 6

Cognitive Disability Case Study: Home and Leisure Accommodations for an Individual After Experiencing a Stroke

Carolyn A. Unsworth

Learning Objectives

On completion of this chapter, the reader should be able to

- Describe, in general terms, the "therapeutic" approach a clinician and an ergonomist may take when working with a client who has a cognitive disability.
- Understand the analyses a clinician and an ergonomist may choose when working with a client who has a cognitive disability.
- Understand the interventions a clinician and an ergonomist may offer when working with a client who has a cognitive disability.
- Understand how a clinician and ergonomist may evaluate the effectiveness of interventions for a client who has a cognitive disability.

Key Words

Cognitive rehabilitation
Occupational therapy
Ergonomics
Neglect
Memory

Abstract

This chapter presents a case study that illustrates clinically based ergonomics for a client with a cognitive disability. The chapter opens with brief reviews of the cognitive difficulties that clients may experience following stroke, and the systems approach in ergonomics in relation to clients with cognitive disabilities. The fictitious clinical case of Mr. Taylor describes a man whose main cognitive limitations are decreased short-term memory, left-side neglect (also known as *unilateral neglect*), and some spatial relations difficulties. This case study explores suitable home and leisure adaptations and activity methods for Mr. Taylor, such as rearranging the home environment, providing an arrow system to increase left-turn taking and a stand for one-handed card playing, and assigning use of a detailed diary to aid memory. The chapter concludes with approaches that can be used to evaluate the outcomes of these therapeutic interventions. The evaluation revealed that although a return to work for Mr. Taylor is not feasible at this stage, he has made significant gains in his ability to care for himself, and carry out simple community daily living tasks.

Introduction

Stroke and Cognitive Disabilities

A stroke, or cerebrovascular accident, can cause a sudden onset of neurologic deficits following ischemia to an area of the brain. Stroke is one of the foremost causes of disability among older adults (Kelly-Hayes, 1989), and stroke-related disability involves significant use of health and community services. The American Heart Association (1991) estimated that each year approximately 550,000 Americans will have a stroke, and it has been documented that at any one time approximately 3 million people in the United States have a stroke-related disability that requires ongoing management and care (Agency for Health Care Policy and Research, 1995). Costs associated with diagnosis and treatment of stroke, and with lost productivity, exceed $30 billion each year (Matchar et al., 1994).

After a stroke, an individual may experience residual motor, sensory, cognitive, perceptual, behavioral, or emotional disabilities. Cognitive and perceptual disabilities (Arnodottir, 1991; Grieve, 1993) that may result from stroke include

- Apraxia (the inability to carry out skilled, purposeful movements)
- Impulsivity
- Loss of insight
- Disorders of simple and complex perception (the inability to recognize objects, and understand the relationship between objects)
- Body or spatial neglect (the inability to attend to a hemispace or body side despite intact sensory abilities)
- Disorders of memory
- Difficulties with executive functions (this includes planning, decision making and judgment, reasoning, monitoring and regulating, and evaluation of performance)

In the United States, approximately 17% of patients who have had a stroke enter inpatient rehabilitation to help them regain the abilities required to resume their everyday lives (Agency for Health Care Policy and Research, 1995). The case study in this chapter presents a man who was admitted to a private physical rehabilitation facility following a stroke.

Review of the Systems Approach for Clients with Cognitive Disabilities

Performance enhancement and fatigue control are two of the main objectives of an ergonomic intervention (Anderson, 1995). When using an ergonomic approach to working with a client with a cognitive disability, therapy aims and methods of assessment and treatment are similar to those used within other frameworks. However, if using an ergonomic approach, then the clinician often works within a systems theory framework.

A system may be defined as "a complex of interacting elements" (von Bertalanffy, 1968, p. 42). Furthermore, it has been described as "a set of objects together with relationships between the objects and between their attributes" (Hall & Fagen, 1968, p. 81). To understand any system, the components and their relationships require examination. Hence, therapy focuses on the client, the client's environment, and the interface between these two. Pheasant (1991) describes a "person-machine system" as one in which a person feeds information into a machine or task by tools, a device or controls, then receives information via a display or any sensory feedback. *A systems theory framework* views the client as interacting in a task, within an occupation or activity, within their social and environmental context.

Using this systems framework, ergonomics focuses on designing the tasks, tools, or environment to fit the capabilities and limitations of the user or client. As the client may continue to improve during the rehabilitation process, these designs may go through several alterations before the client reaches his or her maximal functional status. In addition, tasks, tools, or the environment may need to be designed to provide successful use while still challenging the client cognitively or physically so that further functional improvements are promoted. Therefore the designer must collaborate closely with the therapist during the design process. There can be considerable overlap between the roles of the therapist and ergonomist. For example, therapists use ergonomic principles when they use cueing or chunking techniques to assist a client with memory problems. Similarly, ergonomists may use therapeutic principles when using progressively more demanding job assignments (activity grading) during a return-to-work regime. In general, the ergonomics approach is to alter the environment to fit the person, and if that cannot be achieved then training is used. In contrast, the therapeutic approach seeks to assist the person to regain skills to interact successfully with the environment. If a person is not able to regain the level of function required to manage independently, then environmental modifications are considered.

Case Study: Mr. Taylor

Mr. Taylor, a 59-year-old man, was referred for occupational therapy as part of a 3- to 5-week inpatient rehabilitation program following a stroke. He was also referred for physical therapy and neuropsychologic evaluation. He is currently in week 4 of his rehabilitation, and the team anticipates discharging him at the end of the week. He has made steady progress during his stay and is looking forward to returning home. Given that Mr. Taylor is due to be discharged to his home, therapy is now focused on ensuring a successful transition from hospital to home, and investigating the possibilities of his returning to work.

Service Providers

A registered occupational therapist (OTR), a trained and certified occupational therapy assistant (COTA), and an ergonomist worked with this client. As discussed above, in many cases, the roles of these professionals overlap, and this is appropriately noted in the text. Some of the services provided by the OTR are unique, whereas other services could be provided by health professionals such as a speech-language pathologist or neuropsychologist. Together, the ergonomist and therapist work with the client to achieve maximum independence. This may be done by a combination of the following techniques: (1) assisting the client to fit in with the existing task/environment (clinically this is referred to as *remediation*), and (2) by ergonomics or modifying the task/environment to suit the abilities of the client (clinically this is referred to as *compensation*).

Results of Analysis and Formal Assessment

The analysis section provides details of Mr. Taylor's abilities and limitations through the use of a series of standardized and nonstandardized assessments. Table 6-1 summarizes the methods used in this case and the personnel involved. The times of these assessments are noted, given that therapy goals and patient performance change over the course of rehabilitation. Typically, an ergonomist works with a nondisabled population; the clinician contributes specialized skills for assessing the abilities and limitations of a person with a disability. Appropriate subject matter experts (SMEs) were consulted during the analysis.

Medical History

Mr. Taylor, who was previously in good health, experienced a right hemisphere cerebrovascular accident (stroke) 5 weeks ago. He was admitted to an acute care facility where a computed tomography (CT) scan revealed a moderate-sized lesion in the parietal lobe with some frontal involvement following an infarction in the middle cerebral artery. Five days after his admission, he was discharged to a freestanding rehabilitation facility. Currently, Mr. Taylor is able to walk independently with distant supervision. This means that for safety reasons, a person needs to monitor Mr. Taylor's walking from a distance (i.e., does not need to walk next to him). He has a flaccid left arm (hypotonic, or low muscle tone), with some swelling in the hand and pain in his shoulder. Following medical investigations, shoulder-hand syndrome (a form of reflex sympathetic dystrophy [RSD]) was diagnosed.

Mr. Taylor's main area of difficulty is in cognition. No behavioral problems are noted; however, Mr. Taylor does seem subdued and staff therapists are watching for signs of depression. Mr. Taylor has been advised by his physiatrist not to drive after his release from hospital.

Social History and Family Issues

Mr. Taylor lives with his wife and the youngest of their three children, Sally, who is 20 years old. Their two older children are married and live in other states. Mrs. Taylor works part time at the local school as a secretary-receptionist. They live in a comfortable apartment approximately 13 miles from Mr. Taylor's workplace. Mrs. Taylor has expressed concern regarding their medical insurance, her husband's ability to return to work, and their financial future if he is unable to work. She is also concerned that "mentally he is not the same." She feels that his lack of understanding as to the nature of his problems makes him hard to talk to. She is concerned about safety issues with his neglect and his eagerness to return to driving.

Table 6-1. Assessment Modes

Method	Conducted by
Family interview with wife and daughter	Could be conducted by the clinician or the ergonomist; in this case it was conducted by the clinician.
Medical record review	Conducted by the clinician; relevant findings shared with the ergonomist.
Strengths and limitations assessment	
Interview Mr. Taylor	Can be conducted by the clinician or ergonomist; it was conducted by the clinician.
Functional Independence Measure (Hamilton, 1987)	Administered by various members of the clinical team, at an accredited rehabilitation facility.
Arnodottir OT-ADL Neurobehavioral Evaluation (A-ONE; Arnodottir, 1990)	Can only be administered by registered occupational therapists certified in A-ONE assessment.
Functional Activities Questionnaire (Pfeffer et al., 1984)	The therapist gave this to Mrs. Taylor to complete.
Environmental assessments	
Introductory telephone call to Mr. Taylor's workplace	Can be conducted by the ergonomist or clinician; the ergonomist conducted this assessment.
Work-site assessments:	Both can be conducted by the ergonomist or the clinician; in this case, the ergonomist carried out the work visit and assessments.
• Americans with Disabilities Act Work-Site Assessment (Aja, Jacobs, & Hermenau, 1992)	
• Job Analysis During Employer Site Visit (Demore-Taber, 1995)	
Leisure assessment: The Interest Checklist (Kielhofner, 1985)	Can be conducted by the ergonomist or occupational therapist; it was done by the occupational therapist.
Home site evaluation	Routinely conducted by an occupational therapist before a client's discharge from rehabilitation; an ergonomist may also do a home evaluation. In this case, it was done by both team members.

Financial Situation

Mrs. Taylor reports that their financial commitments include paying off the mortgage on their apartment, assisting their youngest daughter to pay for college tuition, meeting their health insurance contributions, and covering normal household running expenses. The Taylors had expected to pay off the mortgage on their apartment within the next 2 years. Their health insurance plan is held with Mr. Taylor's company and will cover the majority of his current medical expenses. However, Mrs. Taylor is concerned that if he is unable to return to work, they will need to fund their own health insurance. She is prepared to work full time if Mr. Taylor is unable to work and believes that the school where she works will be able to accommodate this. They would then be able to take out health insurance through the school.

Work History and Job Evaluation

Mr. Taylor was the foreman at a medium-sized import company. He has worked for the company for 20 years, working his way up to his present position. Mr. Taylor's job involves overseeing the work of six employees who move floor stock, completing paperwork for incoming and outgoing orders, managing inventory on the computer system, and preparing weekly summary reports for his manager. He enjoyed his work, states that he would like to return, and that he feels he is ready now to return to work.

The ergonomist called his employer at the end of week 2 of his rehabilitation. This call revealed that Mr. Taylor was well liked at work and that he was a valued employee. His employers were hopeful that he would be able to return to work soon. At the beginning of week 3 of Mr. Taylor's rehabilitation, an Americans with Disabilities Act Work-Site

Assessment (Aja, Jacobs, & Hermenau, 1992) and a job analysis were undertaken by the ergonomist during an employer site visit (Demore-Taber, 1995). These were conducted to establish the demands of his job, without Mr. Taylor's presence.

The results of these assessments indicated that, although Mr. Taylor's job was not physically taxing, it was quite intellectually demanding. Cognitive skills required to carry out the job included organizational skills, computer skills, information synthesis, memory, problem solving, and navigating a complex, multilevel work environment full of obstacles. The work environment presented many hazards, including different levels and elevated surfaces (platforms for transport loading and unloading), as well as moving objects (such as trucks and forklifts). In addition, Mr. Taylor's job demands he work with little supervision. The therapist and ergonomist explained to his employer that at this stage, Mr. Taylor was not ready to return to work, and that it was uncertain if he would be able to return in the future. The therapist explained the nature of Mr. Taylor's current limitations, and the ergonomist stated that if Mr. Taylor was to return to work they would be able to make suggestions as to how to modify the environment to assist Mr. Taylor to do his job.

Home and Leisure

Home Visit. The OTR and ergonomist conducted a home visit with both Mr. and Mrs. Taylor at the beginning of week 4 of therapy. The purpose of the visit was to consider the suitability of the floor plan given Mr. Taylor's neglect and safety issues. Many checklists are available to guide a therapist through a home visit. A home site assessment commonly used in Massachusetts was adopted (Appendix 6-1). The home visit revealed few problems with a return home for Mr. Taylor. A summary of the problems and recommended ergonomic solutions is provided in Appendix 6-1. Some of these solutions are also discussed in the Intervention section of this chapter.

Leisure Interests. The Interest Checklist, as modified by Kielhofner (1985), was used to determine the kinds of leisure pursuits Mr. Taylor had been involved in and those he would like to try. In summary, working through the checklist indicated that

Mr. Taylor was involved in the following activities before his stroke and that he would like to continue with them: home repairs, exercise, driving, yard work and gardening, church activities, radio, walking, car repair, holiday activities, movies, barbecues, reading, traveling, and watching television. Although he had been a social golfer, he expressed a lack of interest in returning to this. Future new activities that interested him included table games, woodworking, leatherwork, and playing cards.

Personal Care Independence

The Functional Independence Measure (FIM) (Hamilton, 1987) is used routinely at the rehabilitation facility to determine each client's level of personal care independence on admission and discharge. Eighteen items are assessed in the following six categories: self-care, sphincter control, mobility, locomotion, communication, and social cognition. The FIM has a 7-point scoring system as follows: 7 = independent; 6 = independent with aids or adaptive equipment; 5 = supervision or set up of the task is required; 4 = minimal physical assistance; 3 = moderate physical assistance; 2 = maximal physical assistance; 1 = dependent on others to do the task.

Mr. Taylor was first assessed using the FIM 8 hours after he was admitted to the facility. The OTR performed an interim FIM assessment at the beginning of week 4 to assist in discharge planning. The findings of this assessment indicate that although Mr. Taylor is independent with supervision (score = 5) or minimal assistance (score = 4) for most personal activities of daily living (ADLs) tasks, he still requires moderate assistance with memory (score = 3). His current FIM score is 91/126.

Instrumental ADL Assessment

Following a suggestion made by the therapist, Mrs. Taylor has spent some time over the last few days with her husband sorting through current bills and financial statements. She has also attended many therapy sessions over the last 2 weeks on her days off. The therapist gave Mrs. Taylor a copy of an assessment called The Functional Activities Questionnaire (Pfeffer et al., 1984) to complete. The purpose of this assessment was for Mrs. Taylor to determine Mr. Taylor's abilities to independently conduct home, domestic, and some community ADLs. The findings of this assessment suggest that Mr. Taylor is largely dependent on others for activities such as managing finances, shopping, meal preparation, getting around the community, playing games of skill, and following the plot of a television show. He currently scores 25; maximum independence receives a score of 0, and maximum dependence receives a score of 30.

Cognitive Assessment

The Arnadottir OT-ADL Neurobehavioral Evaluation (A-ONE) (Arnadottir, 1990) was performed at the beginning of the week 3 of therapy. The assessment results are presented in full in Appendix 6-2. In summary, Mr. Taylor's main difficulties are

- Decreased attention and short-term memory
- Left-side body and spatial neglect
- Topographic disorientation
- Some spatial relations difficulties (complex perception)
- Some difficulty with the organization and sequencing of tasks
- Limited insight into the nature of his problems, although he does understand the physical problems associated with his left arm

One method of measuring cognitive workload is to have clients rate their perceptions of how hard they are working, or how difficult they perceive an activity to be (Folts, Gianni, & Otonicar, 1995). Although the therapist may consider that there is a considerable cognitive workload associated with Mr. Taylor's day-to-day tasks, Mr. Taylor perceives that there is very little.

Physical and Sensory Assessment

When Mr. Taylor began rehabilitation, assessments revealed mild balance problems in standing, and some mild gait disturbances related to weakened tibialis anterior muscle. During the first 2 weeks of rehabilitation, the difficulties associated with standing balance resolved. Although his gait has improved, on occasion he will stumble when his toe catches the floor or carpet. A sensory assessment revealed no deficits in the right leg, arm, or trunk. Given his neglect, it was not possible to do a sensory assessment on Mr. Taylor's left leg, arm, or trunk. On admission, Mr. Taylor had a flaccid left arm (low muscle tone) with no return of movement. He has since developed RSD in his left arm as noted in his medical history above. This has caused him some pain and discomfort. No return of function has been noted in his left arm over the course of rehabilitation. Given his neglect, this arm is at risk of injury as he tends to allow his hand to bump furniture or walls as he passes; these incidents probably exacerbate the RSD.

Reanalysis and Problem Identification

At the end of week 3 of his rehabilitation program, Mr. Taylor's initial problem list was revised in light of more recent assessments, his progress in therapy, and the need to finalize a discharge plan. Table 6-2 outlines prioritized problem lists from the therapist and Mr. Taylor, and in the third column, their consensus list.

Strengths Identification

Consideration was given to Mr. Taylor's strengths as well in formulating plans for his discharge and continuing rehabilitation. The following were identified:

- Appropriate affect (monitor for signs of depression)
- Friendly outgoing personality
- Supportive wife and family
- Motivated to try tasks
- Steady progress in his recovery over the past 3 weeks of therapy
- Long-term memory
- Able to walk (although he is a little unsteady and may stumble at times)

Prognosis

At this point, it is also relevant to consider Mr. Taylor's prognosis. The term *prognosis* refers to the expected outcome for a patient based on their diagnosis, disabilities, and mediating social factors. Mr. Taylor's current strengths and limitations have been presented above, but these lists are not static. Mr. Taylor will continue to show improvements, as the brain swelling associated with the stroke subsides and other brain areas attempt to compensate for or take over lost functions. The magnitude of this improvement, however, is uncertain. Factors such as Mr. Taylor's age, family support, and motivation point to a continued recovery. However, his neglect has not spontaneously resolved in the first few weeks following his stroke, which suggests that this will be an ongoing problem. It is often difficult for patients to manage independently and safely at work or in the community with a neglect. Knowledge of the patient's expected prognosis assists clinicians to formulate treatment goals and plan therapy at an appropriate level. This information also assists the ergonomist to plan appropriate task-environment adjustments that will work for the patient now and in the future.

Goals and Objectives

When demand exceeds capacity, overload is produced (Pheasant, 1991). In the case of Mr. Taylor, his overload (and fatigue) is often due to his inability to meet the cognitive demands of his environment. The primary goal of therapeutic and ergonomic interventions is to help Mr. Taylor meet the demands of his environment, so that he can independently return to his home and community activities. In considering Mr. Taylor's prognosis, the decision was made that a return to his job as a foreman was unlikely for some time, if at all. Therefore, therapy was focused on home and community, rather than work activities.

As a final analysis, the OTR and ergonomist assessed Mr. Taylor's home environment (presented in Appendix 6-1) for potential problems. The therapist prepared a list of all the tasks that would be difficult for Mr. Taylor and, in collaboration with the ergonomist, devised a series of ergonomic solutions to ensure that Mr. Taylor will find his way around his home and manage independently there.

For the purposes of this chapter, problems 1, 2, 5, 8, and 9 were selected from the therapist/client collaborative list on Table 6-2. Behavioral objectives were set for these problem areas at the beginning of week 4. These objectives are presented in full in Table 6-3 and follow the "who, given what, does what, how well" written format.

Table 6-2. Problem Lists

Therapist-generated list
  Occupational performance component problems:
  1. Reduced insight to problems
  2. Left neglect/decreased attention
  3. Reduced short-term memory
  4. Some spatial relations difficulties
  5. Fatigue
  6. Reflex sympathetic dystrophy (RSD) in left upper extremity
  Occupational performance area problems:
  7. Environment/home layout
  8. Lack of independence in domestic and community activities of daily living (ADLs)
  9. Identifying meaningful work and play activities after discharge

Mr. Taylor's list
  1. Not walking very well
  2. Doctor says I can't drive
  3. My left arm hurts
  4. I get a bit tired
  5. Go back to work

Therapist/client collaborative list
  1. Neglect: environment/home layout/walking activities—e.g., not attending to doorways and furniture on left, and stumbling (spatial relations)
  2. Neglect: not attending to people and things on the left side in general
  3. Not being able to drive
  4. Pain in left arm/hand, RSD
  5. Decreased memory
  6. Explore what my problems are and what that means for my future
  7. Tiredness
  8. Identifying meaningful work and play activities post discharge
  9. Lack of independence in domestic and community ADLs

Design Intervention

This section explores the kinds of intervention, and environmental modifications necessary for Mr. Taylor to return home. Ergonomic implementation strives to match the environment, product, or activity to the person. An effective match is one that encompasses working efficiency, comfort, ease of use, health, and safety (Rice, 1995; Pheasant, 1991).

Table 6-3. Objectives, Treatment Solutions, and Outcomes for Each Problem Area

Behavioral Objectives*	Remediation Technique/ Ergonomic Solution-Compensation (ESC)	Outcome Summary
Problem 1: Left turns and some topographic disorientation while walking		
Mr. Taylor, given maps and maze activities, and home modifications, including an arrow system, will become more aware of his neglect, and begin to compensate. At the end of his inpatient hospital stay, he will be able to successfully find his way from his room to OT and find his way around his house.	Remediation: Many techniques have been tried ESC: Floor mazes to improve concentration; red arrows at left turns; maps listing turns	Performance is inconsistent; attention to the left deteriorates as he fatigues Responded well to red arrow prompts for left turns; using them, independently found his way to OT Although performance deteriorates with fatigue, success rate is 85% for left turns using arrow prompts.
Navigating doorways and furniture while walking		
Given a small wrist bell, will be alerted to his left neglected arm if it bumps furniture or doorways so that he can attend to that arm as evidenced by no cuts or bruises on his left hand.	Remediation: Attach bell to left wrist bracelet; see if ringing as he walks or bumps objects will bring his attention to his left arm and minimize damage	Walking does not ring bell loud enough to draw Mr. Taylor's attention. He does notice the sound when he bumps his hand. Drawbacks: other therapists find the bell intrusive, and inappropriate for an adult Option: The Taylors may choose to continue use of the bell at home.
Spatial relations and stumbling while walking		
Given perception-improving exercises and physical cues (such as white strips on steps), will be able to more accurately judge depth perception on floor surfaces so that the number of times he stumbles is reduced to once per week.	Remediation: range of activities, including tabletop construction activities and woodworking ESC: install internal and external entrance rails on the right; paint a white strip on the edge of each step	Construction and woodworking activities to improve perception were successful, demonstrated by unassisted task completion. Mr. Taylor is now independent when walking inside. Although cautious, he manages the hospital steps (with white line painted at end of each step). Lacking these cues in the community, Mr. Taylor uses a foot slide method to assist him. For safety, he does need a companion when walking outside.
Problem 2: Neglect, attending to the left in general		
Given verbal cueing from his therapist, wife, and others and taught a "turn and scan method" will be able to find items and attend to people more consistently at the end of a 1-week period.	Remediation: "turn and scan method"; verbal cueing A discussion was held with his wife to ensure she sets up activities, or places important information, on his right side.	Mr. Taylor has not responded well to this approach. His limited insight makes it hard for him to self-cue to scan left. He is better able to attend to information on the left if given cues such as the arrows or signs on the bulletin board to scan to the left.
Neglect, in reading		
Miss fewer words on the left side of page (less than 10 per page)	Remediation using ESC principles: To prompt a return to the far left margin during reading tasks, a red ribbon is placed down the left margin (attached with a U-hold) to trigger self-cueing.	His reading has improved significantly with the red ribbon technique—an ergonomic solution (misses only two or three per page).

Problem 5: Reduced short-term memory

Given computer memory tasks and games; a diary and real-life tasks such as banking will increase his short-term memory so that he is able to do the following:

Independently set up the computer for use

Reach the medium level of Memory Castle (Sunburst Communications, 1986)

He is taught to trace each line with his finger to locate this red ribbon, which indicates the start of a line.

To reinforce scanning to a red ribbon, one has been attached to the far left side of the computer screen. The React computer program (Gianutsos & Klitzner, 1981) has also been used.

His performance on programs such as React has greatly improved, as evidenced by the results printout showing an initial score on of 7.51 seconds improving to 1.6 seconds 3 weeks later.

Steady progress has been made during Mr. Taylor's rehabilitation. He can independently set up the computer for use.

His performance on memory tasks such as the card game Concentration and Memory Castle (Sunburst Communications, 1986) has improved significantly. Mr. Taylor and the occupational therapist graphed his computer results from Memory Castle for 4 weeks to demonstrate this improvement. He has progressed from the easy level of this program to the medium level and can remember 11 items.

Independently use his diary, by the time of his discharge

He is independent in the use of a memory notebook/diary to record information to assist his memory. However, limited insight means he does not always recognize when to use the notebook.

Problem 8: Identifying leisure activities

Will be able to engage in at least three recreational activities during the final week of his hospital stay, and will be able to participate in at least four recreational activities after his discharge

Four activities were identified:

1. Woodworking

He enjoyed woodworking very much and he seemed to feel comfortable working with the supervisor. He does require supervision in the workshop given safety considerations (due to neglect and memory).

2. Card games

Mr. Taylor enjoys playing cards and his ability to engage in this activity has improved. However, he is not yet at the level of playing in local community clubs. He was given the suggestion to organize his family, friends, and relatives for friendly card evenings on a regular basis.

3. Watching a movie and television

He successfully follows the plot with the aid of his memory notebook. On occasion, when engrossed in the plot, he may forget to make note of important points. He will continue to go to the cinema with his wife, who is aware of the importance of discussing the movie afterwards, both for pleasure, and to ensure retention of information.

Table 6-3. *Continued*

Behavioral Objectives*	Remediation Technique/ Ergonomic Solution-Compensation (ESC)	Outcome Summary
	4. Planning a weekend trip	Mr. Taylor successfully planned two weekend trips: one to Nantucket Island, MA, with the assistance of the occupational therapist, and a trip to Camden, ME, which he planned independently.
Problem 9: ADLs, domestic and community		
Given familiarization with the OT kitchen, arrows for left turns, and written memory prompts attached to the refrigerator, will be able to make his lunch each day with distant supervision from the COTA	Lunch preparation: Mr. Taylor and the COTA developed a routine of making lunch each day. A standard lunch consists of a bagel with salad filling, fruit, cookies, and coffee. The COTA taught him how to use an unfamiliar kettle. Two red arrows have been placed on kitchen cupboards at eye level on corners to prompt left turn taking. Mr. Taylor was initially prompted verbally to scan to the left to find items in the refrigerator. Now a simple sticker is hung on the front of the shelf as a prompt. Mr. Taylor will take this prompt home.	Mr. Taylor is independent in making his lunch each day. Initially the COTA felt Mr. Taylor supervised from a distance. However, the COTA felt Mr. Taylor was safe in the kitchen at this level of task (there were minimal safety considerations as there was no cooking, and the kettle switched off automatically). Mr. Taylor continues to use prompts such as red arrows and cue cards. It is anticipated that these will also be used at home. Mrs. Taylor is aware of his progress in this area and will reinforce these skills at home. On occasion, he does forget where he is in a task, but is usually able to return to the task without assistance.
ADLs, banking		
Given banking activities from the *Cognitive Rehabilitation Workbook* (Dougherty, 1993), real-life banking tasks with the therapist, written notes in his diary that he can refer to if needed, and given success in other treatment objectives listed above, will be able to successfully manage the families checking account and make withdrawals from the local bank or automatic teller machine	Remediation: Initially, banking and money management tasks from *Cognitive Rehabilitation Workbook* were used. These are graded from simple (red) activities through to more sophisticated tasks (blue). Mr. Taylor and the OTR have planned an electronic and counter service banking activity as part of their community outing. It is anticipated that Mr. Taylor will continue to use his neighborhood bank where he is known. ESC: The ropes used to guide traffic in the bank should suffice to lead him to the teller. The ergonomist will work with Mr. Taylor to enable him to do phone banking and approach the bank to devise a simplified computerized banking procedure for Mr. Taylor.	Although Mr. Taylor managed the actual banking tasks with only minor prompting, he did have significant difficulties getting about in the community due to his neglect. In a controlled environment such as the hospital, or his home, Mr. Taylor has sufficient cues to manage. In the community, however, his neglect 1. Places him in danger when he is a pedestrian in traffic, and 2. Although he knows the area, his inability to consistently make left turns means he is often unable to locate his destination (e.g., the bank). He therefore requires a companion when on community outings.

*Problems numbered according to their placement in Table 6-2.

OT = occupational therapy; OTR = registered occupational therapist; COTA = certified occupational therapy assistant.

Given Mr. Taylor's limited insight and the goal of his discharge home, we focused on problems relating to modification of his environment, as follows (numbered according to their placement in Table 6-2):

1. Neglect: walking activities, including navigating his home environment
2. Neglect: not attending to people and things on the left side in general
5. Decreased memory
8. Identifying leisure activities
9. Domestic and community ADLs

The intervention section also presents the two different approaches that are taken by a clinician and an ergonomist. A clinician usually takes a three-pronged approach to intervention or treatment:

- Remediation—working with the client on deficit areas to overcome limitations
- Education—making sure that the client and his or her family are aware of the client's limitations, strengths, and prognosis
- Compensation—modification of task or environment to enable the client to be independent

Ergonomists play an important role in client and family education, but their particular strength is in the third area: modifying or redesigning the task or environment to suit the client. This is usually called an *ergonomic solution;* thus the intervention section for Mr. Taylor specifies whether the intervention is a treatment (remedial) or an ergonomic solution (compensatory).

Treatment Timetable

It was decided that Mr. Taylor would attend occupational therapy twice each day for the final week of his therapy program: a 1-hour morning session and a 2-hour session in the afternoon. In the morning session he would be treated individually by the OTR, and in the afternoon he would work with the COTA with supervision from the OTR.

Treatment Strategies

Treatment strategies must be understood and adopted by all team members when working with a client who has cognitive problems. They consisted of the following:

- Reinforce, in a supportive way, Mr. Taylor's limitations and strengths, giving consideration to his limited insight. Encourage Mr. Taylor to identify areas in which he experiences difficulties and successes.
- Provide a supportive, nonconfrontational environment for Mr. Taylor. He does not respond well if confronted with his weaknesses.
- Conduct treatment activities within Mr. Taylor's fatigue limit, and use a graded program to extend this.
- Reinforce methods and tasks through repetition.
- Give verbal praise for effort and performance.
- Assist Mr. Taylor to transfer skills acquired in one environment, or on one task, to other environments and tasks to enhance generalizability.
- Grade activities with respect to therapist input, time spent in the activity, environmental distractions, and task complexity.
- Provide opportunities for success through activities.

Ergonomic Solutions and Treatment Activities

Table 6-3 provides a broad view of the discharge plan objectives, remediations, and compensations (environmental and task modifications) chosen to address problems 1, 2, 5, 8, and 9 summarizes the outcome for each. The methods and activities used to assist Mr. Taylor are detailed below.

Problem 1: Walking Activities

In summary, the following recommendations were made for his home environment: apply red floor arrows to assist left turn taking; install internal and external entrance rails on the right; paint a white strip on the edge of each step; use erasable bulletin boards in the kitchen to prompt memory; upgrade lighting; remove all throw rugs; rearrange furniture (remove unnecessary small tables that clutter walking areas); adapt bathroom to assist independence (install bath seat and grab rails as documented in Appendix 6-1).

Therapy time was used to ensure Mr. Taylor became familiar with these ergonomic solutions so he could use these systems at home. For example, floor mazes were constructed in the therapy department and corridor to encourage Mr. Taylor to concentrate on where he walks. These were constructed with furniture, draft stoppers, and miniature bean bags. Red arrows were placed at turn points as prompts for Mr. Taylor to choose a left turn if appropriate. He was given instruction maps with all turns listed, and asked to find his way to a predetermined target. This system of red arrows for turns has also been set in place for Mr. Taylor to find his way from his room to the OT department.

Navigating Doorways and Furniture. Mr. Taylor developed RSD and complains of shoulder-hand pain. This is exacerbated when he does not attend to the left side of door frames and objects and consequently hits his arm. Although a "look left" campaign was mounted, this did not prove successful. After several discussions with Mr. Taylor and his wife, it was decided to attach a bell bracelet to Mr. Taylor's left arm for a trial period to determine if the ringing as he walked or bumped objects would alert him to attend to his arm.

Stumbling (Spatial Relations). A range of remedial activities were conducted with Mr. Taylor to reduce perceptual problems. Table-top construction activities and woodworking tasks were used with success.

Mr. Taylor did have some problems in judging depth and distance, particularly when walking on stairs and walking about the community. Ergonomic compensatory methods were used as a trial to determine if performance would improve: white lines were painted at the edge of each step of the hospital fire escape stairs (to cue Mr. Taylor regarding depth perception), and at the beginning and end of ramps. Mr. Taylor has a flight of steps at the entry of his home, so this method may also be used at his home. A community shopping and banking task was planned during the week to practice. When walking in the community, Mr. Taylor's main problems are not attending to information coming from the left (including traffic, roads, and shops) and stumbling on uneven ground and on single steps. Although white lines are not found on the edge of many steps in the community, Mr. Taylor was taught to carefully attend to visual cues, such as

changes in surface texture or color and cracks, as indications of steps or uneven ground. He was also taught to slide his right foot along each step to locate its edge. He does need a companion when walking in the community for safety, and to find his way around.

Problem 2: General Left-Side Neglect

People and Things on the Left Side. Remediation techniques such as the "turn and scan method" have been used over the last 3 weeks to help Mr. Taylor locate objects and notice people. As his neglect is primarily visual, he does attend to people when they approach him to gain his attention. Verbal cueing from his therapist, his wife, and others was used to assist Mr. Taylor locate objects he cannot "find" when carrying out ADLs.

Reading Activities. Treatment-remediation (using ergonomic principles): Mr. Taylor required a prompt to return to the far left margin when moving down a line during reading tasks, and he tends to miss some words. Currently, he is being taught to self-cue by placing a red ribbon down the left margin (attaching it with a U-hold) before commencing a reading task and to trace each line with his finger to locate this red ribbon, which indicates the start of a line. A discussion was held with his wife to ensure she sets up activities, or places important information, on his right side.

Computer Tasks. Treatment-remediation (using ergonomic principles): To reinforce scanning to a red ribbon, one has been attached to the far left side of the computer screen. The React computer program (Gianutsos & Klitzner, 1981) has also been used. In this program, a dot appears at random times and places on the screen. The patient must scan the screen to attend to all dots and react by pressing the space bar. The computer prints out the number of correct responses and the time taken to respond.

Problem 3: Reduced Short-Term Memory

Memory-Improving Programs. Remedial activities (using some ergonomic principles) included a memory program similar to the one outlined in Parente and DiCesare (1991, pp. 147–162). Key components in assisting a client improve short-term memory include working on the following:

- Attention: "I don't get it." Not paying adequate attention is the reason we often forget information. You have to understand something before you can remember it. Make sure the patient understands the information before the therapist works with him or her to remember it.
- Interest: If we are interested in something, this increases our attention, and therefore, our chances of remembering it. Ensure the context is relevant.
- Visualization: "I can see it." The patient is taught to produce an image or picture of what he or she is trying to remember.
- Chunking: Chunk information. Use acronyms and acrostics (making words or phrases out of the first letters of the items to be remembered also helps make the items meaningful). Creating a logical story line can also assist a client to recall information.
- Organization: Organization makes a difference in your ability to remember. Most of the information in your memory is organized in some way. Teach the patient to organize information: the more purposefully it is organized when learning it, the easier it will be to remember. Organization includes making patterns, and grouping by categories.
- Association: "That reminds me." Association refers to relating the material you want to remember to something you already know. Use comparisons or contrasts.

Activities used included:

- Card games such as Concentration (in which picture cards are placed face down and turned over in pairs: identical cards are removed from the pool).
- Computer games such as Memory Castle (Sunburst Communications, 1986). These programs are excellent for trying out different memory strategies with clients. Mr. Taylor found that the logical story line worked well to assist his memory. It is important to generalize computer activities to the real world. Hence, like the knight in Memory Castle, Mr. Taylor was sent on graded scavenger hunts to locate a set of items, and on errands for the department to increase his short-term memory skills.

Diary (Journal) Use. Mr. Taylor was asked to use a diary as a memory notebook. The steps used to introduce a diary include (1) Acquisition: learning the parts of the diary and how to use it. (2) Application: learning when and where to use the memory book. (3) Adaptation: using the memory book in functional settings (Sohlberg & Mateer, 1989). The diary was introduced as a compensation technique, however, as most people use some form of diary, this is not seen as unusual. During Mr. Taylor's final week of therapy, the emphasis was on ensuring Mr. Taylor recorded appropriate information, and that he used his diary at appropriate times to retrieve information.

New Skill Acquisition. Mr. Taylor was required to learn how to set up the occupational therapy department computer for cognitive skills retraining. The OTR and Mr. Taylor recorded these steps to assist him in the future to remember information and therefore learn new skills.

1. Consolidate prior computing skills first. Discuss the computer that Mr. Taylor used at work, the frequency of use, the steps involved and where it was used. Draw on these past skills.
2. Plan out his steps before doing task. Mr. Taylor wrote down the steps involved in setting up the computer. This should reduce anxiety regarding the task, use more than one sense, and therefore improve performance.
3. Have the computer set up in a distraction-free environment.
4. Minimize memory demands by trying to eliminate some of the memory and new learning demands of the task, providing an introduction list, for example. He can tick off the points as he does them.
5. Have a written checklist for occurrences that are out of the ordinary. He will require some training and repetition to remember to look at his checklist.
6. Direct his attention to external cues for prompting memory: labels on keyboard, green switch at the back of the computer for "on."
7. Encourage mental rehearsal.
8. Encourage Mr. Taylor to suggest or confirm strategies that may be helpful.
9. Repetition plus; Mr. Taylor is to set up the computer each day this week.

Problem 4: Identifying Suitable Activities

Mr. Taylor was not to return to work immediately (if at all); thus it was important to ensure that he would have sufficient recreational pursuits to enhance his quality of life. The leisure assessment revealed a range of activities in which Mr. Taylor was interested.

Woodworking. The woodworking supervisor in the OT department worked with the COTA under direction of the OTR to assist Mr. Taylor in engaging in woodworking activities. Mr. Taylor chose to make a shoe rack for his wife. The therapist taught him how to use a bench clamp so he could work one-handed. The supervisor and Mr. Taylor devised a plan to construct the shoe rack, and used a task list as a memory prompt. A woodworking club was located through Veterans Affairs (VA), and it was decided that he would be able to attend weekly following his discharge and would use taxis to go to and from the center. The OTR arranged a referral to the woodworking supervisor at the VA center and will also assist in formulating written memory prompts.

Activity 2: Card Games. Mr. Taylor and the therapist looked at simple group and solitary card games. Learning these new skills was a challenge for Mr. Taylor given his short-term memory problems. However, using notes in his diary as a prompt he was able to play gin rummy and solitaire with only minimal prompting from the therapist. The ergonomist selected a one-handed card holder from the Independent Living Foundation. The local community house in the area where Mr. Taylor lives holds regular card nights. However, Mr. Taylor is not at the level of playing the games held there, such as bridge. The ergonomist and the therapist decided that attendance at this activity would be re-evaluated toward the end of Mr. Taylor's outpatient program. It was decided that the therapist would devise a graded entry program to the bridge group, if this was indicated.

Activity 3: Movie and Television Viewing. In the past, Mr. Taylor and his wife were regular movie-goers. Mr. Taylor also enjoyed watching television. His short-term memory problems mean that he currently has some difficulty following a complex plot,

or determining how the events in a movie fit together. The OTR or COTA watched programs of 20, 30, and 60 minutes in length with Mr. Taylor and paused at regular intervals to recap events and the plot. Mr. Taylor was encouraged to write main plot events in his notebook. Over time, Mr. Taylor's ability to pay attention to, encode, and retrieve information relating to the film has improved (during the film, and recall of the film later the same day and the next). The therapist is now using normal feature length videos and stops the tape only once in the middle to ask Mr. Taylor to provide a summary of events. His recall of events 4–5 hours after the film has improved such that he is able to recall approximately three-fourths of the plot and significant events.

Activity 4: Planning a Weekend Trip to Nantucket. Mr. Taylor worked with the OTR to plan a weekend trip with his wife during the early fall. In the past, Mr. Taylor planned many weekend trips like this, although they had never visited Nantucket. Mr. Taylor and the therapist decided they would need to:

1. Plan a budget.
2. Plan transportation. Obtain the Hyannisport Ferry timetable (from Cape Cod to Nantucket Island).
3. Obtain the AAA Massachusetts guide and identify suitable accommodation, points of interest to visit, cafes and restaurants to suit the budget.
4. Write an itinerary for the weekend (leaving Friday night and returning Sunday, including all travel times).
5. Write a packing list of things to take.

This model for planning a 3-day weekend trip was then entered into his diary. Using the same model, Mr. Taylor was then able to plan a weekend trip to Camden, Maine, with minimal prompts for the majority of tasks.

Problem 5: Domestic and Community ADLs

Difficulties with these tasks related to the underlying skill deficits identified above, primarily his one-sided neglect and memory.

Lunch Preparation. Mr. Taylor and the COTA developed a routine of making lunch each day. The purpose of this was to increase Mr. Taylor's independence in caring for himself at home during the day while his wife is at work. A standard lunch consists of a bagel with salad filling, fruit, cookies, and coffee. Neglect is more of a problem with this task than memory. However, learning how to operate the kettle (different than the one Mr. Taylor has at home) did take several days. Two red arrows have been placed on kitchen cupboards (at eye level) on corners to prompt left turn taking. Mr. Taylor was initially prompted verbally to scan to the left to find items in the refrigerator. Now a simple sticker is hung on the front of the shelf as a prompt. Mr. Taylor will take this prompt home. Occasionally, he does forget the stage he is up to in a task, but he is usually able to return to the task without assistance.

Banking and Money Management. Mr. Taylor previously managed the family budget and would like to regain these skills. Although he has many of the skills necessary for this, his wife has volunteered to check calculations and transactions before he completes transactions at the bank. Initially, banking and money management tasks from the Cognitive Rehabilitation Workbook (Dougherty, 1993) were used. These are graded from simple (red) activities through to more sophisticated (blue) tasks. Mr. Taylor and the OTR have planned to do electronic and counter service banking activities as part of their community outing. It is anticipated that Mr. Taylor will continue to use his neighborhood bank where he is known.

In the bank, an existing device would be used as an ergonomic device: The ropes set up to guide traffic should suffice to lead him to the teller. The ergonomist will work with Mr. Taylor to enable him to do telephone banking and approach the bank to devise a simplified computerized banking procedure for Mr. Taylor.

Re-Evaluation

The treatments and ergonomic solutions listed above were implemented during Mr. Taylor's final week as an inpatient at the rehabilitation facility. On the last day of his program, the OTR and ergonomist evaluated Mr. Taylor's progress over the past week and the therapy program overall (see Table 6-3). This enabled them to develop the final discharge plan with Mr. Taylor and his family. To evaluate the outcome of the therapeutic and ergonomic interventions three approaches were used.

Re-Examination of Behavioral Objectives

Objectives were set for each problem area. The "how well" component of the objective provides the expected outcome of treatment activities for each problem area. In Table 6-3, objectives are listed in one column with a summary of outcomes in a column to the right. Patient gains are often the result of the total input from all professionals, and hence, ergonomic versus therapeutic outcomes have not been separated in Table 6-3.

Reassessment Using Standardized Instruments

Of the assessments used with Mr. Taylor, only the FIM was readministered on discharge. At the time of discharge he was independent with supervision, and with some verbal prompts from his wife for most self-care tasks. He required supervision only for walking (for safety). Although he has made several gains over his rehabilitation in terms of FIM-social cognition, this remains his weakest area of functioning. Outpatient therapy will continue to target performance in these areas. Overall, his FIM score was raised from 71 to 103 out of a total 126 over the course of his 4-week inpatient rehabilitation.

The A-ONE (Appendix 6-2) was administered for the first time at the beginning of the third week of therapy, and it was determined that he should be reassessed using this tool at 3 months following discharge.

Interview with Mr. Taylor and His Family

Mr. Taylor is very pleased overall with his rehabilitation and is delighted to be able to return home. He maintains that he should have been discharged earlier and that he is able to return to work. Mrs. Taylor seems aware of her husband's problems and limited insight and is very supportive. She has expressed great sadness at the changes the stroke has brought to their lives, but she is very pleased with his rehabilitation program and his gains over the past 4 weeks. Although Mrs. Taylor recognizes that her husband is not able to drive, Mr. Taylor is persistent in his desire to resume this activity.

Discharge Plan

It was arranged for Mr. Taylor to attend occupational therapy as an outpatient at the rehabilitation facility twice per week, and to attend a woodwork program at the VA center. The OTR will consult with the ergonomist at 3 months after discharge to review the success of environmental modifications and changes to tasks, and will determine if any further changes at home or in the community are required. Mr. Taylor is eager to return to work and very frustrated that this has been advised against. The plan is for the physiatrist, OTR, and ergonomist to review this situation with Mr. Taylor at 3 and 6 months after discharge. His employer has been informed of this and of the possibility of a graded return-to-work program for Mr. Taylor, if it is appropriate in the future. It was also arranged to review his ability to drive at 3 and 6 months after discharge. However, unless his neglect resolves, Mr. Taylor will not be able to return to driving. Mrs. Taylor is to commence full-time duties at her place of work next month, and feels less concerned about the family's financial status.

Conclusion

This chapter examined clinical and ergonomic interventions for a client with cognitive deficits following a stroke. The case study demonstrates how an OTR and ergonomist can work together to provide quality services to a client with cognitive disabilities. Although the case presented was for a man who had a stroke, a similar approach could be taken with clients who have cognitive disabilities as a result of a head injury, Alzheimer's disease, a mental illness, or an intellectual disability.

References

Aja, D., Jacobs, K., & Hermenau, D. (1992). *Americans with disabilities act work site assessment.* Boston: Author.

American Heart Association. (1991). *Heart and stroke facts.* Dallas: Author.

Agency for Health Care Policy and Research. (1995). *Post stroke rehabilitation guidelines.* No. 95–0662. Washington, DC: U.S. Government Printing Office.

Anderson, M.A. (1995). Ergonomics: Analyzing work from a physiological perspective. In S.J. Isernhagen (Ed.), *The comprehensive guide to work injury management.* Gaithersburg, MD: Aspen.

Arnadottir, G. (1990). *The brain and behaviour: Assessing cortical dysfunction through activities of daily living.* St. Louis: C.V. Mosby.

Demore-Taber, M. (1995). Job analysis during employer site visit. In K. Jacobs, & C. Bettencourt (Eds.), *Ergonomics for therapists* (pp. 237–244). Boston: Butterworth–Heinemann.

Dougherty, P.M., & Radomski, M.V. (1993). *The cognitive rehabilitation workbook* (2nd ed.). Gaithersburg, MD: Aspen.

Folts, D.J., Giannini, A.J., & Otonicar, B. (1995). Cognitive workload. In K. Jacobs, & C.M. Bettencourt (Eds.), *Ergonomics for therapists.* Boston: Butterworth–Heinemann.

Gianutsos, R., & Klitzner, C. (1981). *Handbook: Computer programs for cognitive rehabilitation* (Vol. 1). Bayport, NY: Life Science Associates.

Grieve, J. (1992). *Neuropsychology for occupational therapists.* Oxford: Blackwell Scientific Publications.

Hall, A.D., & Fagen, R.E. (1968). Definition of system. In W. Buckley (Ed.), *Modern systems research for the behavioral scientist* (pp. 81–92). Chicago: Aldine.

Hamilton, B.B., Granger, C.V., Sherwin, F.S., et al. (1987). A uniform national data system for medical rehabilitation. In M.J. Fuhrer (Ed.), *Rehabilitation outcomes. Analysis and measurement* (pp. 137–147). Baltimore: Brooks.

Kelly-Hayes, M., Wolf, P.A., Kase, C.S., et al. (1989). Time course of functional recovery after stroke. The Framingham Study. *Journal of Neurological Rehabilitation, 3,* 65–70.

Kielhofner, G. (Ed.). (1985). *A model of human occupation. Theory and application.* Baltimore: Williams & Wilkins.

Matchar, D.B., McCrory, D.C., Barnett, H.J.M., & Feussner, J.R. (1994). Medical treatment for stroke prevention. *Annals of Internal Medicine, 121,* 41–53.

Parente, R., & DiCesare, A. (1991). Retraining memory: Theory, evaluation, and applications. In J.S. Kreutzer, & P.H. Wehman (Eds.), *Cognitive rehabilitation for persons with traumatic brain injury. A functional approach* (pp. 147–162). Baltimore: Brookes.

Pfeffer, R.I., Kurosaki, T.T., Chance, J.M., et al. (1984). Use of the Mental Function Index in older adults: Reliability, validity, and measurement of change over time. *American Journal of Epidemiology, 120,* 922–935.

Pheasant, S. (1991). *Ergonomics, work and health.* London: MacMillan Press.

Rice, V. (1995). Ergonomics: An introduction. In K. Jacobs, & C. Bettencourt (Eds.), *Ergonomics for therapists* (pp. 3–12). Boston: Butterworth–Heinemann.

Sohlberg, M.M., & Mateer, C.A. (1989). Training use of compensatory memory books: A three-stage behavioral approach. *Journal of Clinical Experimental Neuropsychology, 11,* 871–891.

Sunburst Communications (1986). *Memory Castle* [computer program]. Pleasantville, NY: Author.

von Bertalanffy, L. (1968). *Organismic psychology and systems theory.* Worcester, MA: Clark University Press.

Suggested Reading

Abreu, B.C., & Toglia, J.P. (1987). Cognitive rehabilitation: A model for occupational therapy. *American Journal of Occupational Therapy, 41,* 439–448.

Baron, J.B., & Sternberg, R.J. (1987). *Teaching thinking skills: Theory and practice.* New York: Freeman.

Bennett, T.L. (1987). Neuropsychological counseling of the adult with minor head injury. *Cognitive Rehabilitation, 5,* 10–15.

Bracy, O.L. (1983). Theories of cognition and brain function: Alexander Luria. *Cognitive Rehabilitation, 1,* 15–17.

Carter, L.T., Howard, B.E., & O'Neill, W.A. (1983). Effectiveness of cognitive skill remediation in acute stroke patients. *American Journal of Occupational Therapy, 37,* 320–326.

Carter, L.T., Olivera, D.O., Duponte, J., & Lynch, S.V. (1988). The relationship of cognitive skills performance to activities of daily living in stroke patients. *American Journal of Occupational Therapy, 42,* 449–455.

Katz, N. (1992). *Cognitive rehabilitation: Models for intervention in occupational therapy.* Boston: Andover Medical Publishers.

La Pointe, L.L., Katz, R.C., & Kraemer, I. (1985). The effects of stroke on appreciation of humor. *Cognitive Rehabilitation, 3,* 22–24.

Pollens, R.D., McBratnie, B.P., & Burton, P.L. (1988). Beyond cognition: Executive functions in closed head injury. *Cognitive Rehabilitation, 6,* 26–32.

Smart, S. (1988). Computers as treatment: The use of the computer as an occupational therapy medium. *Clinical Rehabilitation, 2,* 61–69.

Van Deusen, J. (1993). *Body image and perceptual dysfunction in adults.* Philadelphia: Saunders.

Wilson, S.L. (1987). Cognitive assessment in clinical rehabilitation. *Clinical Rehabilitation, 1,* 257–263.

Zoltan, B. (1996). *Vision, perception, and cognition: A manual for the evaluation and treatment of the neurologically impaired adult* (3rd ed.). Thorofare, NJ: Slack.

Appendix 6-1

Home Site Assessment

Home Site Assessment *

Name of client:	Mr. Taylor	**Therapist:** OT and Ergonomist	
Address:	Massachusetts		
Date of Assessment:	15/6/95		

I.   General Information

a. Type of residence:

Apartment/Condo: √   House_____

Number of floors: _3 - Taylors live on the 2nd floor_

Stairs: Yes √   No ___

    If yes, number and total height in inches: _1-2nd floor 8'2"_
    outside _5 stairs_   inside _14 stairs_

Is a Stair Glide needed: Yes ___ No √____

Ramp: Present_____Recommended ___ Not Required √____

    If yes, how long _____
    (1 inch slope per 12 inches of ramp is recommended; the ht of stairs is used to
    determine length of ramp)

Elevator: Yes ___ No √____

    If yes, does it have accessible controls?_____
    (no higher than 48 inches from the floor)
    If yes, is the door width at least 36" wide? _____

b. Approach to residence:

Parking: On street √_____Driveway_____Parking lot_____

Handicapped-designated parking: Yes ___ No √_____

Is the space adequate for parking and transfer from the car: Yes √   No ___

(need minimum of 4 feet beyond car to open door to transfer)_____

Is the path accessible from parking to entrance? (Comment on the curbs, terrain,
incline, width of paths and other potential obstacles)

Pathway from street to porch is paved and level. Curb from street to sidewalk. No
obstacles.

c. Entrances

Number: Description	entrance #1	entrance #2	
Type of door	wooden hinge door	wooden hinge door aluminum screen door	
Width-min. = 32" ideal = 36"	34"	32"	
Direction of Swing	Inwards	Screen out Door inwards	
Ht. of handles/locks	39" 43"	Door 36" 53"	Screen 45"
Thresholds no more than 1/2"	1/2"	1/2"	
Railings (L or R)	On L side of door	None	
Outside avail. space need 18" more than door width in space opposite door hinge (if opens out)	4 x 8'	4 x 5'	
Inside avail. space can wc move thru once door is opened	4 x 3' - ground entrance 4 x 5' - 2nd floor entrance	4 x 3' - ground entrance 4 x 6' - 2nd floor entrance	

* Source unknown. This home site assessment is used with students in Occupational Therapy Schools in
New Hampshire and Massachusetts.

II.   Interior of Residence

a. Sketch of existing and modified floor plan including bathroom, kitchen, hallways, living room, bedroom and key appliances, obstacles, and all doors attached.

b. Specific measurements

Room 1st or 2nd floor	kitchen 2nd	living 2nd	dining 2nd	bedroom 1 2nd	bathroom 2nd	T.V. room 2nd
size						
floor cover	lino & polished wood	polished wood	polished wood	polished wood	linoleum	polished wood
threshold ht.						
door width min. 32", ideal 36"	30"	30"	29"	29"	271/2"	29"
turning space 5' radius or 3' T	N/A Not in a	N/A wheelchair	N/A	N/A	N/A	N/A
obstacles present	N/A	N/A	N/A	N/A	N/A	N/A
location & ht of telephone - 42" on wall		hall table 26"		on top drawer storage unit - 35"		
light switch ht. 48" max.	48"	49"	54"	49"	54"	50"

c. Hallways: Width?   _35"_____

(need 32" with turning radius of 5' or 3' T space)

Obstacles?   _2 tables_____

d. Bedroom:

1. bed

    a. Bed size: Twin_____Full_____Queen √_____King_____

    b. Mattress: Firm √_____Soft_____Water_____Platform_____

    c. Height from floor? _24"_____

    d. Is the bed stable for transfers? _Yes_____

2. closet

    a. Door: Swings _Out____ Slides _N/A_____

    b. Width?   _27"_____

    c. Rod height?   _56"____ (should be between 36" - 48" from floor)

    d. Shelf ht?   _61"____ (max. is 54") shelf depth? _12"_____ (max. is 16")

e. Bathroom:

1. Bathroom floor plan with key measurements:

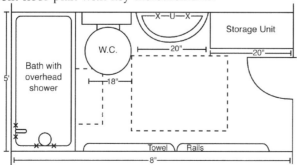

2. Toilet:
   a. ht. from floor to rim with seat up? _14"_ (19-20" is ideal)
   b. are grab bars present? _No_

3. Bathtub _√_ Shower _in bath √_ if shower stall, measurements? _____
   a. are grab bars present? _No_ feasible _√_
   b. faucet height? _30"_ (no more than 48")
   c. glass doors _____ shower curtain _√_

4. Sink: Freestanding _____ Wall hung _√_ Vanity attached _x_

   a. height of sink?   _33"_ (no more than 34" high)
   b. depth to wall?   _17"_ (not more than 27" from wall)
   c. clearance for knees under sink?   _√_ (need 31")
   d. is the mirror at a functional ht?   _√_ over sink
   e. are the towel racks at a reachable level? _√_
   f. is the storage and/or counter space accessible? _√_

f. Kitchen
   1. Kitchen diagram with the refrigerator, stove, and sink. "Working triangle" provided.

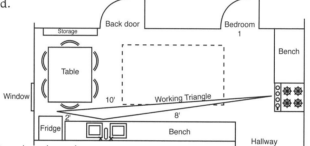

   2. Counters/cupboards
      a. height of counter tops? _32"_ (no more than 34" from floor)
      b. height of cupboards? _45"_ (no more than 48" from floor)
      c. depths of counters? _24"_ (no more than 27" deep)
      d. Is there free space to move wc under counter tops? _N/A_

   3. Comment on the client utilization of the following items; consider controls, height and accessibility.
      a. table _ht 29" x top 30" x 50"_ (ideally 31" high & no more than 42" to reach across)
      b. sink _7" deep / 36" high / 22" to reach faucet_ (ideally 6 1/2" deep & 24" to reach faucet)
      c. cupboards (#) _8 + 4 overhead/above sink / 4 overhead oven bench_
      d. stove _36" high_
      e. oven _door opens down_
      f. microwave _standard size. Located on bench next to stove_
      g. refrigerator _handle 34" from floor / freezer 39" from floor_
      h. freezer _accessible_
      i. other _N/A_

g. Living room
   1. Accessible for leisure / social activities?
   Middle sized room. Most furniture is towards perimeter except coffee table.
   Similar layout in T.V. room.

h. Laundry Location
In basement. Wife does laundry.

SUMMARY OF PROBLEM/ACTION/COST

PROBLEM AREA	RECOMMENDED ACTION	ESTIMATED COST
1. House Entrance: There are 5 steps to the front entrance and 14 stairs inside to their unit. Mr. Taylor is unsteady on stairs. All railings are on L. Due to inability to use L arm (hemiparesis & neglect). The rails are not of assistance.	Install rails on R side at entrance. Install a handrail on R side for internal entrance stairs. Paint white line on the edge of each step.	$400.00
2. Floor Coverings: Throw rugs located in all rooms. Mr. Taylor is at increased risk of falling by tripping over these (particularly with L leg).	Remove throw rugs.	
3. Kitchen: Mr. Taylor has difficulties remembering how to operate microwave.	Provide laminated chart with instructions and pictoral guides.	$5.00
4. Back Entrance: No railing on R side. Difficult to attach railing to R side due to method of construction. Poor lighting. Uneven tread on stairs.	Do not use this entrance, except in emergency. Upgrade light fittings.	$50.00
5. Room Access: Mr. Taylor tends to ignore L turns into rooms. Thus, when going from the living room to the toilet, he may not be able to locate the bathroom door. He may not attend to each of the door openings in the house, depending if he is walking towards the living room or bedroom 1.	Using temporary sticker paper in red, cut out arrows, and stick these on the floor to lead into rooms. These arrows may be removed in the future if not needed. 	$20.00
6. Obstacles: Furniture: Mr. Taylor may bump into the lounge & T.V. room small tables (in center of the room). Hallway tables.	Remove small tables or push up against a wall. Remove hall table, leave telephone table. Put edge pads on tables.	
7. Safety Issues: No smoke detectors installed.	Purchase & install smoke detectors in kitchen & hallway near front entrance.	$80.00
8. Bathroom: Mr. Taylor is unsteady when standing to shower and needs to sit down. Support required when entering/ exiting bath. Occasionally needs assistance when getting up from toilet.	Purchase & install bath board/seat. Grab rail installed on R wall of shower & backwall of shower. Install grab rail on R side of toilet.	$90.00 $70.00 $70.00 $70.00
	Total	$855.00

Summary of Tasks to Be Undertaken by Whom

Occupational therapist:

- Design and place floor stickers
- Advise on rail and bath seat purchase and location
- Provide microwave instruction chart

Mrs. Taylor:

- Purchase smoke detectors
- Remove rugs
- Push tables to the side of the rooms

Handyperson:

- Install shower seat and rail
- Install smoke detectors
- Install entrance and staircase railing

Original and Modified Home Plan

Patient: Mr. Taylor
Date: 8/15/96

Key:
Rugs marked as - - -
Tables marked as ⊤

Original Plan: Modified Plan:

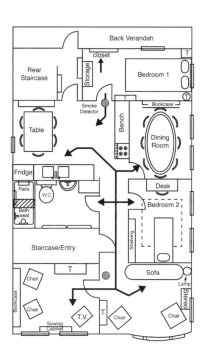

Arnadottir OT-ADL
Neurobehavioral Evaluation
(A-ONE)

Name _____ Mr Taylor _____   Date _____ 6/8/95 _____

Birthdate___ 8/23/1936 _____   Age _____ 59 _____

Gender _____ Male _____   Ethnicity ___ Caucasian _____

Dominance _ Right _____   Profession _____ Foreman _____

Medical Diagnosis:
```
R CVA on 5/20/95 - L Weakness in L.E.          L Neglect
                 - L Loss of function in U.E.  Cognitive deficits
```

Medication: None

Social Situation:
Lives at home with wife and one of his 3 children. Wife is supportive and
wants him to return home. She seems insightful to his current difficulties.

Summary of Independence:
Although Mr Taylor is able to complete most personal ADL tasks with supervision,
or some occasional minor assistance, he is not independent in domestic or
community ADL's due to his cognitive difficulties including neglect, memory
difficulties, spatial relations difficulties, and (possibly) problems with
topographical disorientation. It is anticipated that these difficulties will
impact significantly on his ability to return to work.

FUNCTIONAL INDEPENDENCE SCORE (optional)

FUNCTION	TOTAL SCORE	% SCORE
Dressing	15/20	75
Grooming and hygiene	24/24	100
Transfer and mobility	15/20	75
Feeding	20/20	100
Communication	7/8	88

List of Neurobehavioral Impairments Observed:

SPECIFIC IMPAIRMENT	D	G	T	F	C
Motor Apraxia					
Ideational Apraxia					
Unilateral Body Neglect	✓	✓	✓		
Somatoagnosia					
Spatial Relations		✓		✓	
Unilateral Spatial Neglect	✓	✓	✓		
Abnormal Tone: Right					
Abnormal Tone: Left	✓	✓	✓	✓	
Perseveration					
Organization	✓				
Topographical Disorientation			✓		
Other					
Sensory Aphasia					
Jargon Aphasia					
Anomia					
Paraphasia					✓
Expressive Aphasia					

PERVASIVE IMPAIRMENT	ADL
Astereognosis	
Visual Object Agnosia	
Visual Spatial Agnosia	
Associative Visual Agnosia	
Anosognosia	
R/L discrimination	
Short–Term Memory	✓
Long–Term Memory	
Disorientation	
Confabulation	
Lability	
Euphoria	
Apathy	
Depression	✓
Aggressiveness	
Irritability	
Frustration	

PERVASIVE IMPAIRMENT	ADL
Restlessness	
Concrete Thinking	
Decreased Insight	✓
Impaired Judgment	
Confusion	
Impaired Alertness	
Impaired Attention	✓
Distractibility	
Impaired Initiative	
Impaired Motivation	
Performance Latency	
Absent mindedness	
Other	

Use (√) for presence of specific impairments in different ADL domains (D = dressing, G = grooming, T = transfers, F = feeding, C = communication), and for presence of pervasive impairments detected during the ADL evaluation.

Summary of Neurobehavioral Impairments:

Unilateral body and spatial neglect present during most ADL tasks. This compromises safety. He has low tone throughout L arm – although it is possible that spasticity may develop. He has difficulty finding his way around the hospital – compounded by his neglect of left turns. Short term memory problems are compromising learning. Reduced insight.

Treatment Considerations:

Life relevant tasks necessary to engage Mr Taylor's interest.
Activities that facilitate transfer of training.
Select therapy activities that appear work related (in terms of Mr Taylor's job as a foreman).
Graded program.

Occupational Therapist: Dr Carolyn Unsworth

A-ONE certification Number: US-9X-0XX

A-ONE Part I
Functional Independence Scale and
Neurobehavioral Specific Impairment Subscale

Name ___Mr Taylor_____ Date ___6/8/95_____

INDEPENDENCE SCORE (IP):

4 = Independent and able to transfer activity to other environmental situations.
3 = Independent with supervision.
2 = Needs verbal assistance.
1 = Needs demonstration or physical assistance.
0 = Unable to perform. Totally dependent on assistance.

NEUROBEHAVIORAL SCORE (NB):

0 = No neurobehavioral impairments observed.
1 = Patient is able to perform without additional information, but some neurobehavioral impairment is observed.
2 = Patient is able to perform with additional verbal assistance, but neurobehavioral impairment can be observed during performance.
3 = Patient is able to perform with demonstration or minimal to considerable physical assistance.
4 = Patient is unable to perform due to neurobehavioral impairment. Needs maximum physical assistance.

LIST HELPING AIDS USED:

PRIMARY ADL ACTIVITY   SCORING   COMMENTS AND REASONING

DRESSING	IP	SCORE				Inconsistent performance in
Shirt (or dress)	4	3	(2)	1	0	] attending to L arm
Pants	(4)	3	2	1	0	] sits to complete tasks
Socks	(4)	3	2	1	0	]
Shoes	(4)	3	2	1	0	
Fastenings	4	3	2	(1)	0	Unable to manipulate feelings
Other						with L arm/hand

NB IMPAIRMENT	NB	SCORE				
Motor apraxia	(0)	1	2	3	4	
Ideational apraxia	(0)	1	2	3	4	
Unilateral body neglect	0	1	2	(3)	4	Dressing L arm
Somatoagnosia	(0)	1	2	3	4	
Spatial relations	(0)	1	2	3	4	
Unilateral spatial neglect	0	1	2	(3)	4	Doesn't attend to therapist on L side
Abnormal tone: Right	(0)	1	2	3	4	
Abnormal tone: Left	0	1	2	(3)	4	
Perseveration	(0)	1	2	3	4	
Organization/Sequencing	0	(1)	2	3	4	
Other						

Note: All definitions and scoring criteria for each deficit are in the Evaluation Manual.

Functional Independence Scale and Neurobehavioral Specific Impairment Subscale cont.

PRIMARY ADL ACTIVITY   SCORING   COMMENTS AND REASONING

GROOMING AND HYGIENE	IP	SCORE				COMMENTS
Wash face and upper body	④	3	2	1	0	
Comb hair	④	3	2	1	0	Misses L side on some occasions
Brush teeth	④	3	2	1	0	
Shave/make up	④	3	2	1	0	Has a beard & moustache
Continence/toilet	④	3	2	1	0	Supervision for transfers
Bath	④	3	2	1	0	Supervision for transfers
Other						

NB IMPAIRMENT	NB	SCORE				
Motor apraxia	⓪	1	2	3	4	
Ideational apraxia	⓪	1	2	3	4	
Unilateral body neglect	0	①	2	3	4	
Somatoagnosia	⓪	1	2	3	4	
Spatial relations	0	①	2	3	4	
Unilateral spatial neglect	0	①	2	3	4	
Abnormal tone: Right	⓪	1	2	3	4	
Abnormal tone: Left	0	①	2	3	4	
Perseveration	⓪	1	2	3	4	
Organization/Sequencing	⓪	1	2	3	4	
Other						

TRANSFERS AND MOBILITY	IP	SCORE				
Sitting up in bed	④	3	2	1	0	
Transfers to/from bed (chair)	④	3	2	1	0	
Maneuver around	4	3	2	①	0	Difficulty taking L turns
Toilet transfers	4	③	2	1	0	Supervision for safety
Tub transfers	4	③	2	1	0	Supervision for safety
Other						

NB IMPAIRMENT	NB	SCORE				
Motor apraxia	⓪	1	2	3	4	
Ideational apraxia	⓪	1	2	3	4	
Unilateral body neglect	0	1	2	③	4	L arm in danger of injury during
Spatial relations	⓪	1	2	3	4	transfers
Unilateral spatial neglect	0	1	2	③	4	
Abnormal tone: Right	⓪	1	2	3	4	
Abnormal tone: Left	0	1	2	③	4	
Perseveration	⓪	1	2	3	4	
Organization/Sequencing	⓪	1	2	3	4	
Topographical disorientation	0	1	2	③	4	Problem is compounded by inability
Other						to take L turns

Functional Independence Scale and Neurobehavioral Specific Impairment Subscale cont.

List of Neurobehavioral Impairments Observed:

OTHER	ADL
Motor Apraxia	
Ideational Apraxia	
Unilateral Body Neglect	✓
Somatoagnosia	
Spatial Relations	✓
Unilateral Spatial Neglect	✓
Abnormal Tone: Right	
Abnormal Tone: Left	✓
Perseveration	
Organization	✓
Topographical Disorientation	✓
Other	
Wernicke's Aphasia	
Jargon Aphasia	
Anomia	
Paraphasia	
Broca's Aphasia	
Other	

Comments:

REFER TO TEXT

FUNCTIONAL INDEPENDENCE SCORE (optional)

FUNCTION	TOTAL SCORE	% SCORE
Dressing		
Grooming and hygiene		
Transfers and mobility		
Feeding		
Communication		

Treatment Considerations:

Occupational Therapist: Dr Carolyn Unsworth

A-ONE certification Number: US-9X-OXX

Functional Independence Scale and Neurobehavioral Specific Impairment Subscale cont.

PRIMARY ADL ACTIVITY   SCORING   COMMENTS AND REASONING

FEEDING	IP	SCORE				
Drink from a mug	(4)	3	2	1	0	
Use fingers/sandwich	(4)	3	2	1	0	
Use fork or spoon	(4)	3	2	1	0	Uses a spork (combined fork/spoon)
Use knife	(4)	3	2	1	0	Uses a rocker knife
Other						

NB IMPAIRMENT	NB	SCORE				
Motor apraxia	(0)	1	2	3	4	
Ideational apraxia	(0)	1	2	3	4	
Unilateral body neglect	(0)	1	2	3	4	Eats one-handed
Spatial relations	0	(1)	2	3	4	Orientation to knife to food
Unilateral spatial neglect	(0)	1	2	3	4	Generally attends to all food on
Abnormal tone: Right	(0)	1	2	3	4	plate
Abnormal tone: Left	0	(1)	2	3	4	Doesn't seem to impair performance
Perseveration	(0)	1	2	3	4	
Organization/Sequencing	(0)	1	2	3	4	
Other						

COMMUNICATION	IP	SCORE				
Comprehension	4	(3)	2	1	0	Occasional prompting required
Speech	(4)	3	2	1	0	

NB IMPAIRMENT	NB	SCORE (0 = absent, 1 = present)				
Wernicke's aphasia / Sensory aphasia	(0)	1				
Jargon aphasia	(0)	1				
Anomia	(0)	1				
Paraphasia	0	(1)				On occasion only
Perseveration	(0)	1				
Broca's aphasia / Expressive aphasia	(0)	1				
Dysarthria	0→(1)					Some very occasional slurring
Other	(0)	1				

Results from specific sensory and motor tests:

N/A

A-ONE Part I
Neurobehavioral Pervasive
Impairment Subscale

Name _____Mr Taylor_____ Date _____6/8/95_____

Scoring criteria: Circle one
0 = Impairment is absent
1 = Impairment is present

Pervasive signs may be observed or noted in any Activities of Daily Living (ADL) domain, according to specific instructions in the manual.

NEUROBEHAVIORAL IMPAIRMENT	NB SCORE				COMMENTS AND REASONING
AGNOSIA					
1. Tactile/astereognosis: Right/Left side?	0	1			Not able to assess L side
2. Motor impersistence	0	1			
3. Visual object agnosia	0	1			
4. Visual spatial agnosia	0	(1)			
5. Associative visual agnosia	0	1			
6. Anosognosia	0	1			
BODY SCHEME DISTURBANCES					
1. Right/Left disorientation	0	(1)			on left side
2. Body part identification	0	(1)			on left side
EMOTIONAL/AFFECTIVE DISTURBANCES					
1. Lability	0	(1)			on rare occasions gets teary
2. Euphoria	(0)	1			
3. Apathy	(0)	1			
4. Depression	0	(1)			Showing some signs
5. Aggression	(0)	1			
6. Irritability	(0)	1			
7. Frustration	(0)	1			
8. Restlessness	(0)	1			
COGNITIVE DISTURBANCES					
1. Concrete thinking	0	(1)			Present during some calculations
2. Decreased insight	0	(1)			for ADL problems
3. Impaired judgment	0	(1)			Difficulty using feedback
4. Confusion	(0)	1			
OTHER DYSFUNCTIONS					
1. Impaired alertness	(0)	1			
2. Impaired attention	0	(1)			
3. Distractibility	0	(1)			
4. Impaired initiative	(0)	1			
5. Impaired motivation	(0)	1			N.B. monitor, however, if signs
6. Performance latency	(0)	1			of depression persist
7. Absentmindedness	(0)	1			
8.					

Neurobehavioral Pervasive Impairment Subscale continued:

NEUROBEHAVIORAL IMPAIRMENT   NB SCORE   COMMENTS AND REASONING

MEMORY DISTURBANCES					
1. Short-term memory loss	0	①			Impairs ADL's
2. Long-term memory loss	⓪	1			Recalls majority of information
3. Disorientation	⓪	1			prior to stroke concerning
4. Confabulation	⓪	1			family, workplace. Many details

of specific work activities are
not recalled.

Summary:

The following pervasive neurobehavioral deficits manifested during daily living
activity: visual spatial agnosia, R/L disorientation, body part identification,
emotional lability and some depression, concrete thinking, decreased insight,
impaired judgment, distractibility and some short-term memory loss.
Task performance and independence in ADL's is affected by these deficits.

Section III

Ergonomics for Special Populations

Chapter 7

Ergonomics for Special Populations: An Introduction

Shrawan Kumar and Valerie J. Berg Rice

Learning Objectives

On completion of this chapter, the reader should be able to

- Understand the need for anthropometric, strength, cognitive, and functional ability databases.
- Comprehend the usefulness of such databases for design of equipment and environments.
- Recognize the need for applied research to prevent injuries and promote safety and health.
- Realize the value of usability testing of medical, rehabilitation, and consumer products.
- Become acquainted with an ergonomic approach for profiling and describing task demands and the ability of disabled populations to meet those demands.

Key Words

- Special populations
- Function
- Task analysis
- Disability

Abstract

The need for and benefits of quality ergonomics when working with special populations is potentially greater than with nondisabled populations. Their quality of life can be influenced to a greater extent. In accordance, databases should be developed and used for designing environments for special populations. Design should consider injury prevention, productivity enhancement, ease of use, and acceptability to the particular population that will use the product, be it medical or rehabilitation equipment, a consumer product, or tools in a work setting. An approach to applying ergonomic principles for special populations is introduced to help match task requirements with the functional capabilities of special populations. This approach also challenges the definitions of who may be considered disabled versus enabled by promoting the use of design concepts to alter task requirements. It is hoped that this methodology will be used to benefit the lives of the individuals within special populations.

Introduction

Application of ergonomics to special populations has unique challenges. Although ergonomics touches the lives of every man, woman, and child each day, its impact is often not recognized. This is in part because ergonomics is not a causal factor; rather it is a modifier. One can do most any task without appropriately designed ergonomic equipment; however, the task should be accomplished more easily and efficiently when ergonomic principles are applied to design. Universal incorporation of ergonomics in our lives would require extreme effort and be very expensive and therefore continues to be overlooked. Cost, effort, and nonessential status generally result in only fair application of ergonomic principles at work,

Table 7-1. Percentage of Disabled People by Gender

Country	Year	Age Group	Both Sexes	Male	Female
Egypt	1976	All ages	0.3	0.4	0.2
Pakistan	1981	All ages	0.5	0.4	0.5
Peru	1981	All ages	0.2	—	—
Poland	1978	All ages	7.1	—	—
Turkey	1975	All ages	1.5	1.7	1.2
Australia	1981	All ages	13.2	—	—
Austria	1976	All ages	20.9	19.9	21.8
Canada	1986	All ages	13.2	12.7	13.8
China	1987	All ages	4.9	—	—
FRG	1983	All ages	—	11.8	9.8
Japan	1980	≥18 yrs	2.4	—	—
Philippines	1980	≥18 yrs	4.4	5.1	3.7
Spain	1986	≥18 yrs	15.0	14.8	15.7
United Kingdom	1985–1986	≥16 yrs	14.2	12.1	16.1

Source: Extracted from DISTAT. (1988). *United Nations disability statistics data base*. New York: United Nations.

home, and leisure. However, when dealing with a population with diminished abilities in regard to their task or environmental requirements, the application of ergonomics can make a substantial difference in quality of life.

Disabilities have been reported in most communities around the world. Their prevalence seems to vary between 0.2% in Peru to 20.9% in Austria based on figures extracted from Disability Statistics Database (DISTAT, 1988; Table 7-1). However, it must be pointed out that due to a lack of uniform definition of disability, and social and cultural stigma attached to disability in many countries, the figures reported by the United Nations (1990) are thought to be conservative. Furthermore, the methods of reporting, data collection, and analyses may also vary from country to country. Regardless of the method of calculation, the size of the disabled population is considered to be large. In Canada alone, 3.3 million people are estimated to have some disability—constituting 14.3% of the total population of the country (Statistics Canada, 1990). As early as 1979, in a study for the Veteran's Administration, Grall estimated that 62.5 million people in the United States suffered from some disability (Grall, 1979). This constituted 30% of the entire population of the United States! Perhaps because of a greater acceptance of disability in American society, residents may not be deterred from reporting their disabilities, as they might be in other countries. According to the Committee on a National Agenda for the Prevention of Disabilities (Pope, 1991), one in

seven Americans has disabling conditions, and more than 43 million Americans have physical or mental disabilities (Bello, 1991).

The scenario described above poses a challenge to society. Most facilities, processes, and products have been designed to the standards obtained from a 35-year-old, able-bodied man. A man's capabilities are likely to be in their prime at that age; therefore, use of such design information for persons with disabilities will affect and perhaps even hamper their functional abilities.

There is a need for a scientific database for individuals with functional impairment regardless of the cause of that impairment. The database needs to include anthropometrics, strength, cognitive functioning, and especially functional abilities. One argument against such a proposition is the diversity among disabled populations—as if there were no diversity among able-bodied populations. Until the functional *abilities* of special populations are identified, suitable products will not be developed on a consistent basis. One population that has received more attention in recent years is the geriatric population; however, a commensurate increase in research for the disabled has not occurred. Even with the increased attention paid to the problems associated with cumulative trauma, and the emphasis on prevention of injury due to poor posture (as well as other risk factors), little attention has been paid to this special population.

Work, home, and leisure design requirements differ for individuals with disabilities as compared to requirements for able-bodied populations, and they will vary according to the handicapping condition. Also, the design of medical and rehabilitation equipment should be tailored to those who will use them (medical practitioners, patients, and primary caregivers). Ergonomists study slip and trip injuries to identify prevention strategies. In a similar manner, Gaal, Rebholtz, Hotchkiss, and Pfaelzer (1997) studied wheelchair rider injuries and identified design and selection criteria to prevent such injuries. Ergonomists are employed by sportswear companies to assist in developing and evaluating footwear for athletes. In a similar manner, Reiber et al. (1997) recently published a study for a different special population—evaluating footwear for patients with foot insensitivity resulting from diabetes.

There are three major areas of concern in regard to ergonomics and special populations. First, a database of information describing basic characteristics of special populations is needed to assist with overall design strategies for special populations, although some designs will have to be client-centered for a particular individual. Second, research is needed to investigate and prevent injuries and illnesses of special populations, such as evaluating reinjury statistics of persons with a prior back injury. Third, application of usability testing for medical and rehabilitation devices will enhance the use of these devices, and promote the function of their users.

Responding to these three concerns by incorporating ergonomics into rehabilitation and clinical settings will enhance the function and productivity of special populations. To obtain optimal results of ergonomic application, one has to have relevant information and an appropriate strategy of intervention.

An Ergonomic Approach for Special Populations

The Disability Concept

We all can understand and recognize the concept of disability. However, due to a lack of precise standards, boundaries become somewhat fuzzy. Most of the people who may consider themselves normal in an overall sense may harbor some disabilities that may not affect them in a significant way. In an effort to explain this, Kumar (1989, 1992) described an ability-disability continuum. In fact, it is hard to identify a

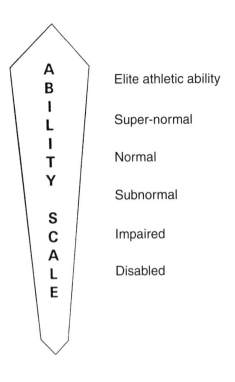

Figure 7-1. Ability-disability continuum. (Reprinted with permission from S. Kumar. [1992]. Rehabilitation: An ergonomic dimension. *International Journal of Industrial Ergonomics, 9,* 97–108.)

discrete point among most human functions where a line can be drawn between ability and disability (Figure 7-1). Therefore, it is essential to develop a standard or a reference against which function can be compared to determine ability from disability.

The World Health Organization (1980) in its publication, International Classification of Impairments, Disabilities, and Handicaps (ICIDH) defined disability as follows: "A restriction or lack of ability (resulting from impairment) to perform an activity in the manner or within the range considered normal for a human being." Therefore, a disability is a functional limitation or activity restriction, probably caused by an impairment. In the foregoing definition and explanation the comparator reference is anchored on who is considered normal for that attribute (to address the concept clearly, only one disability is being considered rather than a compound situation with multiple disabilities). Considering the variability among "normals," questions arise regarding which values should be taken to be

Table 7-2. Nature of Disabilities and Percent Among Disabled with Category of Disability in Canada

Nature	Percent (not in labor force)		Description
	One Disability	Multiple Disabilities	
Mobility	60	67	Limited in ability to walk, move from room to room, carry an object for 10 m, or stand for long periods
Agility	45	67	Limited in ability to bend, dress or undress oneself, get in and out of bed, cut toenails, use fingers to grasp or handle objects, reach, or cut own food
Seeing	59	74	Limited in ability to read ordinary newsprint or to see someone from 4 m, even when wearing glasses
Hearing	51	67	Limited in ability to hear what is being said in conversation with one other person or two or more persons, even when wearing a hearing aid
Speaking	48	69	Limited in ability to speak and be understood
Other	63	71	Limited because of learning disability or emotional or psychiatric disability, or because of developmental delay
Unknown	40	—	Limited but nature unknown

Source: Modified from Statistics Canada. (1990). The Health and Activity Limitation Survey. *Highlights: Disabled persons in Canada.* (Catalogue No., 82–602). Ottawa.

normal—mean or fifth percentile or any other. Furthermore, if a disabled person can perform a task with an assistive device, should that person be considered disabled or normal?

Profiles of Disability

In defining disability, the criterion is function or lack thereof. Function can be determined by an assessment of task demands, along with an assessment of an individual's ability to meet those demands. If the demands of the task can be lowered, then many people who are considered disabled (for that task) will suddenly become enabled. Therefore, in applying ergonomics principles to special populations, two complementary strategic steps will be very useful. First, one should develop the functional profiles of disability groups and grades among those groups. Second, the functional demands of tasks should be lowered by design to enable more people to accomplish the task, without sacrificing the quality of the product or outcome. These profiles should be developed based on ability rather than disability. The Disability Compendium has described seven classes of disability (Table 7-2). The ICIDH has listed about 250 individual disabilities, which are divided into nine broad categories (WHO, 1980). The broad categories in turn are divided into as many as 10 subcategories, some of which are further divided. Thus, considerable information on the nature of disability exists. From an ergonomic standpoint, it would be prudent to develop an *ability* profile of people in these categories.

Various disability measuring schemes have been proposed in the literature, including Bowling, 1989; Wade, 1992; Duckworth, 1983, 1995; Martin et al., 1988; Slater et al., 1974; Bird et al., 1993; Gorter, 1993; and Haley et al., 1989. One of the conceptually simplest ways of measuring disability is by simple classification as proposed by ICIDH (WHO, 1980), and as accomplished by Bowling (1989). However, this tends to be tedious and for many purposes not very useful (Duckworth, 1995). Among other methods of measurements, Wade (1992) based his approach on neurologic rehabilitation. Duckworth (1983, 1995), and Martin et al. (1988) have advocated a questionnaire survey method of measuring disability. Simeonsson et al. (1995) have argued that functional measurement to document individual characteristics would be of value. Such representative measures have been focused on global impairment (Bird et al., 1993), physical dis-

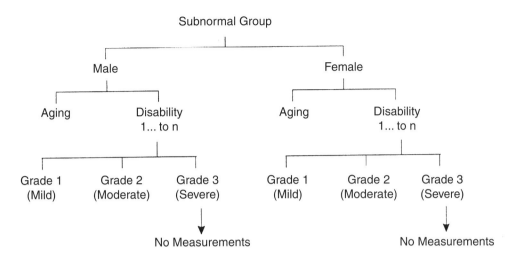

Figure 7-2. Categories of disabilities. (Reprinted with permission from S. Kumar. [1992]. Rehabilitation: An ergonomic dimension. *International Journal of Industrial Ergonomics, 9,* 97–108.)

ability (Gorter, 1993), and motor functions (Haley et al., 1989). The field of disability is vast and diverse; thus, only well-conceived and systematic efforts will bring sufficient generalizability.

In approaching the application of ergonomics for special populations, it may be desirable to classify clients by appropriate categories of disability (Figure 7-2; Kumar, 1996). Following this, one should proceed to determine an ability profile for individuals. Kumar (1992) broadly divided the functional attributes in three groups: physical, psychological, and social. Once the domain in which a deficiency lies has been identified, efforts should be concentrated on that domain. A functional activity rarely requires only one trait or ability, even though it may challenge one trait more than others. Thus, a clear determination of traits of interest will be of value.

For a given task with a physical capacity component, an individual will be required to have some degree of range of motion, strength, endurance, and motor coordination. However, the kinematics and kinetics of a disabled person could deviate from those of persons without disabilities. A painful injury can affect more than one variable in the execution of a task, and each variable can be affected to a different extent, when compared to the preinjury state. Therefore, the physical capacity to do any task must be assessed multidimensionally, consid-

ering all relevant variables involved. For example, a simple task of moving an object from point A to point B will require an individual to move within a particular range of motion, use of some level of force to overcome resistance, and attain a velocity of motion.

For testing an individual's range of motion, one method would be to measure joint movement as described by Kumar (1992) and represent the motions as shown in Figures 7-3 and 7-4. Following the determination of range of motion, the strength capabilities available at the given joint should be measured. This can be done in isometric, isokinetic, or isotonic modes. Once the strength has been determined, a relationship between the individual's range of motion and his or her strength also becomes quite important, due to concurrent requirement for both as presented in the Figure 7-5. Many occupational tasks involve repetitive motions or differing motions, and there may be an optimum speed of operation for enhanced productivity. A simultaneous consideration of all three factors (range of motion, strength, speed) can provide a comprehensive picture of the capability of the individual in physical domains (Figure 7-6). Such a profile will allow one to categorize the individual with disability into a functional group. It is essential that functional groupings be based on functional criteria. A standardized description of such

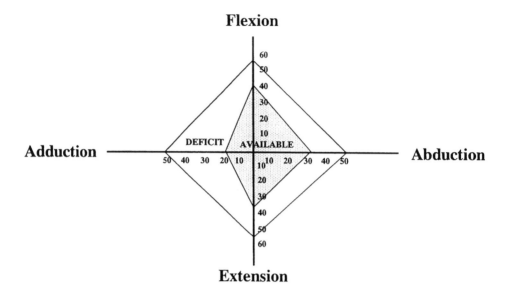

Figure 7-3. A hypothetical drawing showing available range of motion and the deficit. (Reprinted with permission from S. Kumar. [1992]. Rehabilitation: An ergonomic dimension. *International Journal of Industrial Ergonomics, 9,* 97–108.)

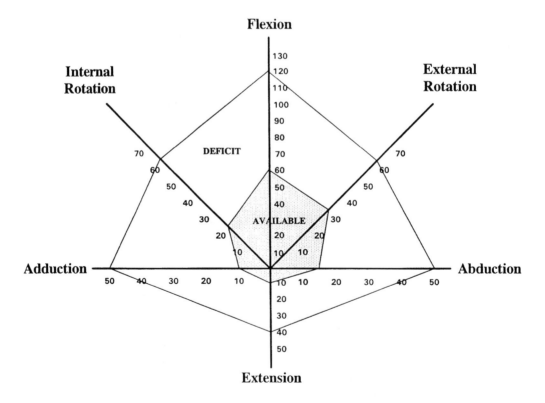

Figure 7-4. A hypothetical representation of available range of motion and deficit of a joint. (Reprinted with permission from S. Kumar. [1992]. Rehabilitation: An ergonomic dimension. *International Journal of Industrial Ergonomics, 9,* 97–108.)

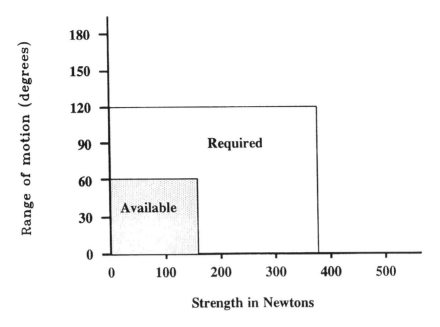

Figure 7-5. A depiction of available and required strength and range of motion. (Reprinted with permission from S. Kumar. [1992]. Rehabilitation: An ergonomic dimension. *International Journal of Industrial Ergonomics, 9,* 97–108.)

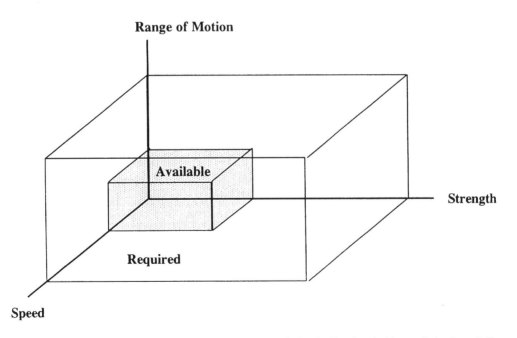

Figure 7-6. A depiction of required and available traits for a hypothetical task. (Reprinted with permission from S. Kumar. [1992]. Rehabilitation: An ergonomic dimension. *International Journal of Industrial Ergonomics, 9,* 97–108.)

functional groupings for future reference and allocation will become strategically important and valuable information. After categorizing this functional profile, the person's abilities will have to be compared against the task requirements on a quantitative level. Such an exercise will allow the evaluator and the individual to determine reserves or deficiencies, if any. The determination of the degree of reserve is thought to be essential from the standpoint of continued safety and optimal operation on the given task by a given individual. The difference between the boundary lines of the task demands and the individual's capability will be a quantitative measure of deficiency. However, if the task demand is lower than that of the patient capability, the difference will represent the reserve of the individual. According to these principles, it will be essential to determine other physical and physiological variables such as endurance, aerobic capacity, dexterity, and precision to determine the physical task capability. Based on the same principles, Kumar (1992) also outlined determination of the psychological and social work capability, to arrive at a total functional profile of the individual with a disability.

Functional Demands of Tasks

The next strategic step is to develop a profile of task demands of standard tasks. These may begin from basic activities of daily living, to intermediate, and on to advanced activities of daily living. Once the functional profiles and the demands of the tasks are developed and categorized, they can be matched to determine the functional capability of the categories and grades of particular groups. The task demands can also be matched with the functional profiles of individuals to determine their ability to handle particular task demands.

After such comparisons, the ergonomic effort should be to reduce the task demands to the maximum extent possible and compare them once again with the functional capabilities of the functional groups profiled above. This will clearly indicate the further inclusion of people with lesser capability in groups that have been enabled to perform the required jobs. For example, the information could be used to design a structured living environment that requires less strength, less complex task requirements, and provides both physi-

cal and cognitive assistive devices for a developmentally disabled population. A consideration of development of appropriate assistive devices to enable additional groups of people to perform such tasks is the final stage. Likewise, after the task demands are compared with the functional profiles of an individual, the information could be applied to designing work and living environments that enable individuals to function at their highest ability level, and therefore, perhaps be considered able-bodied, rather than disabled.

Conclusion

The application of ergonomics with special populations should mirror that with nondisabled populations. That is, databases of information should be developed and used to design environments, equipment, products, and procedures for situations in which special populations can benefit. Design concepts should be explored to prevent injury and illness and enhance productivity and ease of use for special populations. Usability testing procedures should be applied to specialized medical and rehabilitation equipment to further their usefulness and acceptability for the populations that use them. By bringing these areas to attention, it is hoped that readers will recognize the needs, embrace them, and put them into action.

A potential method for applying ergonomic principles with special populations has been introduced. First, special populations would be classified according to their levels of functional ability. Following a task analysis, the functional abilities of the population could then be matched the task demands and be used to design the work, home, or leisure environment to fit the population or individual. It is hoped this methodology will be used for—and will benefit the lives of—the individuals who constitute special populations.

References

Bello, M. (1991). Preventing disability demands new thinking: Looking toward a national agenda. *News Report, XLI(3)*, 2–4.

Bird, H.R., Shaffer, D., Fisher, P., et al. (1993). The Columbia Impairment Scale (CIS): Pilot findings on a measure of global impairment for children and adolescents. *Inter-*

national *Journal of Methods in Psychiatric Research, 3,* 167–176.

Bowling, A. (1989). *Measuring health.* Milton Keynes, UK: Open University Press.

DISTAT (1988). *United Nations disability statistics data base.* New York: United Nations.

Duckworth, D. (1983). *The classification and measurement of disablement.* London: Her Majesty's Stationery Office, 77.

Duckworth, D. (1995). Measuring disability: The role of the ICIDH. *Disability and Rehabilitation, 17,* 338–343.

Gaal, R.P., Rebholtz, N., Hotchkiss, R.D., & Pfaelzer, P.F. (1997). Wheelchair rider injuries: Causes and consequences for wheelchair design and selection. *Journal of Rehabilitation Research and Development, 34(1),* 58–71.

Gorter, K.A. (1993). Survey methods for the assessment of physical disability among children. *Disability and Rehabilitation, 15,* 47–51.

Grall, T.B. (1979). *A feasibility study of product testing and reporting for handicapped consumers.* New York: Veterans Administration.

Haley, S.M., Hallenborg, S.C., & Gans, B.M. (1989). Functional assessment in young children with neurological impairments. *Topics in Early Childhood Special Education, 9,* 106–126.

Kumar, S. (1989). Rehabilitation and ergonomics: Complementary disciplines. *Canadian Journal of Rehabilitation, 3,* 99–111.

Kumar, S. (1992). Rehabilitation: An ergonomic dimension. *International Journal of Industrial Ergonomics, 9,* 97–108.

Kumar, S. (1997). Aging, disability and ergonomics. In S. Kumar (Ed.), *Perspectives in rehabilitation ergonomics* (pp. 1–33). London: Taylor & Francis.

Martin, J., Meltzer, H., & Elliot, D. (1988). *The prevalence of disability among adults.* (OPCS survey of disability in Great Britain, Report 1). London: Her Majesty's Stationery Office, 59.

Pope, A.M., & Tarlov, A.R. (Eds.). (1991). *Committee on a National Agenda for the Prevention of Disabilities, Division of Health Promotion and Disease Prevention.* (Summary and recommendations available from the committee: [National Institute of Medicine, phone 202-334-1716] or the full report is available from the National Academy Press.) Washington, DC: National Academy Press.

Reiber, G.E., Smith, D.G., Boone, D.A., et.al. (1997). Design and pilot testing of the DVA/Seattle footwear system for diabetic patients with foot insensitivity. *Journal of Rehabilitation Research and Development, 34,* 1–8.

Simeonsson, R.J., Chen, J., & Hu, Y. (1995). Functional assessment of Chinese children with the ABILITIES index. *Disability and Rehabilitation, 17,* 400–410.

Slater, S.B., Vukmanovic, C., Macukanovic, P.O., et al. (1974). The definition and measurement of disability. *Social Science and Medicine, 8,* 305–308.

Statistics Canada. (1990). The Health and Activity Limitation Survey. *Highlights: Disabled persons in Canada.* (Catalogue No., 82–602). Ottawa.

United Nations. (1990). *Disability statistics compendium.* New York: Department of International Economic and Social Affairs Statistical Office, Series Y;4.

Wade, D.T. (1992). *Measurement in neurological rehabilitation* (p. 10). London: Oxford University Press, 10.

World Health Organization. (1980). *International classification of impairments, disabilities, and handicaps* (reprint, 1993). Geneva: Author.

Chapter 8

Physical Disability Case Study: An Ergonomics Approach to Workstation Design for Paraplegics

Biman Das

Learning Objectives

On completion of this chaper, the reader should be familiar with

- Structural anthropometric measurements and three-dimensional isometric strength profiles of male and female paraplegics.
- Application of the above information to workstation design optimizations for such a population.

Key Words

Anthropometric measurements
Isometric strengths
Workspace

Abstract

Structural anthropometric measurements were determined for male and female paraplegics. The data would be useful for the design of industrial workstations especially for such a population. The three-dimensional isometric strength profiles of male and female paraplegics were determined for pull, push, push-up, and pull-down exertions in the normal, maximum, and extreme workspace reach envelopes. The study measured how anthropometric workspace reach distances, horizontal and vertical angles, and gender would affect the stated maximum voluntary isometric strengths. The information would be helpful in workstation design optimizations. A computerized isometric-strength measurement system was designed and constructed for the study.

Introduction

An ergonomics approach to workstation design envisions an appropriate matching of worker capabilities and work requirements. The physical size, shape, and strength of the individual will greatly affect the physical dimensions of the workstation and the tasks capable of being performed. For the design of the workstation, it is essential that the controls, materials, tools, and equipment requiring manual operation be placed in an area that can be used efficiently and safely by most of the user population. Small changes in the physical dimensions in the workspace can have considerable impact on worker productivity and occupational safety and health (Tichauer, 1975). The aim of an ideal industrial workstation design is to eliminate harmful postures and to minimize the design imposed stresses on the user. Inadequate posture resulting from an improperly designed workstation can cause static muscle efforts, which eventually results in acute muscle fatigue, decreased performance and productivity, and increases work-related injuries (Corlett et al., 1982).

For the design of an industrial workstation, reliable and accurate anthropometric measurements for both able-bodied and wheelchair-bound individuals are required. However, similar data are not readily available for paraplegics. One of the main factors limiting the application of engineering anthropometry is the paucity of practical, standardized methods for measurement of disabled individuals and therefore the lack of measurement on that population (Hertzberg, 1972). Das and Grady (1983) used previously collected structural anthropometric data and made adjustments for applied industrial elements such as slumped posture and variances in shoes and clothing. They were able to present normative data for industrial workstation design for able-bodied populations. This has addressed the problem noted by Hertzberg (1972); however, it does not deal with the needs of all individuals for employment, such as physically challenged individuals who require a wheelchair for mobility or paraplegics.

Industrial workers are required not only to reach but also to exert force to perform tasks in the workplace. Tasks must be arranged so the worker is able to reach the controls and tools and operate them efficiently to accomplish the required job. Thus, knowledge of both functional reach and human strength must be incorporated into an industrial workstation design. Overexertion injuries in industry account for more than 25% of the lost time (National Institute of Occupational Safety and Health [NIOSH], 1981). Consequently, strength measurement plays an important role in the recommended hiring process for jobs involving physically strenuous work, like manual materials handling (Keyserling et al., 1980; Kroemer, 1983). With the increased incidence of soft-tissue injuries and the pressure for maximum efficiency, it is imperative that workstation design give due consideration to human strength.

It is often assumed that an able-bodied worker and a seated paraplegic worker are equivalent and capable of the same amount of work. The stability of a paraplegic is significantly less than that of an able-bodied person, due to limited muscular control of the back and legs and limitations caused by the wheelchair itself. Consequently, strength profiles of paraplegic individuals should be studied in their reach envelopes for optimum design of a workstation.

Most studies to date have concentrated on analyzing able-bodied populations, ignoring any differences associated with physical disabilities. Although approximately 200,000 workers in the United States are paraplegic (Buchanan & Nawoczenski, 1987), no studies have developed a model representing the strength capacity of paraplegic individuals. Lacking such a model, paraplegics usually must accommodate themselves—with few adaptations—to standard workspace areas, regularly experiencing discomfort (Abdel-Moty & Khalil, 1989). Paraplegics are notably subject to additional factors affecting strength capacity, such as those related to mobility, spasticity, and sensation difference, in addition to basic location and exertion-direction definitions. Given the intensive muscular training associated with both genders using manual wheelchairs, strength comparisons by gender may need to be revised before application to paraplegics. Furthermore, the stability constraints associated with lower limb paralysis, including wheelchair stability and vertical displacement of the body's center of gravity, would potentially have drastic effects on spatial strength tendencies, especially relative to able-bodied populations.

The absence of proper workstation design information or data specifically for paraplegics may prolong accommodation and frustrate individuals going through accessibility programs (Canadian Standards Association, 1990). An incompatible workstation design can handicap an individual or, worse, predispose the worker to musculoskeletal injury of the upper extremities. Any injury of this nature would affect the principal means of propulsion and mobility for a paraplegic.

The main objectives of this chapter are to present the results of the experimental studies dealing with

1. Structural anthropometric measurements for male and female paraplegics
2. Isometric strength profiles in the workspace for male and female paraplegics

Structural Anthropometric Measurements for Paraplegics

The existing design guidelines for paraplegics are often based on the information provided by Floyd et al. (1966) or modeled from information obtained from an able-bodied population (Pheasant, 1986). Nowak (1989) provided anthropometric data gathered from a population that had a variety of lower limb dysfunctions, but no classification of the level or type of dysfunction was reported. Kozey and Das (1992) determined the current sources of anthropometric information used in design guidelines for paraplegics and identified large differences in the reported anthropometric dimensions. These differences were attributed to the nature and degree of physical impairments, sample sizes, measurement definitions, and measurement techniques. It would be difficult to apply the existing anthropometric data to industrial workstation design, even for a specific physical dysfunction. Therefore, further investigation is needed to generate anthropometric data for paraplegics, specific to industrial applications, by using a reliable measurement system. The main aim of the experimental study was to determine reliable and accurate structural anthropometric measurements for male and female paraplegics to enlarge and update the information concerning paraplegics for industrial workstation design.

Method

Subjects

For this investigation, the subjects consisted of 42 males and 20 females with spinal cord injuries (SCI). They were recruited through the provincial (Nova Scotia) branch of the Canadian Paraplegic Association. Additional sources of contact were through special groups and local advertisement. Before participating in this investigation, all subjects were informed as to the nature of the study. They were required to sign a document of informed consent. The demographic information and analysis and the classification of the level or type of dysfunction are presented subsequently under Results.

Procedure

A total of 16 structural anthropometric dimensions were measured for both males and females in this investigation: (1) seated stature, (2) eye height, (3) shoulder height, (4) forearm height, (5) knee height, (6) toe height, (7) maximum reach height, (8) overhead reach, (9) normal reach, (10) radial arm reach, (11) maximum reach, (12) trunk depth, (13) bideltoid width, (14) acromion width, (15) elbow width, and (16) overall length. The measurements were obtained from slide film taken of the subjects while they maintained a working or slump posture. The measurements were taken in the Clinical Locomotor and Functional Laboratory, Nova Scotia Rehabilitation Centre, Halifax.

The subjects were instructed to change into clothing that would allow for easy palpation of underlying bony landmarks. Then they were positioned in the area designated for the photogrammetric procedure. Small (15-mm) reflective markers were placed on the subjects over the appropriate bony landmarks. Two 35-mm cameras were positioned and synchronized to operate from one remote position. Slides were taken of the right and front views of the subjects while they were seated in their wheelchairs. Each subject was positioned in a normal reach position (both right and left upper limbs), a maximum reach position (right upper limb only), and an overhead reach position (right upper limb only). Two plumb lines were placed in the field of view of the cameras. One line was placed in the sagittal plane of the subject, in line with the subject's right side. The second line was placed in the frontal plane, in line with the left acromion. Each line was marked with a reference line marker, which was later used for scaling the projected images.

The subjects were constrained in their seated position in the following manner. The subjects were first asked to assume a "normal comfortable" position, as if they were in front of a desk or work area. After the subjects had assumed this position, a tripod and neck support apparatus were placed behind the subject such that the neck support just made contact with the subject. Then the subject was instructed to maintain contact with the neck support for all the subsequent slides. After taking the slides, a vertical measure (in millimeters to the nearest 1 mm) from the floor to a seat reference point (SRP) was taken using a standard measuring tape. This value was used to relate all vertical structural dimensions to the seat.

Data Collection and Analysis

The processed slides were projected to one-half real image size and the appropriate landmarks were manually digitized. The digitized values were entered into a computer database. Subsequently, they were scaled and the anthropometric dimensions were determined. The demographic data were statistically analyzed using pair-wise Student's t-tests with a critical value of 0.05. For the paraplegic population, the level or type of dysfunction was recorded. For the anthropometric data, the fifth and ninety-fifth percentile values were determined using standard statistical procedures.

Table 8-1. Demographic Data of Paraplegic Subjects

	Men	**Women**
Number of subjects	42	20
Age (years)		
Range	22–64	20–63
Mean	39.2	37.3
SD	12.1	12.7
Time in wheelchair (years)		
Mean	11.2	12.7
SD	8.7	13.2

Results

The subjects' demographic information and analysis are presented in Table 8-1. Based on the sample of 42 males and 20 females, the mean ages of the males and females were 39.1 and 37.3 years, respectively. For the males, the ages ranged from 22 to 64 years, and for the females the ages ranged from 20 to 63 years. The mean number of years in a wheelchair for the males and females was 11.6 and 12.7 years, respectively.

The results of the pair-wise Student's *t*-test between the males and females showed that there was no significant difference ($p > 0.05$) in terms of their age and time in the wheelchair (Table 8-2). In other words, the male and female samples were similar for the stated criteria.

Table 8-3 shows the classification of the level or type of dysfunction. The majority of the subjects had a dysfunction at the T5 or T12 location (30 males and nine females), followed by the C5 or T4 location (eight males and two females). Spina bifida caused dysfunction in one male and four females.

For the selected 16 structural anthropometric measurements or dimensions, the mean, standard deviation, fifth, fiftieth, and ninety-fifth percentile values and overall minimum and maximum values for the males and females were determined (Tables 8-4 and 8-5). There were statistically significant differences ($p < 0.05$) for the structural anthropometric dimensions between the males and females for all dimensions, except the toe height and knee height values. The mean, range, and standard deviation (SD) values of seated stature for males were 848, 656–1,011, and 70 mm, respectively (see Table 8-4). The corresponding values of seated stature for females were 752, 601–858, and 64 mm, respectively (see Table 8-5). Thus, there were significant differences between the males' and females' seated stature values. Similar inferences could be made for the other structural anthropometric measurements. Overall the measurements of males were significantly higher than those of the females, as expected.

The mean forearm height for the males was 210 mm, whereas the knee height was 199 mm, for a difference of 11 mm. Similarly, the values for the females were 181 and 172 mm for the forearm and knee heights, respectively, a difference of just 9 mm. These values revealed that there would not be sufficient space between the forearm and knee to provide a work bench or table top of adequate thickness. Thus the alignment of paraplegics at a workstation would require different considerations than the able-bodied population because of the small differences between these measurements. The conventional postural alignment principle of the able-bodied population could not be followed.

Conclusions

Structural anthropometric measurements (16 in all) were determined in terms of mean, standard devia-

Table 8-2. Comparative Analysis of Age and Time in Wheelchair Between Male and Female Paraplegics: Student's *t*-Test

	Degree of Freedom	**Calculated Student's *t* Value**	**Tabulated Student's *t* Value***
Age (years)	34	0.53	2.03
Time in wheelchair (years)	26	0.66	2.06

*The tabulated values for 5% (two-tailed).

tion, fifth, fiftieth, and ninety-fifth percentiles, minimum and maximum values, based on a sample of 42 males and 20 females. The demographic and the level or type of dysfunction of the paraplegic subjects were provided. No significant difference was found between the male and female subjects in terms of their age and time in the wheelchair. Significant statistical differences in 14 anthropometric dimensions were found between males and females, except for the vertical height of knee and toe. Due to small differences in the vertical height of the knee and forearm of 11 and 9 mm for male and female paraplegics, respectively, it would be inappropriate to use dimensions based on an able-bodied population for paraplegics.

Table 8-3. Classification of Level or Type of Dysfunction of Parapalegic Subjects

Location of Lesion and Type of Dysfunction	Frequency	
	Men	Women
CF/T4	8	2
T5/T12	30	9
L1/L5	2	2
Spina bifida	1	4
Friedreich's ataxia	—	1
Arthritis	—	1
Cerebral palsy	—	1
Muscular dystrophy	1	—
Total	**42**	**20**

Isometric Strength Profiles in the Workspace

In the creation of the ideal workstation, several factors are involved, one of which is user reach capability. Accurate reach capability data are essential to ensure that all hand-operated controls or tasks are located where they can be reached and operated efficiently. For the upper body, the three-dimensional workspace has been divided into three contiguous regions in areas of increasing distance from the worker. These have been classified as the "normal," "maximum," and "extreme" reach envelopes. The normal workspace is closest to the body, being circumscribed by the horizontal lower arm pivoting about a relaxed vertical arm. The maximum workspace is circumscribed during movement of the fully extended arm about the shoulder. The extreme workspace is reached when the movement of the trunk extends the reach of the fully extended arm (Farley, 1955; Squires, 1956; Das & Grady, 1983). Another factor that impinges on the creation of the

Table 8-4. Structural Anthropometric Measurements for Male Paraplegics with Respect to Seatpan

Dimension	Mean	SD	Fifth	Fiftieth	Ninety-Fifth	Minimum	Maximum
Seated stature	848	70	734	848	963	656	1,011
Eye height	735	67	496	735	717	456	745
Shoulder height	572	63	468	572	676	414	750
Forearm height	210	62	108	210	312	73	390
Knee height	199	49	118	199	280	55	289
Toe height	−226	71	−343	−226	−109	−430	−103
Max. reach height	607	67	496	607	717	456	745
Overhead reach	1,243	104	1,072	1,243	1,415	945	1,450
Normal reach	488	27	444	488	532	435	549
Radial arm reach	631	35	573	631	689	543	728
Maximal reach	853	45	779	853	926	758	987
Trunk depth	240	25	198	240	281	203	318
Bideltoid width	510	35	452	510	568	434	593
Acromion width	396	26	354	396	439	344	448
Elbow width	626	57	533	626	720	523	720
Overall length	1,127	64	1,022	1,127	1,216	985	1,246

Note: All dimensions in millimeters.

Table 8-5. Structural Anthropometric Measurements for Female Paraplegics with Respect to Seatpan

Dimension	Mean	SD	Fifth	Fiftieth	Ninety-Fifth	Minimum	Maximum
Seated stature	752	64	647	752	857	601	858
Eye height	645	60	546	645	744	523	760
Shoulder height	510	53	423	510	597	386	629
Forearm height	181	46	105	181	257	81	271
Knee height	172	52	86	172	258	74	283
Toe height	−199	64	−304	−199	−94	−291	−92
Max. reach height	502	79	372	502	632	346	645
Overhead reach	1,090	87	947	1,090	1,234	906	1,226
Normal reach	450	24	411	450	490	386	480
Radial arm reach	581	33	526	581	635	498	632
Maximal reach	768	43	697	768	839	689	832
Trunk depth	182	23	143	182	220	139	221
Bideltoid width	469	53	383	469	556	402	593
Acromion width	355	39	291	355	418	291	434
Elbow width	593	78	465	593	721	448	728
Overall length	1,063	87	920	1,063	1,206	894	1,290

Note: All dimensions in millimeters.

ideal workplace is user strength capability. To ensure optimal workplace layout, it is imperative that the operator's strength profile be determined. The strength profile of a person under specified conditions is essential for the design of tools (their weight, ease of use), controls (type of grip required, spatial placement), and equipment—in other words, the workstation.

Studies have shown that horizontal distance and vertical height exertion significantly affect the force that can be exerted, both in static and dynamic strength tests (Chaffin & Park, 1973; Davis & Stubbs, 1977). However, these studies have not attempted to relate anthropometric reach space envelopes to the strength data obtained. Researchers have measured strength at varying elbow angles (Hunsicker, 1955), fractions of mean reach for the population (Davis & Stubbs, 1977; Kumar, 1991), or fixed distances (Mital & Faard, 1990). Measurement locations have not been determined by individual functional reach regions. For optimum workstation design a link must be established between an individual's ability to reach and exert force.

In the past, lift exertions have been studied most frequently. Many tasks performed in industry require pull, push, push-up, and pull-down of objects. Thus, pull, push, push-up, and pull-down

radial exertions should be studied for optimum workstation design. Such radial exertions vary differently with horizontal distance and height (Hunsicker, 1955). Strength profiles of paraplegic individuals should be studied in their reach envelopes for optimum design of a workstation. Also, women on the average are approximately one-third weaker than men. The main purpose of this investigation was to measure isometric pull, push, push-up, and pull-down strength profiles of male and female paraplegics in the normal, maximum, and extreme workspace reach envelopes to facilitate workspace design optimization. The experimental study for the determination of isometric strength profiles in the workspace was carried out in two parts that dealt with: (1) pull and push strengths and (2) push-up and pull-down strengths. Basically the experimental approach was similar in both the cases.

Isometric Pull and Push Strength Profiles of Paraplegics in the Workspace

The experimental method, experimental results, and conclusions of this investigation are described below. Subsequently, a similar procedure will be followed in describing the study dealing with the determination of isometric push-up and pull-down strength profiles of paraplegics in the workplace.

Method

Subjects. The subjects consisted of eight men and eight women who were paraplegics of working age. All were residents of Nova Scotia and used a manual wheelchair for mobility. The average age of the male subjects was approximately 37 and the average number of years since injury was approximately 14. The average age of the female subjects was approximately 35 and their average number of years since injury was approximately 13. Spinal lesions among the subjects occurred between L1 and T4, with two cases of spina bifida.

Strength Measurement System. A specially designed computerized strength measurement system was used for data collection (Figure 8-1; Black, 1994). The essentials of the system relevant to the present study are highlighted here. The apparatus was specially designed to record isometric strength and stability data at adjustable angles and distances. The subjects used their own wheelchairs, which were secured from rolling on a special platform. Wheelchair and body stability were monitored using sensors that were connected through an auditory alarm to the computer. Instability was recorded when either a wheel of the chair broke contact with the floor, or when the subject's buttocks lost contact with the chair cushion. All measurement sessions were conducted in the Nova Scotia Rehabilitation Centre, Halifax.

Procedure. Each measurement session consisted of (1) measuring individual anthropometric and wheelchair characteristics and (2) recording radial maximum isometric strength exertions of the right hand for 5-second periods. All subjects were told to pull (or push) as hard as they could without jerking. Pull and push exertions alternated at each test location, although the ordering of these locations was randomized among subjects. A rest period of at least 1 minute separated each exertion to ensure muscle fatigue recovery. Each test series for a subject lasted approximately 3 hours. To control for stability, subjects were not permitted to lean or grab onto any fixed object (including any portion of the wheelchair) during exertions. Otherwise they were free to assume the posture they felt was most effective for force generation.

Data Collection and Analysis. Radial pull and push isometric exertions were measured for each of 32 locations defined by reach level (normal, maximum, and extreme), vertical angle (ϕ) relative to the elbow (normal reach) or shoulder (maximum and extreme reaches), and horizontal angle (θ) relative to the right shoulder in slump posture (Table 8-6). Reach envelope, ϕ angle, θ angle, direction of exertion, and gender were the independent variables; recorded strength was the dependent variable.

The measurement locations were defined along the outside limit of each individual's normal, maximum, and extreme reaches. The normal reach envelope was defined by the comfortable reach of the lower arm with the upper arm relaxed (Squires, 1956; Das & Behara, 1995). The maximum reach was limited by the outstretched arm (Farley, 1955). The extreme reach was defined by the limiting reach of the outstretched arm with extension of the torso without losing stability.

Recorded ϕ angles ranged from work-surface height ($\phi = -20$ degrees in maximum and extreme reaches, or $\phi = 0$ degrees in normal reach) to 0, 45, and the vertical 90 degrees (for maximum and extreme reaches only). Radial θ angles were recorded from the frontal plane on the right hand side ($\theta = 0$ degrees) for maximum and extreme reaches only, to 45, 90, and 135 degrees for all reach levels.

Raw-strength data were collected using a Durham Instruments MLP force transducer and transferred via a low pass filter to a 386 SX personal computer for recording and subsequent analysis. Strength and stability sensors were sampled at 10 Hz throughout the 5-second exertion. Following the completion of a measurement series, maximum values for each condition were calculated.

Results

The data had revealed that overall women exerted 73% the force of men. Different variations in strength occurred depending on each of the independent variables, direction, reach, and vertical and horizontal angles. Thus results are presented by combinations of independent variables, beginning with separate discussion of male pull and push

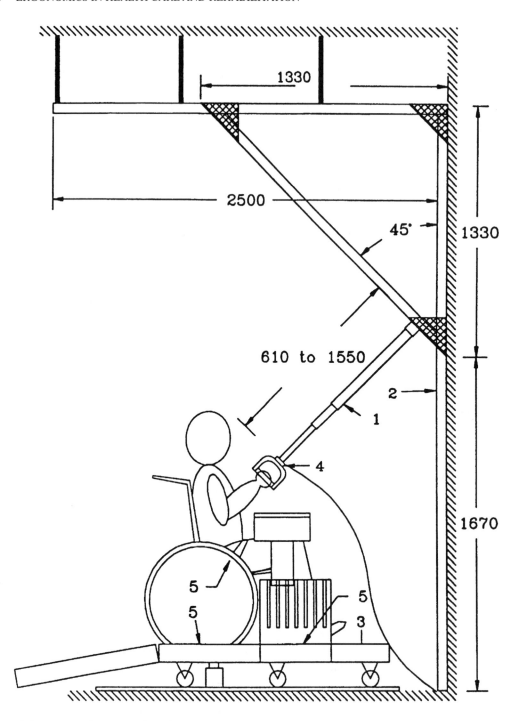

Figure 8-1. A computerized isometric (pull and push) strength measurement system for paraplegics. All dimensions in millimeters. (1 = extendible arm; 2 = supporting track; 3 = platform; 4 = force transducer; 5 = stability sensors.)

Table 8-6. Isometric (Pull and Push) Strength Measurement Locations

No.	Level of Reach	Vertical Angle: ϕ Degrees*	Horizontal Angle: θ Degrees
1	Normal	0	45
2	Normal	0	90
3	Normal	0	135
4	Normal	45	45
5	Normal	45	90
6	Normal	45	135
7	Maximum	−20	0
8	Maximum	−20	45
9	Maximum	−20	90
10	Maximum	−20	135
11	Maximum	0	0
12	Maximum	0	45
13	Maximum	0	90
14	Maximum	0	135
15	Maximum	45	0
16	Maximum	45	45
17	Maximum	45	90
18	Maximum	45	135
19	Maximum	90	90
20	Extreme	−20	0
21	Extreme	−20	45
22	Extreme	−20	90
23	Extreme	−20	135
24	Extreme	0	0
25	Extreme	0	45
26	Extreme	0	90
27	Extreme	0	135
28	Extreme	45	0
29	Extreme	45	45
30	Extreme	45	90
31	Extreme	45	135
32	Extreme	90	90

*At normal reach, phi angle was taken relative to elbow height, in line with the shoulder. At maximum and extreme reaches, phi angle was taken relative to the shoulder.

strengths, then female pull and push strengths, and finally comparisons of each.

Male Pull Strength. Table 8-7 shows the average pull strength of male subjects by location. The maximum overall pull strength was 473 N exerted in the extreme reach at the overhead position where the vertical angle ϕ = 90 degrees and the horizontal angle θ = 90 degrees. The minimum overall strength was 158 N occurring in the maximum reach, where ϕ = 0 degrees and θ = 135 degrees. Strengths at maximum and normal reaches increased with increasing ϕ angle, but were least

where θ = 135 degrees. Maximum strength in the normal reach was 239 N at ϕ = 45 degrees and θ = 90 degrees and the corresponding value in the maximum reach was 426 N at ϕ = 90 degrees and θ = 90 degrees.

Male Push Strength. Table 8-8 reveals that men's push strengths were generally weaker in the extreme reach than in normal or maximum reach. The maximum overall exerted strength was 235 N in maximum reach at ϕ = 45 degrees and θ = 45 degrees. The minimum exerted strength was 101 N in the extreme reach at ϕ = 45 degrees and θ = 0

Table 8-7. Pull Strength (Newtons) of Men

φ Degrees	θ Degrees	Normal Reach		Maximum Reach		Extreme Reach	
		Mean	SD	Mean	SD	Mean	SD
−20	0	—	—	203	56	196	42
−20	45	—	—	195	60	181	61
−20	90	—	—	211	76	182	58
−20	135	—	—	192	50	163	57
0	0	—	—	208	49	208	45
0	45	214	45	205	52	194	45
0	90	218	61	215	56	221	55
0	135	207	45	158	40	180	30
45	0	—	—	274	62	263	59
45	45	229	59	250	67	250	69
45	90	239	72	271	76	282	66
45	135	234	53	240	53	237	62
90	90	—	—	426	101	473	115

Note: Overall mean male pull strength = 232 N.

Table 8-8. Push Strength (Newtons) of Men

φ Degrees	θ Degrees	Normal Reach		Maximum Reach		Extreme Reach	
		Mean	SD	Mean	SD	Mean	SD
−20	0	—	—	194	63	199	58
−20	45	—	—	220	44	203	36
−20	90	—	—	181	60	156	44
−20	135	—	—	152	43	131	29
0	0	—	—	212	72	227	80
0	45	224	57	216	71	231	41
0	90	162	56	189	46	170	43
0	135	156	40	131	47	145	42
45	0	—	—	184	88	101	32
45	45	217	53	235	92	154	59
45	90	223	66	233	72	172	76
45	135	205	56	188	45	184	93
90	90	—	—	192	101	125	84

Note: Overall mean male push strength = 185 N.

degrees. The maximum strengths in the normal and extreme reaches were 224 N and 231 N, respectively, both at φ = 0 degrees and θ = 45 degrees.

Male Pull Versus Push Strength. The average male pull strength was 232 N making it on the average 25% greater than the push strength (see Tables 8-7 and 8-8). Pull strength was less changed by increasing reach envelope than by vertical and horizontal angles. However, push strength decreased from normal and maximum to extreme reach and was less affected by vertical angle. Indeed, push exertions were greatest and least at the same vertical angle (φ = 45 degrees), at different reaches and horizontal angles. When comparing strength in normal and maximum reaches, both pull and push

Table 8-9. Pull Strength (Newtons) of Women

φ Degrees	θ Degrees	Normal Reach		Maximum Reach		Extreme Reach	
		Mean	SD	Mean	SD	Mean	SD
–20	0	—	—	155	46	151	45
–20	45	—	—	139	36	142	36
–20	90	—	—	139	39	152	28
–20	135	—	—	138	35	144	45
0	0	—	—	156	37	149	40
0	45	158	46	151	29	142	30
0	90	149	47	145	33	150	34
0	135	151	55	132	35	131	34
45	0	—	—	241	59	236	71
45	45	193	70	214	40	228	60
45	90	186	60	214	51	225	50
45	135	172	52	202	49	205	40
90	90	—	—	284	49	318	50

Note: Overall mean female pull strength = 178 N.

strengths were similar, exertions at normal reach and φ = 45 degrees being weaker than at maximum reach.

Female Pull Strength. Table 8-9 shows women's pull strength was greatest at 318 N in the extreme reach at φ = 90 degrees and θ = 90 degrees. The minimum pull strength was 131 N exerted in the extreme reach at φ = 0 degrees and θ = 135 degrees. The maximum pull strength in the normal and maximum reaches were 193 N at φ = 45 degrees and θ = 45 degrees, and 284 N at φ = 90 degrees and θ = 90 degrees, respectively. Pull strengths in normal reach varied less than either maximum or extreme reach but were on the average less.

Male Versus Female Pull Strength. The female pull strength was overall 77% of the male push strength (see Tables 8-7 and 8-9). The overall maximum values occurred at identical locations (extreme reach, φ = 90 degrees and θ = 90 degrees) for both genders. The minimum values occurred for both at φ = 0 degrees and θ = 135 degrees but was in the maximum reach for males and extreme reach for females. The difference between the maximum and extreme reach values at this angle for females was negligible (1 N).

Female Push Strength. Table 8-10 shows the female push strength was greatest at 172 N in the

maximum reach at φ = 45 degrees and θ = 0 degrees. The minimum force exerted was 84 N occurring in extreme reach at φ = –20 degrees and θ = 135 degrees. The maximum push strengths in the normal reach was 145 N at φ = 0 degrees and θ = 90 degrees. The corresponding value in the extreme reach was 144 N at φ = 45 degrees and θ = 135 degrees.

Female Pull Versus Push Strength. The pull strength among females was 41% greater than push strength on the average (see Tables 8-9 and 8-10). As with males, the female's strength increased with vertical φ angle when pulling, but not when pushing. Pull strength between different reach envelopes did not differ substantially at like angles, whereas push strength decreased in extreme reach, particularly at vertical angles at or above the horizontal. In these positions there was less support from the wheelchair for a push exertion.

Male Versus Female Push Strength. On the average, females pushed at 68% the force of men (see Tables 8-8 and 8-10). The locations of maximum push strength were similar between male and female data, differing only by the degree of horizontal asymmetry. Women were strongest pushing in the frontal plane (θ = 0 degrees), whereas men were stronger 45 degrees toward the front. This may be due to decreased stability associated with narrower chairs used by women than men. The mini-

Table 8-10. Push Strength (Newtons) of Women

φ Degrees	θ Degrees	Normal Reach		Maximum Reach		Extreme Reach	
		Mean	SD	Mean	SD	Mean	SD
–20	0	—	—	145	57	142	68
–20	45	—	—	109	27	135	56
–20	90	—	—	112	22	106	27
–20	135	—	—	92	39	84	39
0	0	—	—	147	65	127	57
0	45	138	29	136	41	122	36
0	90	145	55	140	51	104	36
0	135	101	22	110	39	104	43
45	0	—	—	172	58	118	27
45	45	137	52	158	49	127	57
45	90	136	57	146	49	124	38
45	135	124	58	134	59	144	61
90	90	—	—	122	56	101	38

Note: Overall female push strength = 126 N.

mum push exerted did not occur at the same vertical or horizontal angle for males and females. Males were weakest (101 N) at φ = 45 degrees and θ = 0 degrees and the females were weakest (84 N) below the horizontal at φ = –20 degrees and θ = 135 degrees. In each case, minimum strength occurred at the extreme reach.

Conclusions

Men's maximum isometric radial pull strength was 473 N, which occurred in the extreme reach in the vertical overhead position. Men's maximum isometric radial push strength was 235 N, occurring in the maximum reach at φ = 45 degrees and θ = 45 degrees. Women's maximum isometric radial pull strength was at 318 N in the same overhead extreme reach position as men. On the average women's pull was 77% the value of men's. Women's maximum exerted push strength was 172 N occurring in maximum reach at φ = 45 degrees and θ = 0 degrees. Overall the forces exerted in the reach envelope by the females were 152 N or 73% those of the males. The pull strength was less affected by gender than push strength; women exerted 77% and 68% the strength of men, respectively. The average pull strength was 25% greater than the push strength for men and the corresponding value was 41% greater than push for women.

Isometric Push-Up and Pull-Down Strength Profiles of Paraplegics in the Workspace

Method

Subjects. Wheelchair-mobile paraplegics from the general working population of Nova Scotia, were asked to voluntarily participate in this study. All participants were screened in advance to ensure that none had a recent history of significant physical ailments or were currently on medication. The sample consisted of eight men and eight women of working age in this study.

The average age of the male subjects was approximately 34 and the average number of years since injury was approximately 13. All eight male subjects had spinal cord injuries ranging from C4 to T11. The average age of the female subjects was approximately 34 and the average number of years since injury was approximately 21. Of the women subjects, five were paraplegics with spinal injuries ranging from T10 to L3, two had multiple sclerosis, and one subject had spina bifida.

Strength Measurement System. Each measurement session was conducted using a specially designed computerized isometric strength measurement system (Figure 8-2; Black, 1994; Forde, 1995). Only the essentials of the system relevant

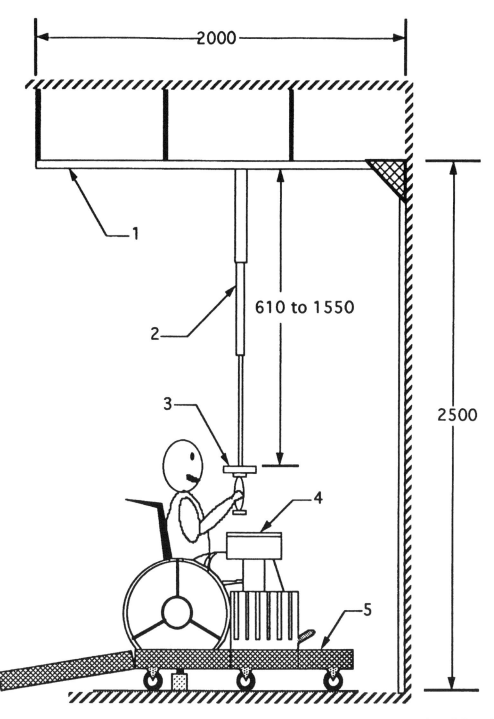

Figure 8-2. A computerized isometric (push-up and pull-down) strength measurement system for paraplegics. All dimensions in millimeters. (1 = supporting track; 2 = extendible arm; 3 = force transducer; 4 = table surface; 5 = rotating platform.)

Table 8-11. Isometric (Push-Up and Pull-Down) Strength Measurement Locations

No.	Level of reach	Vertical Angle: ϕ Degrees	Horizontal Angle: θ Degrees
1	Normal	0	45
2	Normal	0	90
3	Normal	0	135
4	Normal	45	45
5	Normal	45	90
6	Normal	45	135
7	Maximum	−20	45
8	Maximum	−20	90
9	Maximum	−20	135
10	Maximum	0	45
11	Maximum	0	90
12	Maximum	0	135
13	Maximum	45	45
14	Maximum	45	90
15	Maximum	45	135
16	Extreme	−20	45
17	Extreme	−20	90
18	Extreme	−20	135
19	Extreme	0	45
20	Extreme	0	90
21	Extreme	0	135
22	Extreme	45	45
23	Extreme	45	90
24	Extreme	45	135

Note: At normal reach, the angle phi is taken relative to the elbow height in line with the shoulder. At maximum and extreme reaches, the angle phi is taken relative to the shoulder.

to the present study are highlighted. The system basically incorporates three main mechanisms: (1) a stationary track fixed to the ceiling for reach envelope adjustments, (2) an extendible arm to allow for vertical adjustments (ϕ), and (3) a rotating platform to allow for angular adjustments in the horizontal plane (θ). With this system, the subjects do not have to reposition themselves for each measurement location. The subjects used their own wheelchairs, which were secured by wedge-shaped blocks from rolling on the rotating platform.

The system can be further broken down into five main components: (1) an extendible arm with a force transducer and handle attached, (2) a supporting track overhead to locate this extendible arm appropriately for testing, (3) a rotating platform that can locate the subject at specific horizontal angles with respect to the frontal plane, (4) a table surface to simulate a working environment, and (5) a data collection interface.

Procedure. The independent variables in this experiment were: (1) force direction at two levels: push up and pull down, (2) reach envelopes at three levels: normal, maximum, and extreme, (3) vertical (ϕ) angles at three levels: −20 degrees, 0 degrees, and 45 degrees, and (4) horizontal (θ) angles at three levels: 45 degrees, 90 degrees, and 135 degrees. The dependent variable was maximum isometric arm strength.

Isometric arm strength was measured in 24 different locations (Table 8-11). The angle $\theta = 0$ degrees was defined as the horizontal line at shoulder height for maximum and extreme reaches and at the elbow (upper arm parallel to body) for the normal reach, increasing moving upward. The angles used for θ were −20 degrees, 0 degrees, and 45 degrees. Radial angles were set relative to the shoulder point in a slump posture; $\theta = 0$ degrees was defined as the right side of the frontal plane, increasing counterclockwise when viewed from above. The angles used for θ were 45 degrees, 90

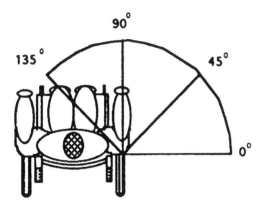

Figure 8-3. Location of horizontal θ angles for all reach levels. Strength measurements taken at 45 degrees, 90 degrees, and 135 degrees.

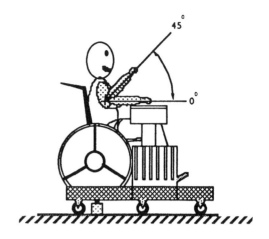

Figure 8-4. Location of vertical φ angles for the normal reach envelope. Strength measurements taken at 0 degrees and 45 degrees.

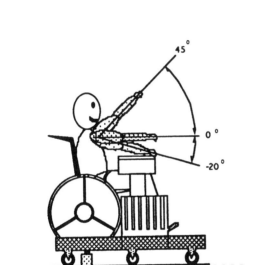

Figure 8-5. Location of vertical φ angles for the maximum and extreme reach envelopes. Strength measurements taken at –20 degrees, 0 degrees, and 45 degrees.

degrees, and 135 degrees (Figure 8-3). Vertical angle φ = 0 degrees was defined as a horizontal plane at the elbow (upper arm parallel to body) for the normal reach (Figure 8-4), and as a horizontal plane at shoulder height for the maximum and extreme reaches (Figure 8-5). A plane aligned with the shoulder joint was used as opposed to the mid-

sagittal plane (passing through the body median) as the reference plane for measurement of symmetry. This plane corresponds to the center of arm rotation and is not affected by anthropometric variations in the distance between the shoulder and midsagittal plane. To best simulate the actual working strength as well as recreate a typical workstation situation, the subjects' strength measurements were taken in their own wheelchairs.

Each measurement session consisted of (1) measuring individual anthropometric and wheelchair dimensions and (2) recording radial maximum isometric strength exertions of the right hand for 5-second periods. A minimum rest period of 45 seconds was given between each trial to overcome the effects of fatigue, if any. All subjects were told to push up or pull down as hard as they could without assuming unnatural postures or jerking on the handle. Push-up and pull-down exertions alternated at each measurement location and were randomized between subjects.

Because of subjects' varying abilities to achieve maximum effort, a mean score of two trials was used to measure isometric strength at each location. Overall posture was constantly monitored visually by the experimenter. On the average, the measurement session per subject took approximately 2 hours to complete.

Table 8-12. Push-Up Strengths (Newtons) of Men

φ Degrees	θ Degrees	Normal Reach		Maximum Reach		Extreme Reach	
		Mean	SD	Mean	SD	Mean	SD
−20	45	—	—	46	19	44	46
−20	90	—	—	51	22	46	40
−20	135	—	—	57	37	34	20
0	45	83	29	44	15	45	29
0	90	115	42	57	24	40	13
0	135	137	61	39	19	32	17
45	45	72	31	67	28	45	27
45	90	93	27	68	32	39	14
45	135	118	44	51	25	47	28

Note: Overall mean push-up strength = 61 N.

Results

The average male push-up and pull-down strengths for all 24 measurement locations are presented in Tables 8-12 and 8-13, respectively, and for the women, in Tables 8-14 and 8-15, respectively. Strength profile trends are given according to gender and force direction (push up or pull down).

Male Push-Up Strength. The maximum push-up strength exertion was 137 N in the normal reach envelope and occurred at vertical angle, $\phi = 0$ degrees, and horizontal angle, $\theta = 135$ degrees (see Table 8-12). The lowest strength exertion recorded was 32 N in the extreme reach at $\phi = 0$ degrees and $\theta = 135$ degrees. The highest push-up strength exertions in the maximum and extreme reaches were 67 N at $\phi = 45$ degrees and $\theta = 90$ degrees and 47 N at $\phi = 45$ degrees and $\theta = 135$ degrees, respectively. Thus the highest male push-up strength was found in the normal reach envelope followed by strength exertions in the maximum reach with strength values in the extreme reach being the lowest. Stated otherwise, the push-up strength had decreased with the increase in reach distance.

Male Pull-Down Strength. The maximum pull-down strength exertion was 151 N in normal reach at location $\phi = 45$ degrees and $\theta = 135$ degrees (see Table 8-13). The lowest strength exertion recorded was 58 N in the extreme reach at $\phi = -20$ degrees and $\theta = 45$ degrees. In the maximum and extreme

reaches, the highest pull-down strengths were 140 and 112 N, respectively, both at $\phi = 45$.degrees and $\theta = 135$ degrees. The maximum pull-down strength exertions for males followed the same trend in the reach envelopes as the male push-up strength.

Male Push-Up Versus Pull-Down Strength. In all except two cases, pull-down strength was noticeably higher than push-up strength. The two exceptions (115 N and 137 N) occurred at measurement locations $\phi = 0$ degrees, $\theta = 90$ degrees and $\phi = 0$ degrees, $\theta = 135$ degrees, both in the normal reach envelope. At these two measurement locations the arm was very close to the body. So it was possible that there was an increase in moment-arm leverage, thus allowing for higher-than-usual push-up strength exertions.

Female Push-Up Strength. The maximum push-up strength exertion was 66 N in the normal reach at $\phi = 0$ degrees and $\theta = 90$ degrees (Table 8-14). The lowest strength exertion recorded was 14 N in the extreme reach at $\phi = 0$ degrees and $\theta = 135$ degrees. The highest push-up strength exertions in the maximum and extreme reaches were 43 N and 26 N, respectively, both at $\phi = 45$ degrees and $\theta = 45$ degrees. The highest strength exertions for female push-up strength were given throughout in the normal reach followed by strength exertions in the maximum and extreme reaches.

Female Pull-Down Strength. The maximum pull-down strength exertion was 80 N in normal reach at

Table 8-13. Pull-Down Strengths (Newtons) of Men

φ Degrees	θ Degrees	Normal Reach		Maximum Reach		Extreme Reach	
		Mean	SD	Mean	SD	Mean	SD
−20	45	—	—	71	21	58	22
−20	90	—	—	78	16	67	23
−20	135	—	—	79	21	67	18
0	45	93	30	73	17	71	30
0	90	94	25	80	17	68	22
0	135	104	24	88	24	79	19
45	45	130	55	127	70	91	31
45	90	139	47	116	37	100	28
45	135	151	48	140	50	112	37

Note: Overall mean pull-down strength = 95 N.

Table 8-14. Push-Up Strengths (Newtons) of Women

φ Degrees	θ Degrees	Normal Reach		Maximum Reach		Extreme Reach	
		Mean	SD	Mean	SD	Mean	SD
−20	45	—	—	33	12	22	11
−20	90	—	—	42	13	24	9
−20	135	—	—	34	15	20	13
0	45	50	15	31	10	22	14
0	90	66	27	38	14	20	7
0	135	64	25	22	5	14	8
45	45	52	21	43	20	26	17
45	90	59	23	41	19	21	8
45	135	64	23	40	15	23	9

Note: Overall mean push-up strength = 36 N.

location φ = 45 degrees and θ = 135 degrees (Table 8-15). The lowest strength exertion recorded was 33 N in the extreme reach at φ = −20 degrees and θ = 45 degrees. The highest strength exertions in the maximum and extreme reaches were 77 and 79 N, respectively, both at φ = 45 degrees and θ = 90 degrees. The female pull-down strength did not follow the general trend of the highest exertions in the normal reach followed by those in the maximum and extreme reaches in descending order. However, the maximum strength values were quite similar in the two reaches.

Female Push-Up Versus Pull-Down Strength. In all but one case, the pull-down strength was notice-ably higher than the push-up strength. The one exception occurred at measurement location φ = 0 degrees, θ = 90 degrees in the normal reach.

Male Versus Female Strengths. Although trends among the two sexes were very similar, males were capable of consistently higher strength exertions. The female push-up strength was, on average, 59% of the average male push-up strength (36 N, Table 8-14, compared with 61 N, Table 8-12). Similarly, female pull-down strength was, on average, 61% of male pull-down strength (58 N, Table 8-15, compared with 95 N, Table 8-13). For all measurement locations, the mean push-up and pull-down strength of males was sig-

Table 8-15. Pull-Down Strengths (Newtons) of Women

φ Degrees	θ Degrees	Normal Reach		Maximum Reach		Extreme Reach	
		Mean	SD	Mean	SD	Mean	SD
−20	45	—	—	41	11	33	11
−20	90	—	—	48	15	41	14
−20	135	—	—	45	13	44	14
0	45	56	13	47	13	42	16
0	90	64	27	55	15	46	15
0	135	66	24	50	14	53	16
45	45	68	20	75	23	65	32
45	90	77	28	77	23	79	28
45	135	80	27	74	24	71	19

Note: Overall mean pull-down strength = 58 N.

nificantly higher than the corresponding values for females.

For pull-down strengths, the highest strength exertions for the males and females were 151 N and 80 N, respectively, at measurement location $\phi = 45$ degrees, $\theta = 135$ degrees in the normal reach. It was possible that this position allowed the subject to use considerable upper-body strength—as opposed to just arm strength—when exerting a downward force.

For both male and female push-up strength exertions, as vertical angle (ϕ) changed, there was no consistent increase or trend in strength values. However, for pull-down strength exertions, there was a clear trend of increasing strength values as the vertical height (ϕ) increased.

Conclusions

The maximum push-up strengths for males was 137 N at measurement location $\phi = 0$ degrees and $\theta = 135$ degrees and for the females was 66 N at $\phi = 0$ degrees and $\theta = 90$ degrees, both in the normal reach. The maximum pull-down strengths for both men and women occurred at $\phi = 45$ degrees and $\theta = 135$ degrees in the normal reach and were 151 and 80 N, respectively. Reach level has a major impact on isometric push-up and pull-down strengths. Strength in the normal reach was noticeably higher than strength exertions in the maximum reach with strength values in the extreme reach being the lowest. Men's overall mean strength was 78 N compared to 47 N for the women. Thus, women had, on the average, approximately 61% of the strength of

the men. Push-up strength is, on the average, approximately 64% of pull-down strength. For both sexes, pull-down strength is noticeably higher than push-up strength.

Summary and Concluding Remarks

Based on 42 male and 20 female paraplegics, structural anthropometric measurements were determined, to assist in the design of industrial workstations for such a population. It was shown that the workstation design based on able-bodied anthropometric measurements would not be suitable for this population.

Based on eight male and eight female paraplegics, three-dimensional isometric strength profiles were determined for pull and push extensions in the normal, maximum, and extreme working reach envelopes. The investigation measured the manner by which workspace reach distances, horizontal and vertical angles, and gender had affected maximum voluntary isometric pull and push strengths among paraplegics. A computerized isometric strength measurement system was designed and constructed for the purpose. Although men were stronger than women, and pull strength was stronger than push strength, each of these groups showed different spatial strength distributions. On average, pull strength in the normal reach was less than in the maximum or extreme reach for both genders, but the push strength was similar in normal and maximum reaches and less in the extreme reach. Pull strength was greatest at the angles closest to the vertical, no matter the horizontal angle. Both push and pull strengths tended to be minimum at θ = 135 degrees, the position that required most twisting of the torso. These results clearly show the importance of strength capabilities in the design and placement of controls in the work area.

Similar isometric strength profiles were determined for push-up and pull-down exertions, based on eight male and eight female paraplegics. For the workstation design of paraplegics, tasks that require high exertions should be placed close to the body with the lower arm angled toward the sagittal plane. Pull-down exertions should be used in preference to push-up exertions wherever practical. Gender ought to be considered when designing jobs or workstations.

Acknowledgments

The contributions made by Dr. John Kozey, Ms. Nancy Black, and Mr. Martin Forde are duly acknowledged in the preparation of this chapter. The research was funded by the Canada Employment and Immigration and the Rick Hanson Man in Motion Legacy Fund. The assistance of the Canadian Paraplegic Association is appreciated.

References

Abdel-Moty, E., & Khalil, T.M. (1989). Computer-aided design and analysis of the sitting workplace for the disabled. In A. Mital (Ed.), *Advances in industrial ergonomics and safety I* (pp. 863–870). London: Taylor & Francis.

Black, N. (1994). *Isometric strength in the workspace reach envelopes of paraplegics,* master's thesis, Department of Industrial Engineering, Technical University of Nova Scotia, Halifax.

Buchanan, L.E., & Nawoczenski, S.A. (1987). *Spinal cord injury: Concepts and management approaches.* Baltimore: Williams & Wilkins.

Canadian Standards Association. (1990). *Barrier free design, a national standard of Canada.* (CSA-B651-M90). Toronto.

Chaffin, D.B., & Park, K.S. (1973). A longitudinal study of low-back pain as associated with occupational weight lifting factors. *American Industrial Hygiene Association Journal, 34,* 513–525.

Corlett, E.N., Bowssenna, M., & Pheasant, S.T. (1992). Is discomfort related to the postural loading of the joints? *Ergonomics, 25,* 315–322.

Das, B., & Behara, D. (1995). Determination of the normal horizontal working area: A new model and method. *Ergonomics, 38,* 734–748.

Das, B., & Grady, R.M. (1983). Industrial workplace layout design: An application of engineering anthropometry. *Ergonomics, 25,* 433–447.

Davis, P.R., & Stubbs, D.A. (1977). Safe levels of manual forces for young males (1). *Applied Ergonomics, 8(3),* 141–150.

Farley, R.R. (1955). Some principles of methods and motion study as used in development work. *General Motors Engineering Journal,* D2-90549, 1–46.

Floyd, W.F., Guttmann, L., Wycliffe-Noble, C., et al. (1966). A study of the space requirements of wheelchair users. *Paraplegia, 5,* 24–37.

Forde, M. (1995). Isometric push-up and pull-down strength in workspace reach envelopes of paraplegics. Unpublished master's thesis, Department of Industrial Engineering, Technical University of Nova Scotia, Halifax.

Hertzberg, H.T.E. (1972). Engineering anthropology. In H.P. VanCott, & R.G. Kincade (Eds.), *Human engineering guide to equipment design* (pp. 467–584) (rev. ed.). New York: McGraw-Hill, Chapter 11.

Hunsicker, P.A. (1955). *Arm strength at selected degrees of elbow flexion* (Technical Report, 54–548). Washington, DC: U.S. Air Force.

Keyserling, W.M., Herrin, G.D., & Chaffin, D.B. (1980). Isometric strength testing as a means of controlling medical incidents on strenuous jobs. *Journal of Occupational Medicine, 22,* 332–336.

Kozey, J., & Das, B. (1992). An evaluation of existing anthropometric measurements of wheelchair mobile individuals. *Proceedings of the Annual Human Factors Association of Canada Meeting,* Hamilton, Ontario.

Kroemer, K. (1983). An isoinertial technique to assess individual lifting capability. *Human Factors, 25,* 493–506.

Kumar, S. (1991). Arm lift strength in work space. *Applied Ergonomics, 22,* 317–328.

Mital, A., & Faard, H. (1990). Effects of sitting and standing, reach distance and arm orientation on isokinetic pull strengths in the horizontal plane. *International Journal of Industrial Ergonomics, 6,* 241–248.

National Institute of Occupational Safety and Health. (1981). *Work practices guide for manual lifting.* Cincinnati, OH: U.S. Department of Heath and Human Services.

Nowak, E. (1989). Workspace for disabled people. *Ergonomics, 3,* 1077–1088.

Pheasant, S. (1986). *Bodyspace: Anthropometry, ergonomics and design.* London: Taylor & Francis.

Squires, P.C. (1956). *The shape of the normal working area.* Report No. 275. New London, CT: U.S. Navy Department, Bureau of Medicine and Surgery, Medical Research Laboratories.

Tichauer, E.R. (1975). *Occupational biomechanics: The anatomical basis of work-place design* (Rehabilitation Monograph No. 5). New York: New York University Medical Center, Institute of Rehabilitation Medicine.

Chapter 9

Gerontology Case Study: Designing a Computer-Based Communication System for Older Adults

Sara J. Czaja

Learning Objectives

On completion of this chapter, the reader should

- Be familiar with the employment of user characteristics in systems design.
- Understand how to use an ergonomic process to identify population characteristics, design a system to accommodate a particular population, implement the design, and evaluate the effectiveness of the system design.

Key Words

Aging
Cognition
Human-computer interaction
E-mail

Abstract

Computer technology offers the potential for improving the quality of life of older adults by providing links to information and services outside of the home. For example, networks such as the Internet allow users to engage in activities such as shopping; access informational databases on a myriad of topics; and communicate with others across a broad geographic region. For these types of applications to be beneficial to older people, systems must be designed to accommodate their needs and abilities.

This chapter discusses a study concerned with designing an electronic message system for older adults. The focus of the chapter is demonstrating how the needs and characteristics of users can be accommodated in system design.

Introduction

Current demographic trends underscore the need to identify strategies that enhance the ability of older people to live independent and productive lives. By the year 2030, people aged 65 and older will represent 22% of the population, an increase of almost 10% since 1990 (U.S. Senate Subcommittee, 1991). The greatest growth rate will occur among people aged 75 and older. For example, by the year 2005, it is anticipated that there will be a 20% growth rate among people over the age of 85 (R. Barr, personal communication, 1996). Thus, there will be vast numbers of older people living in the United States.

Although most older people live active and relatively healthy lives, increased age is typically associated with declines in functional capacity and a propensity to disability through accidents and disease. These impairments can curtail the independence of older people and threaten their ability to live in the community. Currently an estimated 2.8 million older people need some type of help in performing everyday activities, and approximately 5% reside in institutional settings (Office of Technology Assessment, 1985). As the elderly population increases, with people living longer, larger numbers of people will require help. This is significant given the escalating costs of support services and long-term care. An important challenge facing society is the development of systems and interventions that allow older people to live healthy and independent lives. This challenge is particularly compelling for human factors engineers as the focus of the discipline is on designing systems to fit user groups.

It is generally recognized that computer technology offers the potential of improving the quality of life for older people by providing access to information and services (Czaja, 1996). Computer network services can be used to engage in activities such as banking and shopping. Older adults commonly report problems with these types of activities because of transportation problems, restricted mobility, and fear of crime (Nair, 1989). Computers can also be used to increase access to health care services. For example, Holmes, Teresi, and Holmes (1990) demonstrated that computer systems can facilitate interactions between patients and clinicians.

Computers placed in the home can also be used to expand educational, recreational, and communication opportunities for older adults. Large numbers of older people, especially older women, live alone, and many report problems with social isolation, boredom, and loneliness. Software is available for providing instruction in a wide variety of topics, and users are able to access a myriad of databases. Electronic networks also make it easier to maintain ties to family and friends, especially those in a different locale, as well as to form new friendships. SeniorNet, a computer network for seniors, currently has more than 17,000 members and 70 learning sites (SeniorNet, 1995). Finally, computers can be used to augment memory functioning (including reminders of appointments and medication schedules) and to enhance safety and security.

To ensure that the potential benefits of computer technology are realized by older adults, computer systems must be designed so that they are useful to, and useable by, older populations. In other words, the needs and characteristics of older adults must be considered in the design and implementation of computer systems. According to Gould (1988), this requires knowing users and their tasks and actively involving users in the system design process. Current data suggest that older adults are not commonly perceived as active users of technology and are thus overlooked in the design process. A number of studies have shown that although older people are recep-

tive to using technology (Czaja et al., 1989; Jay & Willis, 1992; Dyck & Smither, 1994), they often have more difficulty than younger people acquiring computer skills (Elias et al., 1987; Charness, Schuman, & Boritz, 1992; Czaja et al., 1989) and using computer systems (Frydenberg, 1988; Czaja & Sharit, 1993). Unless the needs of older people are considered in the design and development of technological systems, they are likely to be at a disadvantage in today's complex, technologically rich society.

This chapter presents a study concerned with the design and evaluation of an electronic message system. The goals of the study were to assess the willingness and ability of older adults to use this type of system and to gather information regarding design parameters that enhance system usability for this population. The study was done in collaboration with Bellcore (Bell Communications Research, Morristown, NJ). The intent of this chapter is to demonstrate how the needs and characteristics of user groups, in this case the elderly, can be incorporated in the design of products and systems. The chapter begins with an overview of age-related changes in functional abilities as understanding the characteristics of users is fundamental to successful design. The emphasis is on perceptual and cognitive processes, because these processes were the most relevant to the current study. This is followed by a discussion of the methodology, results, and conclusions. (For a detailed discussion of the results refer to Czaja et al., 1993.)

Age-Related Changes in Perceptual and Cognitive Abilities

As noted by Gould (1988), one of the key features of enhancing system usability is understanding the needs and characteristics of user populations. There are a number of age-related changes in functional abilities that have relevance to the design of computer systems. This section highlights some of these changes. There are many excellent sources of more detailed discussions of these topics (including Birren & Schaie, 1990; Charness, 1985).

Changes in Visual Perception

Age-related changes in visual functioning are important considerations when designing computer systems. Aging is associated with reductions in light sensitivity, color perceptions, resistance to glare, dynamic and static acuity, contrast sensitivity, visual search, and pattern recognition (Kosnik et al., 1988). These changes have an impact on the ability of older people to perform tasks such as reading, driving, and locating targets. For example, survey data collected from a sample of community-dwelling adults, ranging in age from 18 to 100, indicated that older adults had more difficulty than younger adults performing a variety of everyday visual activities. Specifically, they had more trouble with glare, low levels of illumination, and near-vision tasks (such as reading small print). They also reported more problems locating targets amid visual clutter and tracking and processing moving targets, and they need more time to process visual information (Kosnik et al., 1988).

These findings indicate that design of computer screens and keyboards needs special consideration to ensure that older people are able to see and read screen information and identify characters and labels on keyboards. For example, consideration of character size and contrast is especially important for older computer users. Also, as findings from our research indicate, it is also important that keys are easily identifiable and distinguishable.

Changes in Cognition

Age-related changes in cognition also have relevance to the design of computer systems. Aging is generally associated with declines in most component processes of cognition. As summarized by Park (1992), processes that decline with age include attentional processes, working memory capabilities, discourse comprehension, inference formation and interpretation, encoding and retrieval processes in memory and information processing speed. The decline in processing speed is especially significant because reductions in processing speed are believed to contribute to age differences in cognitive performance. Consequently, losses in processing speed not only limit the speed at which older people are able to respond, but also the performance of other cognitive operations that are important to performance of tasks.

Decrements in these component abilities could place older people at a disadvantage in the performance of computer tasks, which are primarily char-

acterized by their information processing demands. For example, one of the primary characteristics of computer tasks is the high demand placed on working memory. Users must learn new concepts and how to attach new meaning to familiar concepts (e.g., *file* and *folder*). They must also learn a new lexicon (Hockey et al., 1989). This case study will demonstrate that these demands often prove difficult for older people.

Age-related changes in attentional and perceptual processes and problem-solving skills may also influence the ability of older people to perform computer tasks. Older adults often have difficulty processing complex, confusing, or inconsistent information and are more likely to experience interference from irrelevant or surplus information (Plude & Hoyer, 1985). These changes in abilities are relevant to the design of interfaces. For example, highlighting significant information and grouping related information is especially important for older people. Also, screen clutter should be kept to a minimum, and incompatibility and inconsistencies within and across applications should be avoided. Finally, the need to memorize commands and complex operating procedures should be kept to a minimum.

In essence, to design computer systems that can be used successfully by older people, it is important to understand the skills and abilities of this user group—they are likely to be different from those of younger computer users. Further it is important to understand the importance to performance of computer tasks of age-related changes in abilities, so that effective design interventions can be identified. The following sections describe a case study in which an effort was made to understand the impact of aging on the performance of a computer task, and an attempt was made to compensate for age effects with modifications in system design. The study represents an example of a user-centered design process for a special population.

Methodology

The methodology adopted for the project was based on a user-centered design approach. The ultimate objective of this approach is to incorporate human issues into the design and development process. The emphasis is on building a system to support users and their tasks. The approach typically involves some form of iterative design during which an analysis of the system is conducted by user groups and evaluators, a product or process is designed according to this analysis, and testing and evaluation (both subjective and objective) of the effectiveness of the product or process is completed. The process is continued until an optimal design is achieved. A key feature of the approach is user involvement in the design and evaluation of a system.

For this project the system analysis was conducted in two phases: laboratory testing and field testing. During laboratory testing, data were collected on user likes, dislikes, and performance problems. The results of this analysis were used to modify the system, and this modified system was then installed in the field. The field testing involved installing the system in the participants' homes for a period of 13 months. The duration of the project was 24 months.

Phase 1: Laboratory Testing

The objective of this phase was to gather some preliminary information on the usability of the system and to identify design problems.

Sample

The sample included 40 women aged 50–95 (mean, 68.2 years) who lived independently in the South Florida community. Half of the participants lived alone, and half lived with a spouse or with somebody else. All of the participants had at least a high school education and the majority (80%) had no prior experience with a computer. Most of the participants (64%) were unemployed, 21% were employed full-time, and 15% worked part-time.

Given that computer tasks involve reading information from screens all participants were required to have at least 20/40 vision, with or without correction. Further, they were required to demonstrate that they were able to use a keyboard. Five of the sample reported that they had some problems with finger dexterity.

System Description

The computer system used in the study was equivalent to a customized personal computer running on a UNIX-based operating system. The hardware consisted of a 15-in. monochrome monitor, keyboard, printer, and modem. For this phase of the project, two systems were set up in the laboratory of the research institute (the Stein Gerontological Institute) in individual cubicles. During the field test, the computer systems were linked to a host computer at the laboratory: a Compaq 386/20 computer, operating a XENIX system that provided multiuser access.

The software, developed by Bellcore, was referred to as "POMS" (Plain Old Message System). Initially it was equipped with a simplified form of e-mail and a simple text editor. As will be discussed, several features were added to the system over the course of the project. The software was designed specifically for people who had limited computer expertise. Thus it was designed so that it was easy to use: Operating commands were minimal and consistent across applications. The system allowed users to send and receive e-mail without needing to log onto a computer, access a program, or perform a series of complex operating commands. Messages were entered into the system via a keyboard and displayed on the screen while they were being created. To send a message the participant simply typed the name of the message recipient after the "To" prompt on the screen. He or she then typed the message and pressed the "return" key to send the message. Messages were received on hard copy via a printer.

System Analysis

As stated, the initial analysis took place in the laboratory. Individuals participated in pairs as they needed to perform a communication task. They were requested to come to the training with a partner, someone with whom they communicated on a regular basis and who would be willing to participate in the project. This was to ensure that some communication would take place when the system was initially installed in the field. Nine of the participants came with partners; the remaining 12 participants were paired into six groups of two. Before interacting with the system, participants were asked to complete a demographic data sheet and a computer attitude questionnaire.

Participants were then provided with an explanation of e-mail and the POMS system. They were introduced to the computer hardware and given practice using the keyboard. They were trained until they demonstrated they could send a message using POMS (in no case was more than 30 minutes of training required).

To evaluate the ability of the participants to use the system, they were asked to complete a series of performance tasks. Specifically each participant was requested to send five messages to the other person and the other person was required to respond to these messages. The messages were to be in the form of a question to stimulate communication and were related to the following topics: hobbies, family, pets, living arrangements, and exercise. The process was then reversed and the message topics were employment, vacation plans, entertainment, politics, and weather. Participants were given a written instruction sheet for the tasks and were observed by a research assistant using a standard observation form. The observational data was used as part of the initial system analysis.

After completion of the communication tasks the participants were asked to complete the computer attitude questionnaire a second time. They were also interviewed regarding their initial impressions of the system and their willingness to use the system once it was placed in their home.

Results and Design Implications

The observational data indicated that the system was relatively easy to learn and use. Of the sample group, 36% required no help during the performance of the communication tasks; 30% ($n = 12$) of the participants required a moderate amount of help; only 10% ($n = 4$) required substantial help during task performance. The most frequent type of help involved reviewing the command procedures and providing information regarding operation of the system. The most frequent questions asked by the participants during training were related to command procedures (e.g., "Do I press this now?"), and the location of specific keys (e.g., "Where is the comma?").

With respect to problems using the system, the most frequently observed problem related to remembering the operating procedures, and most of these problems were related to the need to use the "return" key to input a name into the system. Participants also had problems using the editor to correct mistakes. However, it should be noted that these problems were primarily evident when the participants were initially interacting with the sys-

Table 9-1. Participants' Responses to the Postevaluation Interview

Liked using the electronic message system	100%
Would use a computer if they had one at home	97%
Would like to learn more about computers	97%
Perceived of e-mail as useful	100%
Had difficulty remembering procedures	28%
Had difficulty using the keys on the keyboard	22%
Had difficulty using the keyboard in general	6%
Had difficulty reading the screen	3%
Had difficulty correcting mistakes	28%
Had difficulty using the function keys	23%

tem. They lessened substantially with extended practice. Additional problems related to use of the keyboard, such as difficulty locating keys and using wrong keys.

As shown in Table 9-1, the participants' responses to the interview data were extremely positive. All of the participants indicated that they enjoyed using e-mail and perceived e-mail as useful. Most people indicated they would use a home computer and were interested in learning more about computers. Also, most of the participants found the system easy to learn. They did offer some specific comments on aspects of the system they found difficult. For example, they reported some problems using the arrow keys and using the "return" and "delete" keys. An interesting finding was that the attitudes of the participants toward computer technology became significantly more positive following their interaction with the system. This was an important finding as user attitudes toward technology have an impact on their willingness to use the technology.

On the basis of the observational and interview data several changes were made to the system, including the following:

1. The number keypad and the unused function keys were deactivated to minimize confusion and lessen the opportunity for error.
2. The "caps lock" key was deactivated because it was frequently engaged unknowingly and caused confusion and frustration among the participants.
3. The labels on the unused function keys and numeric keypad were covered to further minimize confusion between used and unused keys.

4. An on-screen prompt was added to remind the participants what to do after the "To" prompt appeared on the screen. This was done to further reduce the requirements for remembering commands.
5. Selection of an alternative printer. The first printer was quiet and several participants commented that they were unable to hear it and thus were unaware that they were receiving a message.
6. The system capabilities were expanded so that the participants could send a message to everyone at once.

Phase 2: Field Testing the System

Sample

The group used for the field test was the same as that for the lab evaluation. However, the sample was reduced from 40 to 36 participants; one participant moved, two became ill, and one decided that she no longer wanted to participate. The geographic range of the sample encompassed both Dade and Broward counties.

System Analysis

As stated, a system was installed on a separate phone line, in each participant's home. Each system was linked to a host system at the lab so that continuous data could be recorded. The system was installed for a period of 13 months.

At the time of installation, all participants were provided with a review of the operating procedures. They were then asked to use the system to send a message to lab staff and to reply to a message from the staff to ensure that they were able to use the system. They were provided with a cue card and they had access to a "hot line" in case of any problems with system operation. Research assistants would attempt to solve these problems over the phone. If this was not possible, home visits would be made. As expected, the number of help requests declined substantially over the course of the project. Many of the problems were related to replacing the paper in the printer.

The system was restricted to e-mail during the first few months after installation. However, other features were added to the system during the course of the project. These features included news, weather information, health information, movie reviews, and horoscopes. The health feature provided information on health-related topics, such as nutrition. For a while, games and community events features were added to the system; however, they were discontinued because they were not used frequently. These applications were developed and maintained by research staff, so it was not considered to be cost-effective to leave them on the system.

Test and Evaluation

Once the system was installed, participants were encouraged to send messages as often as possible. They were provided with a list of the other participants. Initially the lab staff would send regular messages to the participants to ensure that they would become familiar with system and sending messages. After the initial 2 weeks, however, staff members only sent messages if they received one from a participant, or a participant had not sent a message in several days.

The operating procedures were consistent for all features. The participants simply typed the name of the feature they wished to access at the "To" prompt, instead of the name of the person. The features were added gradually, in an incremental fashion, and the participants received training each time a new feature was added to the system.

The participants were asked to complete a system evaluation questionnaire at month 6 of the data collection period and at the end of data collection. The questionnaire assessed perceptions of the system, likes, dislikes, problems, and applications.

The objective performance data included number and types of errors made by users, time spent on the system (overall and per message), frequency of use, patterns of use (e.g., time of day), applications used, and communications patterns. Subjective data included responses to a system evaluation questionnaire. The questionnaire assessed likes, dislikes, problems, and preferences of the users.

Results and Design Implications

Overall, the performance data, which were analyzed over the 13 months, indicated the system was easy to use. The participants committed relatively few

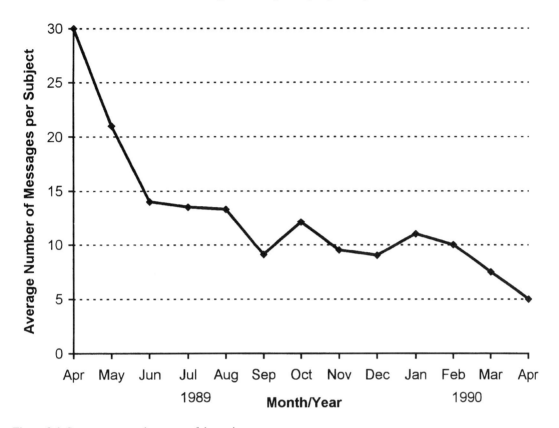

Figure 9-1. System use over the course of the project.

errors per communication session (about two per session). It is interesting to note that the number of errors increased slightly when the new applications were added to the system; however, they declined as the participants became more familiar with the new features.

The most common error was misuse of the "return" key: Participants had difficulty remembering that this key was used to input an address into the system. Participants also confused the function of this key when typing a message and tended to use it to get to the next line, as one would when using a typewriter. In fact, these errors were more common among the better typists. The problems with the "return" key occurred despite provision of the on-screen cue regarding the function of this key. These findings are consistent with the literature on aging and cognition regarding age-related declines in working memory, and ability to modify existing, well-learned concepts. They also point to the need to stress, during training, the differences between the keys used in typ-

ing and those specific computer applications. In addition the interface should be designed to minimize the confusion between typing and text editing.

The second most common error was confusion between the "send" and "cancel" keys. These two keys were in close proximity and identical in size and shape. The data indicated this error was more common among people of low visual acuity. This finding illustrates the importance of clearly differentiating keys through labeling and use of color, size, and shape as codes. This is especially important for older adults given the decline in visual acuity that occurs with age.

As shown in Figure 9-1, use of the system declined over the course of the project. This decline can be attributed in part to a novelty effect—the participants would use a new application frequently on its introduction, but use it less and less as they became familiar with it. Other reasons for decline in use of the system reported by the participants included boredom (due to the limited number of applications on the system), the restricted communication pool, system breakdowns, and being "too busy." People who were unemployed used the system more frequently than those who worked. This suggests that the computer is especially beneficial for people who spend considerable time at home. The findings also suggest that it is important for a system to be equipped with applications that are perceived to be useful by the intended population.

With respect to usage of applications, the data indicated that e-mail, weather information, and health information were the applications most frequently used. When queried regarding the types of applications they would like added to the system, the participants indicated that they would like access to word processing, physician and emergency services, and continuing-education programs. In fact, several of the participants used the system as a word processor by sending e-mail to themselves. Other applications frequently requested were shopping/banking, checkbook balancing, news and weather, and the ability to create personal databases. Interestingly, all of the applications requested were practical in nature rather than concerned with entertainment. As noted, the games feature that was added to the system was removed during the course of the project because it was underused.

When asked what they liked and disliked about the system at the end of the project period, the participants indicated they liked using the system because it allowed them to communicate with others and was interesting and stimulating as well as easy to use. Reasons for using the computer included socialization, the chance to meet new people, the opportunity to learn something new, and experiencing a mental challenge. Consistent with these results, one of the primary dislikes was that the system was too restricted and not challenging enough. Throughout the period of the project the participants constantly requested that new applications be added to the system. The participants also disliked the fact that the system proved vulnerable to breakdowns and that it was sometimes difficult to use the printer.

Overall, 100% of the participants indicated that they found it valuable to have a computer in their home and that they would miss using the system when it was removed (due to cost constraints the systems were only installed for the duration of the project). The majority of the participants (95%)

stated the system was easy to use and that they enjoyed using the system.

In sum, the results indicated that the participants were able to successfully use the system and that the system provided a means for forming and maintaining social contacts and an opportunity to make their discretionary time more meaningful. In fact, the participants produced a cookbook using the system, and organized two luncheons so they could meet one another. These results support the conjecture that home computers can provide older people with a link to the outside world.

Conclusions

The findings from this case study indicate that computers can be used to increase the independence and quality of life of older adults, especially those who live alone or who have restricted mobility. The benefits of this technology could be far reaching given that most older adults live at home, the majority alone. Computer systems can link people to services and information, enhance their safety and security, facilitate social interaction, and provide mental stimulation.

The results also indicate that home computers are feasible for older adults. The participants in our study were both willing and able to operate the computer system. Moreover, they reported that they enjoyed using the system and found it valuable.

Importantly, the study demonstrated the value of the user-centered design approach and underscores the importance of understanding the needs and capabilities of user populations and including the user in the design process. Although the initial system developed for the study was considered by the design team to be easy to use, the participants still had difficulty with certain commands and procedures. The data from the laboratory and field testing identified specific types of problems and difficulties encountered by users; these provided insight into design improvements. The data also indicated preferences of the users with respect to system applications. This type of information is important. The results demonstrated that one of the primary reasons for decreased use of the system was the limited number of applications.

Specifically, our findings show that for computer systems to be easy for older adults to use, operating procedures should be simple and consistent across applications. Further, there should be minimal demands on memory, and complex commands should be avoided. Users should also be provided with a supportive environment and have easy access to help when they experience problems. Additionally, users should be provided with adequate training and support documentation.

Hardware considerations are also important. For example, keys must be clearly labeled and differentiated. As discussed, our subjects commonly confused the "send" and "cancel" keys, which were in close proximity to one another and similar in appearance. Input devices other than a standard keyboard should also be considered. Speech technology or pen-based systems might be particularly useful for this population. In addition, the characters on the screen should be visible and target information such as error messages should be highlighted. Stability of system operation is another important design requirement; one of the most common complaints among our participants was that the system frequently broke down.

Finally, the system should be equipped with practical applications. The data from our study suggest that, in addition to e-mail, these might include word processing, news and weather information, continuing education programs, and health-related information. Older people are unlikely to invest time or money in computer technology unless they perceive it to be beneficial and useful. Gitlin (1995) examined factors influencing the willingness of older adults to use assistive technology. She found that the decision to accept or reject technology is determined by a complex interaction of factors. These factors include human factors such as perceived need; environmental factors such as the physical design of the environment and demands of a task; sociocultural factors such as societal perceptions regarding the use of devices and the design of the device in terms of ease of use, aesthetics, quality, and durability.

The results of this study suggest some general guidelines that can be used to accommodate older people in the design of computer systems. Many questions are still unanswered. For example, issues regarding interface style and input devices are largely unexplored. It is hoped that this chapter will serve to motivate researchers and designers to consider older adults as potential users of products and systems. It is also hoped that the chapter illustrates the importance of involving the user in the design process.

References

Birren, J.E., & Schaie, K.W. (1990). *Handbook of the psychology of aging* (3rd ed.). New York: Academic Press.

Charness, N. (1985). *Aging and human performance*. New York: John Wiley & Sons.

Charness, N., Schuman, C.E., & Boritz, G.A. (1992). Training older adults in word processing: Effects of age, training technique and computer anxiety. *International Journal of Aging and Technology, 5,* 79–106.

Czaja, S.J. (1996). The implications of computer technology for older adults. In W.A. Rodgers, A.D. Fisk, & N. Walker (Eds.), *Aging and skilled performance: Advances in theory and applications* (pp. 201–220). Hillsdale, NJ: Lawrence Erlbaum.

Czaja, S.J., Guerrier, J., Nair, S., & Landauer, T. (1993). Computer communication as an aid to independence for older adults. *Behavior and Information Technology, 12,* 197–207.

Czaja, S.J., Hammond, K., Blascovich, J., & Swede, H. (1989). Age-related differences in learning to use a text-editing system. *Behavior and Information Technology, 8,* 309–319.

Czaja, S.J., & Sharit, J. (1993). Age differences in the performance of computer-interactive tasks. *Psychology and Aging, 8,* 59–67.

Dyck, J.L., & Smither, J.A. (1994). Age differences in computer anxiety: The role of computer experience, gender and education. *Journal of Educational Computing Research, 10,* 239–247.

Elias, P.K., Elias, H.F., Robbins, M.A., & Gage, P. (1987). Acquisition of word processing skills by younger, middle-aged, and older adults. *Psychology and Aging, 2,* 340–348.

Frydenberg, H. (1988). Computers: Specialized applications for the older person. *American Behavioral Scientist, 31,* 595–600.

Gitlin, L.N. (1995). Why older people accept or reject assistive technology. *Generations, 19,* 41–46.

Gould, J. (1988). How to design usable systems. In M.E. Helander (Ed.), *Handbook of human computer interaction* (pp. 757–790). Amsterdam: North-Holland.

Hockey, G.R., Briner, R.B., Tattersall, A.J., & Wiethoff, M. (1989). Assessing the impact of computer workload on operator stress: The role of system controllability. *Ergonomics, 32,* 1401–1418.

Holmes, D., Teresi, J., & Holmes, M. (1990). Computer applications in health care planning and practice. *International Journal of Technology and Aging, 3,* 69–78.

Jay, G.M., & Willis, S.L. (1992). Influence of direct computer experience on older adults attitudes toward computers. *Journal of Gerontology: Psychological Sciences, 47,* 250–257.

Kosnik, W., Winslow, L., Kline, D., et al. (1988). Visual changes in daily life through adulthood. *Journal of Gerontology: Psychological Sciences, 43,* 63–70.

Nair, S. (1989). A capability-demand analysis of grocery shopping problems encountered by older adults. Unpublished master's thesis, Department of Industrial Engineering, State University of New York at Buffalo.

Office of Technology Assessment. (1985, June). *Technology and aging in America* (OTA-BA-264). Washington, DC: U.S. Congress, Office of Technology Assessment.

Park, D. (1992). Applied cognitive research. In F.I.M. Craik, & T.A. Salthouse (Eds.), *The handbook of aging and cognition* (pp. 449–494). Hillsdale, NJ: Lawrence Erlbaum.

Plude, D.J., & Hoyer, W.J. (1985). Attention and performance: Identifying and localizing age deficits. In N. Charness (Ed.), *Aging and human performance* (pp. 47–99). New York: John Wiley & Sons.

SeniorNet. (1995). Welcome to SeniorNet: Introductory brochure. California: Author.

U.S. Senate Subcommittee on Aging, American Association of Retired Persons, Federal Council on Aging, and U.S. Administration on Aging. (1991). *Aging America: Trends and projections.* (FCoA)91-28001. Washington, DC: U.S. Department of Health and Human Services.

Section IV

Industrial Intervention: Musculoskeletal Ergonomics

Chapter 10

Musculoskeletal Ergonomics: An Introduction

Mary S. Lopez

Learning Objectives

On completion of this chapter, the reader should be able to

- Identify the critical elements of an ergonomics program.
- Identify the various types of analyses and surveillance approaches and the appropriate situations for each assessment method.
- Identify the three basic types of ergonomic controls, the basic ergonomic principles that provide a foundation for design solutions, and some basic workstation and task solutions.
- Identify the components of complete medical management.
- Identify general criteria to evaluate each of the program elements and to assess overall program performance.

Key Words

Musculoskeletal ergonomics
Program elements
Program management

Abstract

This chapter provides an overview of the important components of an ergonomic program designed to prevent work-related musculoskeletal disorders (WRMDs) and comply with the Occupational Safety and Health Act (OSHA) ergonomic guidelines (OSHA, 1991, 1995). Components of an ergonomic program include management commitment, analysis of the work site and problem areas (passive and active surveillance), program design issues to manage and alleviate risk factors (controls, medical management, and education and training), and evaluation of program effectiveness. Each area is described in detail, and suggestions for maximizing effectiveness of each element, as well as the program as a whole, are provided. As an additional resource, see the chapter appendix for guiding principles for implement solutions for poor designs, thus reducing risk factors.

Introduction

"How much longer will this take?" he thought as he bent down to pick up another box. They had been working at full speed now for 4 hours. The shipment was much larger than they had expected and everything had to be inventoried, processed, and locked in the special storage containers before they could go home. "That old football injury," he thought again as he felt a nagging and persistent pain in his back. He had been fine for years, but tonight was different. He kept working. Everyone knew how important this shipment was. The company had been struggling to survive, and there had been talk of layoffs. He couldn't afford that. Bills were piling up. The only way he could make ends meet now was to work as much overtime as possible. He looked up again. At least 40 more boxes. It would be after 10 PM before he could get home. "Missed dinner again," he thought as he bent down once more.

The pain kept him awake all night. He could barely get out of bed in the morning. And his leg didn't feel right. He started to worry.

The company doctor sent him to a specialist. "Herniated disk" was all they told him. Off work for 2 weeks. But the leg still felt strange, and he even had trouble sitting in a chair. Surgery. More time off. Physical therapy helped a little, but he would never be able to work at the plant again. When the doctor mentioned "light duty," his boss had just rolled his eyes. He knew it. He was out of options. Permanent disability.

What happened here? This scene has been repeated countless times in U.S. industry. Employees work beyond their capacity, with poor job design, poor workstation design, and poor tool design, which can combine to result in a crippling disability.

But is there a problem warranting national concern? In recent years ergonomics has become a much debated political and economic issue. OSHA has issued citations and fines against business for ergonomic deficiencies under the General Duty Clause (Current Report: Renewed Fight, 1996). OSHA has also published a draft Ergonomic Protection Standard (OSHA, 1995) (patterned after the guidelines for meatpacking plants [OSHA, 1991]), which has met significant opposition from Congress and many businesses (Current Report: Gingrich Urged, 1996). Businesses are concerned about the potentially severe costs of complying with the standard. Ergonomics is often a case of "pay now or pay much more later," and many businesses are choosing to postpone payment, taking the gamble that "later" will never come. Some businesses (Grant & Habes, 1995) have implemented successful ergonomic programs with impressive reductions in workers' compensation payments and lost work time. Preventing WRMDs makes good business sense. The production-related costs of an injured worker far outweigh the medical costs. The business must deal with decreased output, replacement costs, retraining, increased errors, and increased demand on the rest of the work force.

Despite the political and economic arguments for and against ergonomics, injury and illness data indicate trends that cannot be ignored. WRMDs include upper-extremity (UE), neck, back, and leg conditions. Conditions directly related to the workplace account for a significant portion of the injuries and illnesses reported to the Department of Labor (DOL). Sprains and strains accounted for nearly 1 million (44%) of the 2.3 million injuries

and illnesses resulting in lost work time in 1993 (Bureau of Labor Statistics, 1994). Of these sprains and strains, 40% involved the back and other portions of the trunk. Overexertion from lifting, pulling, or pushing heavy objects caused 3 of every 10 workers' compensation cases. Of all cases, 60% required 1–10 days of recuperation and, on average, there were 6 lost workdays per case. Smith (1995) reported that a Liberty Mutual analysis of workers' compensation claims and costs found that back pain accounts for 16% of all workers' compensation claims and 33% of all costs.

Although UE WRMDs have received considerable attention, they represent only 0.83% of all claims and 1.64% of all claims costs (Smith, 1995). Some of the confusion about the magnitude of the UE MSD problem is related to the coding procedures of the Bureau of Labor Statistics (BLS). Back conditions are coded as injuries, and UE WRMDs are coded as illnesses. The number of reported UE MSD illnesses has increased dramatically; however, they represent a relatively small portion of the overall injury and illness picture.

In 1993, the total compensable cost for U.S. businesses was $563 million for UE WRMDs and $11.4 billion for low back pain claims (Smith, 1995). Perhaps the most disconcerting statistic reported by Smith involved the disability rate from low back pain. The rate increased 14% faster than the growth of the population in 1993.

Why are we seeing this dramatic increase in WRMDs? This question has been debated by numerous experts and leaders in the field and remains an issue of contention. Several changes have occurred in the workplace over the past 15 years. Worker awareness has increased and DOL reporting requirements have changed; however, these factors do not account for all of the increase in WRMDs.

The workplace has become more specialized, automated, and production oriented. Companies have downsized and "right-sized" without changing the output demands. Time issues such as flextime, shift work, and the compressed work week have placed further physiologic demands on our work force. We are seeing the result of many years of deficiencies in the design of work and workstations.

The demographics of the work force are also changing. We have more women, minorities, immigrants, and older workers in the work force. The physical capacity of our work force is changing and, in some cases, declining, due to the "couch-potato" syndrome, the deconditioning occurring at the workplace, and the physical limitations related to gender and age.

Ergonomists and health care professionals are often assigned responsibility for the workplace ergonomics program. Workplace ergonomics programs generally have a twofold focus: modifying the workplace to meet the physical limitations of workers with existing conditions (individual case management) and preventing future work-related injuries and illnesses. This chapter is designed to provide the essential tools to design, implement, and maintain a company's ergonomics program and meet current and proposed OSHA ergonomics program requirements (OSHA, 1991, 1995). The chapter covers global program management and structure issues; analysis techniques, including passive and active surveillance; design approaches and solutions to common problems; and test and evaluation issues and methods, including solution-effectiveness assessment, program justification, and common management issues.

Critical Ergonomic Program Elements

Management Commitment

The most critical element in the prevention of WRMDs is management support and commitment to the ergonomics program. Applying ergonomics to the design of the workplace, jobs, tools, and the environment is good business practice. The goals of ergonomic design are improved production, product quality, and morale along with decreased costs associated with absenteeism, turnover, training, and replacement. The ergonomist must be able to communicate and demonstrate the benefits of the ergonomic approach to gain the necessary support and commitment of management. The final section of this chapter discusses the relevant management issues to address when testing and evaluating ergonomic interventions.

Team Approach: Participatory Ergonomics

Many companies use a team approach to ergonomics. Worker input is essential for well-designed and effective ergonomic solutions. The front-line workers know the job better than anyone else in the company and can address particular nuances of the job in developing solutions. In addition, worker participation improves worker "buy-in" and commitment to the solution (Gjessing, Schoenborn, & Cohen, 1994).

Teams should be small, consisting of workers, area supervisors, maintenance and engineering staff, medical staff, and the plant ergonomist. The teams should be trained to bring them to an acceptable level of ergonomic knowledge. Team-building training and periodic reinforcements are important elements for effective ergonomic teams. It is important to recognize that ergonomic team members will not become ergonomists or experts in the field; however, they will be empowered to recognize and eliminate risk factors. The teams must be allowed access to necessary management information such as the incidence of WRMDs by job series or work area so they can focus and prioritize their efforts. (A *job series* is defined as a particular classification of jobs grouped according to function and similar task demands, such as the designation *clerical workers*, which may include receptionists, data entry workers, etc.)

There needs to be a mechanism for team accountability, ergonomic project documentation and tracking, and communication with all plant employees. Finally, the team should be empowered to make ergonomic changes within specific budgetary constraints. The National Institute for Occupational Safety and Health (NIOSH) identified six critical issues in the team approach to ergonomics: management commitment, training, composition, information sharing, activities and motivation, and evaluation (Gjessing, Schoenborn, & Cohen, 1994).

Analysis

Surveillance

Organized, orderly, and guided analyses are key to successful ergonomics programs. Workplace surveillance identifies, records, and tracks WRMDs. Effective surveillance and subsequent intervention ultimately reduce and prevent WRMDs. As described by the Centers for Disease Control (CDC), surveillance is the "ongoing systematic collection, analysis and interpretation of health and exposure data in the process of describing and monitoring a health event. Surveillance data are used to determine the need for occupational safety and health action and to plan, implement and evaluate ergonomic interventions and programs" (CDC, 1988). The surveillance process includes both passive and active surveillance. These analyses target problem work areas, job series, and tasks for in-depth assessment and intervention.

A balanced workplace ergonomic analysis process has several simultaneously occurring "triggers" to identify potential ergonomic problem areas. These triggers involve both passive and active surveillance. The potential problems are then prioritized and targeted for further assessment and possible intervention. The further assessment may include use of a checklist or detailed assessments or some combination of these approaches. Figure 10-1 presents a diagram of the analysis process.

Passive Surveillance

Passive surveillance is the collection and analysis of data from existing records and data sources for trends or patterns of disease. Some of the best sources of data for trend analyses and the identification of work-related problems include the OSHA log, the plant's clinic records, workers' compensation records, insurance claims, and accident reports.

The data should be collected and analyzed routinely (e.g., quarterly), depending on the extent of the problem. Classifying the WRMD according to the current International Classification of Disease (ICD) is common and allows comparisons among jobs, plants, and industries (NIOSH, 1995b). Tables 10-1 and 10-2 list ICD-9 codes and diagnoses associated with musculoskeletal disorders and work-related conditions.

Incidence, severity, and prevalence rates should be calculated. These rates are calculated based on 100 worker-years per year. The rates should be calculated for all musculoskeletal disorders by body location for each department, job title, work area, or process to target specific problem areas or jobs.

Incidence (new case) rate (per 100 worker-years per year) =

$$\frac{New\ cases\ \text{during past 12 mos} \times 200{,}000\ \text{hrs}}{\text{Work hours during past 12 mos}}$$

Severity (lost work days) rate (per 100 worker-years per year) =

$$\frac{Lost\ work\ days\ \text{during past 12 mos} \times 200{,}000\ \text{hrs}}{\text{Work hours during past 12 mos}}$$

Prevalence (all cases during period) rate (per 100 worker-years per year) =

$$\frac{Total\ cases\ \text{in past 12 mos} \times 200{,}000\ \text{hrs}}{\text{Work hours during past 12 mos}}$$

If the specific number of work hours during the past 12 months is not available, multiply the number of full-time-equivalent employees in each area by 2,000 hours to obtain the denominator (NIOSH, 1995a).

Passive surveillance is limited by the quality of data put into the system. Data may be incomplete, inaccurate, or inconsistent. Data quality can be affected by management's attitudes, perceived or real disincentives to reporting, training provided to the personnel responsible for data input, differences in coding systems and in diagnoses assigned by medical practitioners. Under-reporting of conditions can be a serious problem. Many workers delay seeking medical care and reporting a condition until the condition has become functionally limiting.

Active Surveillance

Active surveillance involves actively seeking information to target and assess problematic workplaces, jobs, and tasks. Active surveillance allows greater sensitivity than passive surveillance. For example, active surveillance might identify symptoms that indicate early or developing WRMDs. Early intervention or prevention programs can be more focused and effective with active surveillance.

Worker Surveys and Questionnaires. Active surveillance can include worker surveys to obtain information on current and past symptoms, such as the duration, intensity, frequency, and anatomic location of symptoms. Worker surveys and questionnaires are generally easy and inexpensive to administer, provide a quick way to identify workers' perceptions of discomfort and the sources of discomfort, and identify problems that otherwise might go unreported. There are numerous worker surveys, questionnaires, and body part discomfort surveys available to the ergonomics team (ANSI, 1996; NIOSH, 1995a;

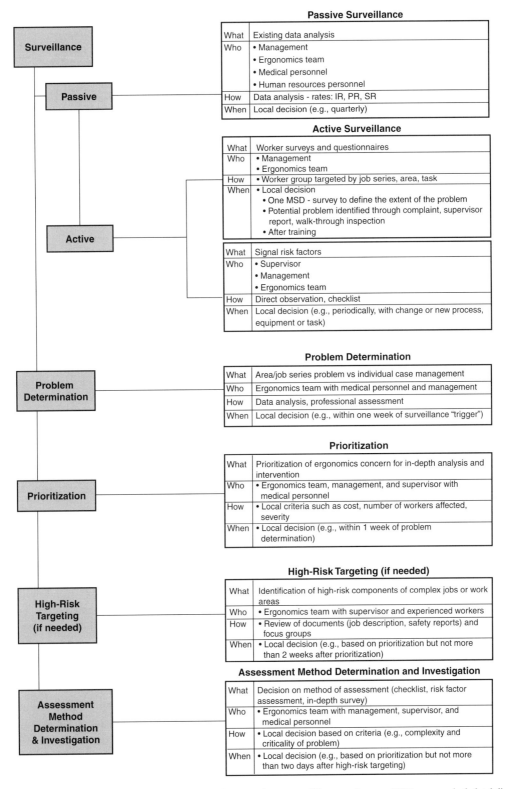

Passive Surveillance

What	Existing data analysis
Who	• Management
	• Ergonomics team
	• Medical personnel
	• Human resources personnel
How	Data analysis - rates: IR, PR, SR
When	Local decision (e.g., quarterly)

Active Surveillance

What	Worker surveys and questionnaires
Who	• Management
	• Ergonomics team
How	• Worker group targeted by job series, area, task
When	• Local decision
	• One MSD - survey to define the extent of the problem
	• Potential problem identified through complaint, supervisor report, walk-through inspection
	• After training

What	Signal risk factors
Who	• Supervisor
	• Management
	• Ergonomics team
How	Direct observation, checklist
When	Local decision (e.g., periodically, with change or new process, equipment or task)

Problem Determination

What	Area/job series problem vs individual case management
Who	Ergonomics team with medical personnel and management
How	Data analysis, professional assessment
When	Local decision (e.g., within one week of surveillance "trigger")

Prioritization

What	Prioritization of ergonomics concern for in-depth analysis and intervention
Who	• Ergonomics team, management, and supervisor with medical personnel
How	• Local criteria such as cost, number of workers affected, severity
When	• Local decision (e.g., within 1 week of problem determination)

High-Risk Targeting (if needed)

What	Identification of high-risk components of complex jobs or work areas
Who	• Ergonomics team with supervisor and experienced workers
How	• Review of documents (job description, safety reports) and focus groups
When	• Local decision (e.g., based on prioritization but not more than 2 weeks after prioritization)

Assessment Method Determination and Investigation

What	Decision on method of assessment (checklist, risk factor assessment, in-depth survey)
Who	• Ergonomics team with management, supervisor, and medical personnel
How	• Local decision based on criteria (e.g., complexity and criticality of problem)
When	• Local decision (e.g., based on prioritization but not more than two days after high-risk targeting)

Figure 10-1. Analysis process. (IR = incidence rate; PR = prevalence rate; SR = severity rate; MSD = musculoskeletal disorder.)

Table 10-1. ICD-9 Codes Associated with Back, Neck, and Lower Extremity Conditions

Code	Condition
333.83	Spasmodic torticollis
720.0	Ankylosing spondylitis
720.1	Spinal enthesopathy
720.2	Sacroiliitis, not elsewhere classified
720.8	Other inflammatory spondylopathies
720.9	Unspecified inflammatory spondylopathy
721.0	Cervical spondylosis without myelopathy
721.1	Cervical spondylosis with myelopathy
721.2	Thoracic spondylosis without myelopathy
721.3	Lumbosacral spondylosis without myelopathy
721.4	Thoracic or lumbar spondylosis with myelopathy
721.5	Kissing spine
721.6	Ankylosing vertebral hyperostosis
721.7	Traumatic spondylopathy
721.8	Other allied disorders of spine
721.9	Spondylosis of unspecified site
722.0	Displacement of cervical intervertebral disc without myelopathy
722.1	Displacement of thoracic or lumbar intervertebral disc without myelopathy
722.2	Displacement of intervertebral disc, site unspecified, without myelopathy
722.3	Schmorl's nodes
722.4	Degeneration—cervical intervertebral disc
722.5	Degeneration of thoracic or lumbar intervertebral disc
722.6	Degeneration of intervertebral disc, site unspecified
722.7	Intervertebral disc disorder with myelopathy
722.9	Other and unspecified disc disorder
723.1	Cervicalgia
723.2	Cervicobrachial syndrome (diffuse)
723.4	Brachial neuritis or radiculitis not otherwise specified
723.5	Torticollis, unspecified
723.6	Panniculitis specified as affecting neck
723.7	Ossification of posterior longitudinal ligament in cervical region
723.9	Unspecified musculoskeletal disorders and symptoms referable to neck
724.0	Spinal stenosis, other than cervical
724.1	Pain in thoracic spine
724.2	Lumbago
724.3	Sciatica
724.4	Thoracic or lumbosacral neuritis or radiculitis, unspecified
724.5	Backache, unspecified
724.6	Disorders of sacrum
724.7	Disorders of coccyx
724.8	Other symptoms referable to back
724.9	Other unspecified back disorders
846	Sprains and strains of sacroiliac region
847	Sprains and strains of other and unspecified parts of back

Table 10-2. ICD-9 Codes Associated with Upper Extremity Conditions

Code	Condition
354.0	Carpal tunnel syndrome
354.2	Cubital tunnel syndrome
354.5	Digital neuritis: mononeuritis multiplex
354.8	Digital neuritis: other mononeuritis of upper limb
354.9	Digital neuritis: mononeuritis of upper limb, unspecified
354.2	Guyon's canal syndrome
	Pronator teres syndrome
354.3	Radial tunnel syndrome
353.0	Thoracic outlet syndrome
	Supinator syndrome
444.21	Hypothenar hammer syndrome
443.0	Raynaud's syndrome (vibration white finger)
715	Osteoarthritis
726.2	Shoulder periarthritis
726.1	Rotator cuff syndrome
726.11	Calcifying tendinitis of shoulder
726.12	Bicipital tenosynovitis
726.31	Medial epicondylitis
726.32	Lateral epicondylitis
726.33	Olecranon bursitis
727.04	de Quervain's disease
727.4	Ganglion cyst (all series)
727.0	Synovitis
727.0	Tendonitis
727.0	Tenosynovitis, unspecified
727.05	Other tenosynovitis of hand and wrist
727.03	Trigger finger
727.2	Specific bursitises of occupational origin
728.4	Game-keeper's thumb (laxity of ligament)
729.1	Myalgia/myositis
840–848	Muscle sprain

OSHA, 1995); these can be adopted to suit the individual organization's needs.

Worker surveys should be conducted periodically: before and after the initiation of new jobs, tasks, tools, or processes; when a worker is hired or transferred (to establish a baseline); or when passive surveillance analysis indicates the presence of, or an increase, in WRMDs.

Active surveillance worker surveys are limited by the workers' comprehension of the survey purpose and questions (including language barriers with some non-English speaking workers) and the accuracy of the workers' responses.

Individual worker's responses to body part discomfort surveys may vary over time; however, when the worker responses are grouped by work area or job, the group responses over time are relatively stable. These surveys can identify problem tasks, tools, or workstations, triggering further in-depth analyses and possibly intervention. The surveys can also be used to assess the effect of ergonomic interventions through distribution before and after intervention.

Supervisor Monitoring: Signal Risk Factors. The area supervisor should assess the work area and tasks for the presence of basic risk factors indicative of potential ergonomics-related problems. The supervisor should reassess the work area and tasks when any significant change occurs (such as new equipment or new work process). OSHA (1995) identified five signal risk factors to trigger further assessment and intervention:

- Performance of same motion or motion pattern every few seconds for more than 2 hours at a time
- Fixed or awkward postures for more than a total of 2 hours
- Use of vibrating or impact tools or equipment for more than a total of 2 hours during a work shift
- Using forceful hand exertions for more than a total of 2 hours at a time
- Unassisted frequent or heavy lifting for more than a total of 1 hour

The presence of a signal risk factor or a WRMD would require, at a minimum, a checklist assessment of the problem job.

Problem Determination

If the surveillance "triggers" indicate a potential ergonomics-related problem, the ergonomics team must determine if the problem exists and the extent of the problem. A surveillance trigger consisting of an increase in incidence rate, of one MSD, or of an employee complaint may represent a false-positive situation—that is, a problem not related to the work area, task, or tools. If the ergonomics team concludes a problem does exist, they must next determine whether the trigger indicates an area-wide or job series–wide problem or only isolated incidents. This determination is important as it will guide further assessment and intervention efforts. An isolated incident—a single

employee with an MSD—requires a case management approach to the problem. The presence of a single WRMD requires further investigation, and may result in a detailed job analysis and intervention.

An area-wide or job series–wide problem requires the team to resolve existing problems and to identify, recommend, and implement workplace changes to prevent the occurrence of future problems.

Prioritization

When prioritizing jobs or work areas for in-depth assessment and intervention, consider the number of workers affected, costs, high incidence or prevalence rates, and case severity. Jobs undergoing major changes in process or in products, or where the interventions can be easily accomplished, should also receive priority consideration.

High-Risk Targeting

Many methods are available for assessing the work environment. If the job is variable (a variety of tasks may be performed by the worker), the ergonomics team must go through a process that helps focus on high-risk tasks. If there are only a few distinct tasks the worker performs daily, the assessment can be easily focused on these tasks.

Many job evaluations require a focus on high-risk tasks. Mechanics generally have a high rate of back injuries; however, the assessment of the mechanics' job is problematic due to the random order of a wide variety of tasks they might perform, based on the repair needs of the vehicle or machinery and the variety of work techniques used among the workers. The task-focusing process uses information from the workers' job description, injury report data, and the input of the workers. The process involves classifying and subclassifying workers according to their jobs and tasks to identify a level at which most of the workers in the group are exposed to the same or at least similar risk factors.

Data on high-risk tasks can be gathered by questionnaire for larger groups or by focus group discussion for smaller groups. Focus groups often provide the most meaningful data. The first step in the focus group process is to identify similar exposure groups. A subgroup of 5–10 experienced workers from the similar exposure group forms the focus group. This subgroup then receives training in the risk factors for WRMDs and typical workstation problems, concerns, and solutions. The focus group should be asked to identify major problem areas, physically demanding high-risk tasks, workstation design problems, and tool and equipment concerns. The discussion can be focused by asking about specific elements of the job description (e.g., a requirement to occasionally lift 75 lb) and injury histories. The focus group workers' familiarity with the job is critical. They can often identify the high-risk tasks, tools, and workstations better than an outside expert can.

Assessment Method Determination and Investigation

Once problem areas or job series have been identified, prioritized, and targeted, the ergonomics team should conduct an in-depth assessment of the work environment. There are three basic components of the work environment: the workstation and physical environment; the task; and the tools, equipment, and containers used in the job. The workstation includes the tables, benches, chairs, stools, mats, vehicle cab, checkout stand, shelves, storage bins, controls, and displays. The physical environment includes the lighting, temperature, and noise level. Task features include work scheduling, pacing, job content (simple, routine or complex, variable), training and autonomy. Finally, the tools, equipment, and containers include hand and power tools, machines, components, keyboards, assembly parts, and boxes.

All of the ergonomic assessment methods focus on the basic risk factors of awkward posture, repetition, duration and recovery time, mechanical compression, vibration, force, and temperature extremes. Acceleration and velocity of dynamic motions have also been identified as risk factors (Marras & Schoenmarklin, 1991). The risk for developing a WRMD increases as exposure to a single risk factor or a combination of risk factors increases. The team can either perform a superficial checklist-based assessment of the problem workstation or task, or it can conduct a detailed assessment of the problem. Regardless of the assessment approach, the team must first

determine the sampling strategy to collect the most representative information in a time-efficient manner.

Basic Risk Factors

Posture. Awkward postures require increased muscle force; contribute to muscle fatigue, tendon fatigue, and joint soreness; and can increase forces on the spine. A method of classifying joint angle stress is presented in Table 10-3, a combination based on a review of published information (Aaras, Westgaard, & Stranden, 1988; Grandjean, 1988) and clinical experience.

Table 10-3 describes the amount of stress placed on a joint in various positions, described in terms of degrees of motion. The joint angles described under severe stress, for example, are thought to have a greater likelihood of leading to musculoskeletal disorders. The joint angle stress is based on position alone and the presence of other risk factors can further increase the possibility of musculoskeletal disorders.

Repetition. Repeated motions using the same muscle groups increase fatigue and muscle-tendon strain. Highly repetitive tasks often prevent adequate tissue recovery from the effects of awkward postures and force. A task is considered repetitive when the cycle time is less than 30 seconds or when one fundamental cycle constitutes more than 50% of the total cycle (OSHA, 1995). The level of risk from repetition varies by body part. High risk for the upper extremity by level of repetition is presented in Table 10-4 (OSHA, 1995).

Force. Forceful exertions increase the physiologic stress to muscles, tendons, and joints. Muscles fatigue faster as the force exerted increases. Force increases with object weight; load distribution characteristics (shifting or bulky loads require more force exertion); object friction (slippery objects require more force); awkward postures; vibration (localized hand tool vibration increases grip forces); and the type of grip (pinch grip places three to four times more force on tendons than power grip).

Mechanical Compression or Contact Stress. Mechanical compression creates pressure over a

Table 10-3. Joint Angle Analysis Criteria

	Optimal (degrees)	Minimal Stress (degrees)	Moderate Stress (degrees)	Severe Stress (degrees)
Neck				
Forward flexion	0–10	11–15	16–20	21–30
Extension	0–5	6–10	11–15	16–20
Rotation	0–15	16–25	26–35	36–45
Side bend (lateral)	0	1–5	6–10	11–15
Back				
Twist	0	1–5	6–10	11–15
Forward bend	0	1–10	11–20	>20
Shoulders				
Side reach	0–5	6–15	16–25	>26
Forward reach	0–25	26–45	46–90	>91
Across body reach	0–10	11–15	16–20	>21
Elbow flexion	60–90	91–105	106–120	121–135
Forearm rotation: pronation/supination	0	1–20	21–35	36–50
Wrist				
Extension	0	1–20	21–35	>36
Flexion	0	1–15	16–35	>36
Deviation	0	1–10	11–15	>16
Hips				
Standing	0	1–5	6–10	11–15
Sitting	90	91–100	101–110	>110
Knees				
Standing	0–95	96–110	111–130	>130
Sitting	0–95	96–110	111–130	>130
Ankles				
Upward flexion	90	89–85	84–80	79–75
Downward flexion	90–105	106–115	116–125	126–135

Table 10-4. Repetition Thresholds: High Risk

Body Area	Repetitions per Minute
Shoulder	>2.5
Upper arm/elbow	>10
Forearm/wrist	>10
Finger	>200

Source: Occupational Safety and Health Administration. (1995). *Ergonomic protection standard* (Draft). Washington, DC: Government Printing Office

small area. Mechanical compression can be caused by hard or sharp objects, the sharp edge of the desk, and small diameter handles. This compression interferes with blood flow and nerve function (Greenberg & Chaffin, 1989; Putz-Anderson, 1990).

Duration. Duration is the amount of time the worker is exposed to a risk factor. Prolonged exposure increases local and generalized fatigue and tissue stress. As the duration of exposure increases, the recovery period increases proportionally.

Vibration. Localized vibration occurs when a part of the body contacts a vibrating object, such as pneumatic, electric, or impact hand tools. Whole-body vibration usually occurs during motor vehicle and larger tool (e.g., jack hammer) operation. Guidelines on the measurement and evaluation of vibration have been published by the American Conference of Governmental Industrial Hygienists (ACGIH, 1995). Detailed vibration assessment requires sophisticated instrumentation; however, the ergonomics team can identify sources of vibration, describe the body parts affected, and compare manufacturer-provided

Table 10-5. Vibration Threshold Guidelines

Total Daily Exposure Duration[a]	Meters/sec^2	Δg[b]
4 hours and less than 8 hours	4	0.40
2 hours and less than 4 hours	6	0.61
1 hour and less than 2 hours	8	0.81
Less than 1 hour	12	1.22

[a]The total time vibration enters the hand per day, whether continuously or intermittently.
[b]$\Delta g = 9.81$ m/sec^2.
Source: Reprinted with permission from American Conference of Governmental Industrial Hygienists. (1995). *Threshold limit values for chemical substances and physical agents and biological exposure indices.* Cincinnati, OH: ACGIH.

information to published standards (Pelmear, Taylor, & Wasserman, 1992).

Acceleration, exposure time and frequency, type of vibration (impact or oscillatory), tool maintenance, and vibration path interact to determine the health impact of the vibration. The ACGIH (1995) identified specific thresholds for hand exposure to vibration (Table 10-5).

Temperature. Low temperatures reduce the dexterity and sensitivity of the hand, increase grip force requirements, and can exacerbate the effects of localized vibration. The ACGIH (1995) recommends temperature limits for bare skin exposure by type of activity (Table 10-6). Gloves are recommended if the worker will be exposed to temperatures below these levels.

Prolonged contact between the bare hand and metal surfaces colder than 59°F (15°C) may impair dexterity and contact with metal surfaces colder than 44.6°F (7°C) may induce numbness (OSHA, 1995).

Quick Assessments—Checklists

Several checklist assessments are available for the ergonomics team. Most of these checklists address the basic recognized risk factors and have a scoring mechanism to quantify risk, although few have established the validity of risk qualification. Checklists are quick and easy to use assessments, requiring a minimum of training. Checklists are limited, however, by a narrow focus on common risk factors and do not cover the entire spectrum of risk factors that may be present at a specific work site. Some checklists focus on a specific element of the work environment, such as a particular

tool or type of furniture, such as a chair. Other checklists examine posture, repetition, and duration factors.

General Workplace Checklists. General workplace checklists examine common workplace issues, such as the workstation, seating, general task features, and administrative requirements. Figure 10-2 provides an example of general workplace checklist.

Assessing Specifics: Hand Tools. Hand tools are used in numerous jobs. Poorly designed tools can be particularly problematic, stressing the entire upper extremity and contributing to WRMDs. Figure 10-3 presents an example of a hand tool assessment checklist developed by Pentikis (1995) based on Greenberg and Chaffin (1989).

Assessing Specifics: Gloves. Gloves are required to protect the hand from physical hazards including chemicals, temperatures, abrasives, and biological contaminants. Gloves reduce dexterity and tactile feedback, causing the worker to increase his or her grip force (Moore, 1994). Working with tight-fitting gloves or bulky gloves also increases the force applied. Proper-fitting gloves in good repair and providing the required protection are critical. The ergonomics team should assess the function, condition, type, and fit of gloves.

Assessing Specifics: Materials Handling. Materials handling problems can be assessed in a variety of ways. Generally, a combination of these methods provide a more complete picture of the problem. These methods include checklists (Figure 10-4) and

Bodily posture (sitting, standing, stooping)

Yes   No

❑   ❑   Does this posture involve much static muscular effort?

❑   ❑   Is the working height correct?

❑   ❑   Is the range of movement of grips and handles anatomically correct?

❑   ❑   Is there enough room to move about?

❑   ❑   Can the work be seen clearly and any instruments read with the body in a natural position?

Seating

Yes   No

❑   ❑   Is the seat correctly adjusted to the working height?

❑   ❑   Does the seat cause aches or pains?

❑   ❑   Is a footrest necessary?

❑   ❑   Is there adequate clearance for feet and calves under chair?

Video Display Terminal Work

Yes   No

❑   ❑   Is the line of sight 15 degrees below the horizon?

❑   ❑   Is display within a circle 10 and 15 degrees in radius around the normal line of sight?

❑   ❑   Is keyboard height (floor to home row) between 23 and 28 inches?

❑   ❑   Is keyboard angle between 5 and 25 degrees?

❑   ❑   Is the angle between the upper arm and forearm approximately 90 degrees?

❑   ❑   Are the hands in approximately a straight line with the forearm?

❑   ❑   Is screen height from floor between 24.4 and 35 inches?

❑   ❑   Is screen angle to vertical at least ±7 degrees (ideal is ±20 degrees)?

Figure 10-2. Ergonomic analysis: general workplace questions.

Table 10-6. Temperature Exposure Limits

Activity	Temperature
Sedentary work	60°F (15.5°C)
Light work	40°F (4.4°C)
Moderate work (fine manual dexterity not required)	20°F (–7.0°C)

Source: Reprinted with permission from American Conference of Governmental Industrial Hygienists. (1995). *Threshold limit values for chemical substances and physical agents and biological exposure indices.* Cincinnati, OH: ACGIH.

standardized assessments of the task and workstation. The critical factors in any assessment of a materials handling task are the distance of the load from the spine, the distance of the load from the floor, any twisting involved in the task, and the frequency and duration of the task (Waters et al., 1993). As the load moves away from the spine and above or below the critical "strike zone" between the thighs and shoulders, the biomechanical stress on the worker increases greatly, potentially increasing the risk of injury. Any twisting decreases the stability of the spine, which also potentially increases the probability of injury (Cailliet, 1988). As the frequency and duration of the task increase, there is less time for the tissues to recover from the physiologic stress, again increasing the probability of injury.

One of the most common standardized approaches to lifting and lowering materials handling assessment is the NIOSH Lift Equation (Waters et al., 1993). This equation is based on studies of human capacities and endurance, biomechanical, physiologic, psychophysical, and epidemiologic data. It calculates the recommended weight limit (RWL) for each lift. The RWL represents the load that the majority of workers (90% of working males and 75% of working females) can

Tool Use and Weight

Yes No

❑ ❑ Is the tool used on a repetitive basis?
        What is the rate of tool use (times/minute)? _____
        How much does the tool weigh? _____

Note: If the tool weight is greater than 25 lb and is used repeatedly, the tool is too heavy. Tools weighing 25 lb or more should not be used more than once every 3 minutes.

Tool Size

Yes No

❑ ❑ Can the fingers wrap around the hand tool?
❑ ❑ Are the handles located under the tool's center of gravity?
❑ ❑ Are high forces needed to operate the tool?
        What is the grip span of the tool (in inches)? _____

Note: An effective grip span for handles is no more than 4–5 inches. If high grip forces are needed for a manually operated (squeezable) handtool, the handle opening should be in the range of 2–3 inches.

Tool Shape

Yes No

❑ ❑ Can both hands easily grasp the tool when it is held?
❑ ❑ Do sharp edges on the tool come into contact with the hands?
❑ ❑ Does use of the hand tool place the wrists in an awkward posture?
❑ ❑ Does use of the hand tool place the arm in an abducted posture?
❑ ❑ Does the tool handle extend past the palm?
❑ ❑ Does the user wear protective gloves?

Note: If the tool handle is too short, or has rough or sharp edges, mechanical trauma to the palms can occur. Gloves reduce mechanical trauma to the hands and often increases the coefficient of friction (e.g., the torque exerted on a screwdriver); however, they decrease manual dexterity and grip strength. Gloves that are too large can significantly increase the force required to handle tools.

Temperature

Yes No

❑ ❑ Is the hand tool used in a cold environment?
❑ ❑ Is the tool handle conductive?

Note: In addition to padding a handle to insulate it, the user can also wear gloves to protect against cold environments.

Tool Vibration

Yes No

❑ ❑ Is vibration exposure present when using the hand tool?
❑ ❑ Is there antivibration padding on the hand tool?
❑ ❑ Does the user wear vibration-damping gloves?

Note: Leather gloves reportedly reduce vibration by 24% and Sorbothane-padded gloves by 45%.

Figure 10-3. Hand-tool assessment checklist.

Distance and Position

Yes No

❏ ❏ Is the horizontal distance from the body to the hands greater than 4 inches?

❏ ❏ Is the object lifted from the floor?

❏ ❏ Is the object lifted above the shoulders?

❏ ❏ Does the object have to be carried? If yes, how far? _____

❏ ❏ Does the object have to be carried up or down stairs?

❏ ❏ Is any twisting of the trunk involved?

Object

Yes No

❏ ❏ Is the object weight more than 25 lb?

❏ ❏ Is the object stable (i.e., no shifting load)?

❏ ❏ Are there good handholds?

❏ ❏ Are mechanical aids available?

❏ ❏ Is repeated lifting/lowering or pushing/pulling required? If yes, how often?

_____

❏ ❏ Is the work machine paced or worker paced?

Work Area

Yes No

❏ ❏ Are there obstacles in the area?

❏ ❏ Is the floor wet or slippery?

❏ ❏ Is the work area well lit?

Figure 10-4. Manual materials handling checklist.

safely lift in a single-person lift. The equation consists of six multipliers and a lift constant of 51 lb. The multipliers are presented in Table 10-7.

The RWL should be calculated for the origin and destination of the lift and for each different lift required in the task. The RWL is then compared to the load actually being lifted in the lift index (LI) calculation. The LI is essentially a hazard index; as the LI value increases, the risk from the lift increases. The optimal value for the LI is 1.0 or less. A lifting index greater than 1.0 suggests the lifting task should be redesigned.

Lift Index Calculation

$$LI = \frac{L}{RWL}$$

L (Load) = Current load weight
RWL = Recommended weight limit

Other methods include the United Auto Workers and General Motors risk factor checklist (1990), the Lumbar Motion Monitor model (Marras et al., 1993), the static strength prediction model (Chaffin & Anderson, 1991), and psychophysically based acceptable lifting guidelines (Snook & Ciriello, 1991). A comparison of three models can be seen in Lavendar et al. (1997).

Assessing Specifics: Prolonged Standing. Prolonged standing, especially on a hard surface, increases lower extremity and back discomfort. If prolonged standing is required, assess the standing surface, shoes, and activity. Antifatigue matting must be at least 0.5 in. thick and made of a firm, resilient material (Redfern & Chaffin, 1988). A wide variety of mats are available to accommodate specific workplace requirements, such as water drainage, static reduction, or chemical resistance. If standing and moving are required, assess the

Table 10-7. NIOSH Lift Equation

$$RWL = LC \times HM \times VM \times DM \times AM \times FM \times CM$$

LC (load constant) = 51 lb (This represents the maximum load allowed under ideal circumstances.)

HM (horizontal multiplier) = 10/H

    H = The horizontal location of the hands from the midpoint between the ankles (in inches). If the horizontal distance is <10 in., then set H at 10 in.

VM (vertical multiplier) = {1 – [0.0075(V – 30)]}

    V = Vertical location of the hands from the floor (in inches).

DM (distance multiplier) = (0.82 + [1.8/D])

    D = The vertical travel distance between the origin and the destination of the lift (in inches). If the distance traveled is <10 in., set D to 10 in.

AM (asymmetric multiplier) = (1 – [0.0032A])

    A = The angle of asymmetry—that is, the angular displacement of the load from the sagittal plane (in degrees). If the asymmetry angle is >135 degrees, then AM will equal zero, indicating the job must be redesigned.

FM (frequency multiplier) = Values from table. For lifting less frequently than once per 5 minutes, set F at <0.2 lifts/min.

CM (coupling multiplier) = Values from table.

Source: T.R. Waters, V. Putz-Anderson, A. Garg, & L.J. Fine. (1993). Revised NIOSH equation for the design and evaluation of manual lifting tasks. *Ergonomics, 36,* 749–776.

workers' shoes for cushioning. Shoe inserts can provide some cushioning for standing and walking tasks. Task requirements during standing should be noted, especially any requirement to operate foot pedals. Using foot pedals while standing can cause extreme and awkward hip and back postures. The team should also note if a sit-stand stool would be feasible given the work situation and task requirements.

Assessing Specifics: Prolonged Sitting. Prolonged sitting can lead to back and lower extremity problems, especially when the chair does not fit the worker or the type of work properly. A chair feature checklist based on the American National Standards Institute (ANSI) Standard (1988) is provided in Figure 10-5.

Assessing Specifics: Lighting. Inadequate lighting or direct or indirect glare can force the worker to assume awkward and fixed postures. Inadequate lighting during inspection tasks or video display terminal (VDT) work often leads to eye strain (Grandjean, 1987). Lighting can be a complex issue in VDT work or any task with a light-emitting display, with factors such as monitor position, angle, and tilt; screen illumination, reflection, luminance balance, and glare usually requiring individual adjustment (ANSI, 1988). Table 10-8 provides recommended lighting levels based on the type of work performed (Sanders & McCormick, 1993). The lighting levels described in Table 10-8 represent the *minimum* acceptable level for each activity. These levels can be measured with a handheld light meter. The levels *do not* indicate the level for maximum worker productivity. The amount of light needed for maximum visual efficiency varies with the task and the worker's age. Lighting issues can be complicated. The team should consider consultation with a lighting engineer for complex or system-wide lighting problems.

Detailed Assessments

Sampling Strategies. The ergonomics team must determine the most appropriate sampling strategy for the tasks of interest. Sampling strategies may be classified as random interval sampling, fixed interval sampling, selected interval sampling, and continuous sampling (NIOSH, 1995a). The type of work performed, the variability of subtasks, the objectives of the assessment, and methodologic constraints determine the choice of sampling strategies.

Continuous work sampling is the most involved approach and requires sophisticated instrumentation and computer assistance; however, this approach provides the most accurate and meaningful data (Wells et al., 1994). Work sampling provides an estimate of the percentage of

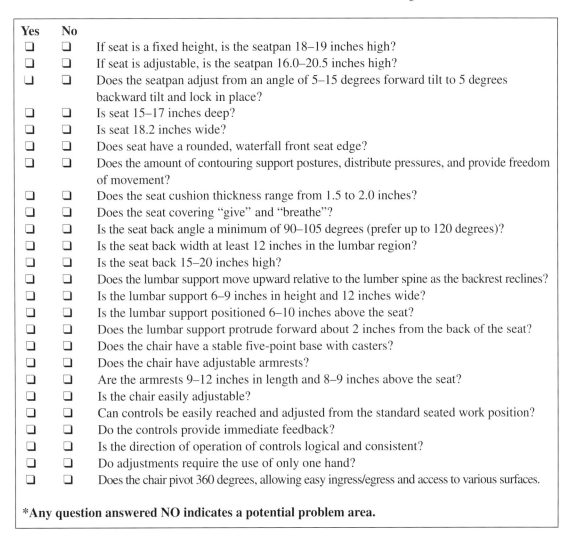

Yes	No	
❏	❏	If seat is a fixed height, is the seatpan 18–19 inches high?
❏	❏	If seat is adjustable, is the seatpan 16.0–20.5 inches high?
❏	❏	Does the seatpan adjust from an angle of 5–15 degrees forward tilt to 5 degrees backward tilt and lock in place?
❏	❏	Is seat 15–17 inches deep?
❏	❏	Is seat 18.2 inches wide?
❏	❏	Does seat have a rounded, waterfall front seat edge?
❏	❏	Does the amount of contouring support postures, distribute pressures, and provide freedom of movement?
❏	❏	Does the seat cushion thickness range from 1.5 to 2.0 inches?
❏	❏	Does the seat covering "give" and "breathe"?
❏	❏	Is the seat back angle a minimum of 90–105 degrees (prefer up to 120 degrees)?
❏	❏	Is the seat back width at least 12 inches in the lumbar region?
❏	❏	Is the seat back 15–20 inches high?
❏	❏	Does the lumbar support move upward relative to the lumber spine as the backrest reclines?
❏	❏	Is the lumbar support 6–9 inches in height and 12 inches wide?
❏	❏	Is the lumbar support positioned 6–10 inches above the seat?
❏	❏	Does the lumbar support protrude forward about 2 inches from the back of the seat?
❏	❏	Does the chair have a stable five-point base with casters?
❏	❏	Does the chair have adjustable armrests?
❏	❏	Are the armrests 9–12 inches in length and 8–9 inches above the seat?
❏	❏	Is the chair easily adjustable?
❏	❏	Can controls be easily reached and adjusted from the standard seated work position?
❏	❏	Do the controls provide immediate feedback?
❏	❏	Is the direction of operation of controls logical and consistent?
❏	❏	Do adjustments require the use of only one hand?
❏	❏	Does the chair pivot 360 degrees, allowing easy ingress/egress and access to various surfaces.

***Any question answered NO indicates a potential problem area.**

Figure 10-5. Ergonomic analysis: chair evaluation.

time the worker spends in awkward postures, on repetitive activities, applying force, exposed to vibration, or using a particular tool or piece of equipment (Keyserling, 1992). The team often considers time-data tradeoffs when choosing the sampling strategy.

Survey Planning and Videotaping. The ergonomics team should have several tools available for the detailed assessment: a video camera to record workers' postures and movements during specific tasks; a tape measure to determine workstation dimensions and reach distances; a timer or stopwatch to measure the duration of a specific task, subtask, or break; and a force gauge or spring scale to measure

push or pull forces or the weight of tools, products, or objects handled.

The videotape is an essential tool in the assessment process. The tapes provide a permanent record of the activity and allow the ergonomist to assess motions and postures in slow motion. Videotapes also serve to enhance ergonomic training and demonstrations. Videotaping guidelines are provided in Table 10-9.

Thorough planning before the site survey is critical. Team members should be assigned specific tasks, including taking workplace measurements, interviewing supervisors and workers, sketching and note taking, videotaping, identifying and measuring risk factors. Schedule the survey when the tasks of interest are being performed and subjects

Table 10-8. Recommended Lighting Levels

Type of Work	Examples	Recommended Light Level*
General	Storeroom	80–170 lux
Moderately precise	Packing, simple assembly	200–250 lux
Video display terminal	Data entry	500–600 lux
Fine work	Reading, writing, bookkeeping, fine work on machines	500–700 lux
Very fine to precise	Technical drawing, watchmaking, testing electrical equipment	1,000–2,000 lux

*1 lux = 0.0929 footcandle.
Source: M.S. Sanders, & E.J. McCormick. (1993). *Human factors in engineering and design.* New York: McGraw-Hill.

Table 10-9. Ergonomic Survey: Videotaping

Presurvey
Check equipment
Obtain approvals and schedule taping
Verify presence of electrical outlets if needed
Verify lighting conditions and bring lighting equipment if needed
Survey
Film job information on a piece of paper at the beginning of the recording
Activate the time/date indicator if the camera has this feature
Select views that will maximize description of movement
Record the worker's whole body posture and entire work area initially
Select views 90 degrees from each other
Film at least 10 cycles if the job is repetitive
If several people perform the job, film two or three employees doing the same job
Focus on overexertion or fatigue conditions
Frame each view with common reference points
If multiple tasks are involved in a process, tape the tasks in order

are available. Every effort must be taken to minimize the disruption to the work and to get a representative "picture" of the tasks.

General Questions. Initially, the ergonomics team should collect basic descriptive workplace information including the number of workers assigned to the area or job; the age and gender distribution of the workers; the length of the workday and daily break schedule; and any special administrative arrangements such as job rotation plans or flex

schedules. Task-related information should also be collected, including its description, objective, percent of time spent on the task daily, and whether the task is continuous or intermittent, machine paced or self paced. If a specific product is produced, the team should identify the product's weight and dimensions; the cost of producing a unit; the production rate and quotas; and the error rate and any error penalties for the workers. Finally, the team should make a sketch of the workstation, identifying dimensions of surfaces, reach distances, clearances, and travel distances. Note locations of equipment, fixtures, and other pertinent features on the sketch.

Specific Task Features. The ergonomics team should assess the special features of the task. These features include the use of hand tools, gloves, materials handling, prolonged standing, prolonged sitting, and exposure to vibration or lighting conditions.

Task Analysis. Task analysis covers many methods used to observe human behavior in a task and record task elements and demands. These elements and demands are compared to human capabilities, to determine if modification, redesign, controls, or automation are required. Task analysis methods include motion analysis, which identifies excessive repetitions and awkward and static postures; timed activity analysis; and time and motion analysis.

During task analyses, tasks are broken into component elements and the elements may be further divided to the motion or micro-motion level. There are five types of information used in task analyses: sequence of activities, duration of activities, frequency of activities, fraction of time (of a person,

	Position	Force	Duration	Repetition	Mechanical Stress	Vibration
Neck						
Back						
Shoulder						
Arm						
Hand/Wrist						
Legs						
Feet						

Figure 10-6. Risk factor analysis.

machine, or work unit) spent in states or activities, and spatial movements.

One of the most useful approaches to ergonomic assessment combines the task analysis methodology with the approach Keyserling, Armstrong, and Punnett (1991) recommended for ergonomic job analysis. Their task analysis records the job, task, work cycle time, and specific component steps in the task. The component steps are then examined for generic risk factors, which include awkward posture, forceful exertion, mechanical compression, repetition, vibration, and duration and recovery time by affected body part. Environmental factors such as temperature extremes and lighting conditions are included in the assessment. This approach requires some qualitative expert judgment as well as comparing observations to specific criteria (e.g., joint angles presented in Table 10-3).

Risk Factor and Body Part Analysis. The task components responsible for identified risk factor exposures can be recorded by affected body part in an analysis grid (Figure 10-6). For example, a mechanic's task of removing a tire requires the subtask of removing the lug nuts. This subtask involves the use of a pneumatic drill to remove the nuts. The subtask exposes the hand to vibration, the hand and arm to forceful exertions, the hand to mechanical compression (depending on

the shape of the handle), and the hand, arm, and shoulder to awkward postures. These exposures are recorded by subtask number for each risk factor identified and body part affected in the analysis grid. This analysis process allows the team to identify the subtasks responsible for high exposures to the risk factors and the body parts most frequently exposed. Generally, intervention strategies are easily identified after this focusing analysis is completed.

Design

Types of Controls

Often, intervention strategies naturally flow from the assessment process. Solutions can be classified as engineering, administrative, or personal protective-equipment controls. Usually, ergonomic solutions involve some combination of engineering and administrative controls. Personal protective equipment is recommended only under specific work conditions.

Engineering Controls

Engineering controls are the most effective method of reducing or eliminating identified risk factors. Workstation design modifications and equipment and hand tool design are based on the physical characteristics (anthropometry) and capabilities of the working population. Engineering controls include workstation design; area layout; equipment design; and tool, handle, and container design.

Administrative Controls

Administrative controls can be used to limit the duration, frequency, and severity of exposure to hazards. Examples of administrative controls include (but are not limited to)

- Reducing the number of repetitions by decreasing production rate requirements and limiting overtime work.
- Reducing the number and speed of repetitions by reducing line or production speed, or by having worker input into production speed; that is, using worker-based rather than machine-based production speed.
- Providing rest breaks to relieve fatigued muscle-tendon groups; the length of the rest break should be determined by the effort required, total cycle time, and the muscle-tendon group involved.
- Increasing the number of employees assigned to the task (e.g., lifting in teams rather than individually).
- Instituting job rotation as a preventive measure, with the goal of alleviating physical fatigue and stress to a particular set of muscles and tendons. (Job rotation should not be used in response to symptoms of cumulative trauma, as this can contribute to symptom development in all employees involved in the rotation schedule rather than preventing problems. Analysis of the jobs used in the rotation schedule should be conducted by trained ergonomic personnel.)
- Providing light or restricted duty assignments to allow injured muscle-tendon groups time to rest, assisting in the healing process. (Light- or restricted-duty assignments should be provided when physical limitations—as identified by a health care provider—allow the worker to return to work performing at less than normal work requirements. The light or restricted work assignment must be assessed by trained ergonomic or health care personnel to ensure the worker is not exposed to hazardous conditions that can interfere with the healing process

or lead to another WRMD. Every effort must be made to provide light- or restricted-duty assignments.)
- Ensuring preventive and regular maintenance of tools and equipment and effective housekeeping tasks are accomplished.
- Monitoring work practices regularly, ensuring proper work techniques are used and adjustments and modifications of schedule or work practices are made as needed.
- Providing a new-employee conditioning period (4–6 weeks, in some situations) for heavier, physiologically demanding tasks.

Personal Protective Equipment

Personal protective equipment (PPE) are devices that serve as barriers between a hazard and the worker. Antivibration gloves are an example of PPE because they act as a barrier between the source of vibration and the hand. PPE should fit properly and should not increase stressors. Braces, splints, and back belts are *not* PPE (NIOSH, 1994). When selecting PPE, potential physiologic hazards should be considered. PPE should be provided in a variety of sizes and accommodate the physical requirements of workers and the job.

Work-Site Design Solutions

Work-site design solutions arise from basic anthropometric and workstation design principles. There are common problems and solutions for a variety of work-site settings and tasks: general work-site design, VDT work; manual materials handling tasks; and tasks requiring hand tools. Basic principles of work-site design and common related problems and solutions are presented in Appendix 10-1.

Selecting the Solution

There are often several possible solutions to non-ergonomic designs. The ergonomics team and management must clearly define the criteria for solution selection. One approach bases solution selection on three criteria: solution effectiveness, timeliness, and employee acceptance (OSHA, 1995). Effectiveness is based on a four-point scale:

4 = risk factors completely eliminated
3 = risk factors mostly eliminated
2 = some risk factors eliminated
1 = few or no risk factors eliminated

Timeliness represents the time required to fully implement the solution and reduce or eliminate the risk factors. If a solution will require a significant amount of time to implement, an interim solution should be implemented.

Employee acceptance of the solution often determines the solution effectiveness and success. Employees must be actively involved in the solution identification and selection process.

Other decision schemes are available or can be developed based on the organization's management philosophies, values, and criteria. Regardless of the method used, the decision process must be clear, documented, supported by the organization, and justifiable. The team must be prepared to explain and justify its recommendation to management *and* workers.

Implementing the Solution

The ergonomics team must ensure appropriate documentation of walk-through and work-site evaluations. This documentation should include the date, areas visited, risk factors recognized, actions initiated, follow-up time frame, and results of the follow-up.

The implementation of solutions should involve a test or trial before full implementation. Mock-ups, sample workstations, or limited changes in work methods can provide information about potential problems and modifications that may be needed. The workers should be directly involved in the solution design, testing, and implementation, whenever possible.

Implementation and follow-up should be carefully planned, scheduled, and documented. Problems, delays, and subsequent actions should also be documented. Clear and relevant criteria should be established to assess the effectiveness of the intervention plan. A tracking log should be used to record activities.

Medical Management

There should be a written plan for the systematic evaluation, treatment, and follow-up of workers with signs and symptoms of WRMDs. This plan should be reviewed and updated on an annual basis. The plan components are discussed in turn below.

Health Surveillance

Health surveillance is often included in the medical management plan. Health surveillance should include a baseline examination, with a medical and occupational history and physical examination of the musculoskeletal and nervous systems for symptoms of MSD.

If a physical examination is required, it should be given only *after* offer of employment has been made, and it must be given to all new or transferred employees rather than selected employees. The Americans with Disabilities Act restricts the scope of the physical examination (Schneid, 1992). Workers assigned to high-risk jobs should receive periodic health surveillance, at least every 2–3 years.

Access and Medical Evaluation

Timely access to care is a critical element in the medical management of WRMDs. OSHA (1995) recommends the worker be evaluated at the earliest possible date, within 5 work days after the onset of symptoms are reported.

The medical evaluation of the worker includes the history of the condition (onset, symptoms, treatments) and the worker's medical history (systemic conditions, trauma, prior MSD). The history should include information about the job conditions, tasks that exacerbate the condition, and recreational activities. The physical examination includes inspection, palpation, range of motion, and sensory, motor, and provocative testing (such as Phalen's test) as indicated.

Treatment

If the medical assessment indicates the condition may be work related, the ergonomics team or another qualified person should be notified to perform a complete ergonomic investigation of the workplace and tasks.

The treatment plan should include medical management of the case as well as the return-to-work plan. The medical management may involve a variety of noninvasive and invasive procedures, including anti-inflammatory medication, therapy, splinting, injection, and surgery.

Splints and braces should be prescribed carefully and clearly. In most cases, wrist splints are not recommended for use during work, unless specifically prescribed by a health care provider. Some businesses have attempted to prevent WRMDs by providing splints for all workers. This approach can cause more problems than it solves. The worker often struggles against the splint to perform the work, which can increase tissue stress and inflammation, exacerbating the condition. The worker may also stress other joints such as the elbow and shoulder, assuming awkward postures to accommodate working with the splint. Wrist splints and back braces are not recommended to prevent injuries.

Return-to-Work Plan

The return-to-work plan is essential: It identifies specific work restrictions, time frames, necessary accommodations, and job assignment recommendations. The ergonomics team should be directly involved in the assessment of the work area and job to accommodate the work restrictions, the identification of necessary modifications, or the identification of temporary work assignments during the recovery period.

The team must verify that the job modifications or temporary assignment reduces or eliminates exposure to the risk factors. This may involve reducing the exposure time, decreasing work pace, redesigning a job or process, eliminating some elements of the work, providing assistive equipment, or retraining.

Complete removal from the work environment is the last resort and should be avoided if possible. Numerous studies have demonstrated that the longer employees are out of work due to injury or illness, the less likely they will return to work (Doyle, Shepherd, & LaFleur, 1993).

Communication with Employer

The health care provider is responsible for communicating findings and treatment plans to the employer. This plan should be clearly written, including the results of the assessment, the treatment plan and specific work restrictions, duration of restrictions, necessary modifications, and reassignment recommendations. The health care provider must observe appropriate confidentiality restrictions, providing only that information which is directly relevant to the work environment.

Follow-Up

Regular contact between the health care provider and management during the recovery period is important. Initially, the worker should be monitored to ensure that the work modifications (or reassignment) have reduced or eliminated the risk factors. If the employee has been removed from the work environment, regular contact is even more important to maintain communication and establish the expectation of returning to work.

Periodic medical reassessments are necessary to determine the response to treatment, the current status of the condition, and any necessary additional treatment or workplace modifications. A final evaluation at the completion of treatment should be performed by the health care provider.

Documentation of all data should be maintained in confidential files. Only the worker, medical personnel, and personnel handling workers' compensation claims should have access to records.

Education and Training

Education and training are essential elements in the ergonomics program. Effective training programs can change the culture of the organization, with front-line workers identifying and resolving many of the work conditions that can lead to WRMDs. Training programs should be initiated if a WRMD has been identified, but proactive training before an injury occurs is optimal.

General Awareness Training

General awareness training should be provided to all employees in problem jobs and their supervisors, every employee involved in high-risk task focusing, and the ergonomics team. The training covers the basic risk factors; causes, signs, and symptoms of WRMDs; means of prevention; proper work methods; employer's ergonomics program and plans; and the procedures for reporting concerns, risk factors, WRMDs, and workplace improvement suggestions. Incorporating examples and pictures of typical work situations in the facility in the presentations and training materials improves the effectiveness of the training. The training should be clear, understandable, and at the appropriate level for the audience.

By the end of the training, employees and supervisors should have an understanding of WRMDs and symptoms, including basic anatomy of the upper limb and back, diseases/potential injuries of upper limb and back, the concept of injuries developing over time (cumulative), and available treatments (OSHA, 1995). They should be aware of the risk factors and causes of WRMDs, such as workplace or job stresses. Workers and supervisors should also be able to recognize early symptoms and understand the necessity of proper work methods. Finally, they should understand and be able to apply ergonomic principles in the prevention and control of injuries.

Specific Training

Job-Specific Training. Job-specific training should be included in the general awareness training and cover the identification of risk factors present in a worker's specific job and the control measures used to deal with these risk factors. Control measures often include the proper, safe use and maintenance of equipment. Personal responsibility should be emphasized in the training. Employees should be encouraged to take action by adjusting their work areas to suit their own needs and by changing their personal habits to prevent discomfort and injury.

Ergonomics Team Training. The course recommended for the ergonomics team and employees involved in workplace assessment, job analysis, and training usually takes 35–40 hours. A site survey exercise is recommended during the course. This experience requires the synthesis and application of the material presented. The survey increases confidence and the probability that these skills will be used after completion of the course. The ergonomics team members should receive periodic continuing education to keep their knowledge and skills at an appropriate level.

The ergonomics team training should develop team members' skills to conduct general training sessions on ergonomics, workstation design, and WRMDs. Although team members will not become ergonomists, they should be able to identify areas requiring further investigation through passive sur-

veillance and be able to conduct worker surveys, administer questionnaires, and interview workers and supervisors to target problem work areas (active surveillance). Finally, team members should be able to conduct basic work-site analyses; contribute to work-site assessments; identify, evaluate, and recommend standard interventions; and contribute to custom-designed or complex interventions.

Testing and Evaluation

Much of the testing and evaluation of an ergonomics program involves establishing relevant and appropriate criteria for the major program elements (analysis and design) and documenting compliance and results. In some cases, general decision criteria that reflect the organization's mission and values may be applied to different program elements (such as financial impact or number of persons or jobs affected). Internal quality audits should document compliance with the criteria and explain any deviation from the organization's standards. Finally, testing and evaluation should examine the overall ergonomics program's performance. A good reference for therapists conducting industrial outcome studies can be found in Schwartz (1997). All programs must be able to demonstrate a valued contribution to the organization or the program should not exist. Good documentation is essential to later outcome evaluation, and elements of documentation are covered below for each portion of the ergonomic process.

Analysis

Passive Surveillance

Passive surveillance should be performed at set intervals (e.g., quarterly) and the results and subsequent actions documented. Thresholds for further action (perhaps one MSD) must be clearly established, justified, and compliance documented. Often the ergonomics team must prioritize work areas, job series, or tasks for further assessment and intervention. The prioritization criteria should be clearly established, justified, and documented. Some companies use cost, numbers of workers affected, incidence, case severity, and criticality of the work area as criteria.

Active Surveillance

Active surveillance is generally triggered by the passive surveillance results. Criteria for the type of active surveillance (worker survey, general checklist, or in-depth survey) should be established, justified, and documented. Again, companies may use cost, numbers of workers affected or incidence, or problem severity or criticality as criteria. When active surveillance is triggered, action should be taken within a set period (quantified, as in within 5 days). The action plan should document the type of action or assessment planned, justification for this choice, the responsible individuals, and the time frame for completion. Results of active surveillance should document dates, actions, findings, and recommendations for further action or closure.

Design

Intervention Plan

If active surveillance identifies a concern, an action plan should be required. The action plan should document and justify the choice of control, either engineering, administrative, PPE, or some combination of these controls. Short-, intermediate-, and long-term plans should be documented and the time plan established. Although full problem resolution may be a long-term process, short-term immediate actions should be taken to temporarily remedy the highest risk situations. Again, criteria to define high risk, prioritize intervention areas, and justify choice of intervention (effectiveness, timeliness, and employee acceptance) should be clearly established.

Follow-up on implemented solutions must occur within a set period from the implementation. Solution effectiveness can be assessed using the same risk factor checklist or assessment methods used to identify the problem area: worker surveys, production and quality improvements, or turnover and absentee rates. Changes in incidence, severity, or prevalence can be used as long-term indicators of solution effectiveness. The ergonomics team should document the dates and results of the follow-up assessment; further action required or planned, responsible parties, and time frame; or problem closure.

Medical Management

Relevant evaluation criteria for medical management define the frequency of and procedures for health surveillance (such as every 2–3 years for high-risk jobs); time limit between the first report of symptoms and medical examination (e.g., 5 days); the return-to-work planning; and communication with employer (time and content requirements). The medical records should document compliance with the established time guidelines, the medical evaluation findings, diagnosis, treatment plan, return-to-work plan, light duty restrictions, and results of communication with the employer. Follow-up evaluation findings and any treatment plan modifications should also be documented.

WRMDs should be reported to the ergonomics team for investigation. The medical management criteria should include a time frame for this reporting and communication guidelines (including close collaboration between the health care provider and the ergonomics team on the workplace assessment, light duty prescription, and return-to-work plan). The health care provider should document compliance with these established criteria.

Education and Training

Criteria should be established to specify who will receive training, the training content by audience, the frequency of training, and the expected outcome (e.g., "workers will be able to identify basic risk factors"). The ergonomics team should plan, schedule, and document the training programs.

Worker Training. Workers should be tested before and after completion of training and should also be observed on the job to evaluate the effectiveness of the training program. The testing and observation should reflect the expected training outcomes. The test should be anonymous; it is intended to evaluate the effectiveness of the training, not employee knowledge. Results of the evaluation should be recorded and, if necessary, training program modifications implemented.

Ergonomics Team Training. When training the ergonomics team itself, a combination of written tests and hands-on tasks should be used both to train the individuals and to evaluate the effectiveness of the training. The tests should cover material presented in the sessions, and the tasks should involve demonstration of workplace evaluation skills (use of checklists, interviews, surveys, hand tools, office equipment, and safe materials handling procedures) and intervention planning. Results of the training should be documented and, if an individual fails to meet an outcome criterion, additional training should be provided to raise expertise to an appropriate level.

Overall Program Objectives and Justification

Every ergonomics program must be able to justify its existence. Programs usually have two basic areas of justification concern: employee health and management issues. Criteria should evaluate the program performance in both areas.

Employee Health

The ergonomics team usually is involved in individual case management and prevention. Each function requires different evaluation criteria. Case management criteria relate directly to case issues, such as the number of cases opened, closed, or reopened.

Success in the prevention function can be demonstrated in accepted rate measurements (incidence, prevalence, and severity) and the number of lost work days or hours. Rate measurement is one of the most commonly used program justification approaches. Unfortunately, most programs do not see a reduction in case rates for 18–24 months after program implementation. In fact, some programs see an initial rise in the new case rate due to increased awareness among the workers. After the initial period, however, the case rate usually falls below previous levels.

"Softer" data are also available to demonstrate program success. These data include repeated employee questionnaires and body part discomfort surveys. Objectively, the ergonomics team can document a decrease in risk factors in the work area or task. Finally, team performance can be assessed by examining the number of surveys performed, training conducted, recommendations made, and per-

Table 10-10. Cost Analysis of Work-Related Musculoskeletal Disorders

1. Wages (hours × payroll rates)
   a. Injured worker
      Days of injury
      Lost time
      Medical visits
   b. Other workers
   c. Other workers' lost time
   d. Overtime/make-up time
   e. Supervisors' time (reports, counseling)
   f. Hiring, training new employees
      Supervisor's time
      Employees' time
   g. Administrative staff time
2. Administrative costs
   a. Equipment damage
   b. Miscellaneous (clean up, repair)

haps most importantly, the number of solutions implemented.

Management Issues and Cost Analysis

Ergonomic program justification is easy when the program is substantiated on an economic basis by comparing program costs and the benefits. The problem the ergonomics team faces is selling management on the program despite the potential initial increase in workers' compensation claims. The team must identify, address, and measure management concerns that can show immediate payoff. These issues include the quality of work, productivity, lost work time, absenteeism, or employee safety, symptoms, or satisfaction.

Most cost analyses examine costs directly related to the WRMD: the medical and workers' compensation costs. However, there are several indirect or hidden costs associated with each WRMD. These costs include hiring and training replacement workers, decreased productivity, and overtime. These costs can equal 3–10 times the medical care costs. A list of these costs is provided in Table 10-10.

Quality of Work and Productivity. Historical information is usually available on production rates, cycle time per number of pieces, error rates, and reject rates. These rates and costs can be compared before and after the solution implementation.

Absenteeism. Look at the cost of relief staffing or lost production. This information can provide a strong case for changes that will lower the absentee rate.

Safety. Based on historical information, develop reasonable predictors of future injuries and project the number and costs associated with injuries. These projections can justify the expense of studying a high-risk job and implementing changes.

Turnover. Compare the costs of employing a new person (recruitment, selection, orientation) with the cost of retraining a current employee to fill a job vacated due to the development of a WRMD in the previous job-holder. For complex jobs, the time to reach proficiency for a new employee will be measured in months, not days. These costs are usually large and therefore desirable to avoid.

Conclusion

This chapter has presented the critical program elements in a comprehensive ergonomics program. Ergonomists may serve as consultants to establish a program, provide education to ergonomic team members, conduct a portion of the program, or serve as program managers. Expert management of the ergonomics program is essential to its success. The ergonomics team must be able to demonstrate that the benefits of the program are greater than its cost to the organization. Even the most technologically advanced program will fail if management issues and justification are ignored. There are some common management causes for program failures (Many Corporate Programs, 1994). These causes include a lack of direction and focus, lack of resources, and lack of coordination among internal company departments such as engineering, medical, and safety. Above all, ergonomists must understand the critical program elements: management commitment, analysis (passive and active surveillance), design (controls, medical management, and education and training), and program evaluation. Integration of these elements creates the comprehensive program necessary for the company to realize the full potential of injury prevention through the proper use of ergonomics in the workplace.

References

Aaras, A., Westgaard, R.H., & Stranden, E. (1988). Postural angles as an indicator of postural load and muscular injury in occupational work situations. *Ergonomics, 31,* 915–933.

American Conference of Governmental Industrial Hygienists. (1995). *Threshold limit values for chemical substances and physical agents and biological exposure indices.* Cincinnati, OH: ACGIH.

American National Standards Institute. (1988). *American national standard for human factors engineering of visual display terminals workstations* (ANSI/HFS Standard No. 100–1988). Santa Monica, CA: Human Factors Society.

American National Standards Institute. (1996). *Control of work related musculoskeletal disorders* (ANSI Z-365, Draft, Part 1). Itasca, IL: National Safety Council.

Bureau of Labor Statistics, U.S. Department of Labor. (1994). *Workplace injuries and illnesses in 1993* (USDL 94–600). Washington, DC: Bureau of Labor Statistics.

Cailliet, R. (1988). *Low back pain syndrome* (4th ed.). Philadelphia: F.A. Davis.

Chaffin, D.B., & Andersson, G.B.J. (1991). *Occupational biomechanics* (2nd ed.). New York: Wiley & Sons.

Centers for Disease Control. (1988). Guidelines for evaluating surveillance systems. *MMWR CDC Surveillance Summaries, 37(S-5),* 1–18.

Current report: Gingrich urged to extend ergonomics ban in any continuing resolution for fiscal 1997. (1996, September 18). *Occupational Safety & Health Reporter,* p. 539.

Current report: Renewed fight for restriction on OSHA rule gearing up as Congress moves on omnibus bill (1996, September 25). *Occupational Safety & Health Reporter,* p. 563.

Doyle, E., Shepherd, S., & LaFleur, B. (1993). *Costs for Department of the Navy civilians due to the Federal Employees' Compensation Act: How much does a case cost?* (Report No. 93–6). San Diego, CA: Naval Health Research Center.

Gjessing, C., Schoenborn, T., & Cohen, A. (Eds.). (1994). *Participatory ergonomic interventions in meatpacking plants.* (DHHS Publication No. 94–124). Cincinnati, OH: DHHS, Publication Dissemination, NIOSH.

Gordon, C., Churchill, T., Clauser, B., et al. (1988). *1988 anthropometric survey of U.S.Army personnel: Methods and summary statistics.* Natick, MA: U.S. Army, Natick Research Development and Engineering Center.

Grandjean, E. (1987). *Ergonomics in computerized offices.* New York: Taylor & Francis.

Grandjean, E. (1988). *Fitting the task to the man* (4th ed.). New York: Taylor & Francis.

Grant, K., & Habes, D. (1995). Summary of studies of the

effectiveness of ergonomic interventions. *Applied Occupational Environmental Hygiene, 10,* 523–530.

Greenberg, L., & Chaffin, D. (1989).*Workers and their tools.* Midland, MI: Pendell Publishing.

Kelly, P.L., & Kroemer, K.H.E. (1990). Anthropometry of the elderly: Status and recommendations. *Human Factors, 32,* 571–595.

Keyserling, W. (1992). Sampling strategies for ergonomic job analysis. Ergonomic Job Analysis Course, Course conducted 6–7 November 1992, Arlington, VA.

Keyserling, W., Armstrong, T., & Punnett, L. (1991). Ergonomic job analysis: A structured approach for identifying risk factors associated with overexertion injuries and disorders. *Applied Occupational Environmental Hygiene 6,* 353–363.

Lavendar, S.A., Oleske, D.M., Nicholson, L., Andersson, G.B.J., & Hahn, J. (1997). A comparison of four methods commonly used to determine low-back disorders risk in a manufacturing environment. In *Proceedings of the Human Factors and Ergonomics Society 41st Annual Meeting* (pp. 657–660). Santa Monica, CA: Human Factors and Ergonomics Society.

Many corporate programs 'floundering' due to poor management. (1994, July 20). *Occupational Safety & Health Reporter,* p. 359.

Marras, W.S., Lavendar, S.A., Leurgans, S.E., et al. (1991). The role of dynamic three-dimensional trunk motion in occupationally-related low back disorders: The effects of workplace factors, trunk position, and trunk motion characteristics on risk of injury. *Spine, 18,* 617–628.

Marras, W.S., & Schoenmarklin, R.W. (1991). Quantification of wrist motion in highly repetitive, hand-intensive industrial jobs. Biodynamics laboratory, Department of Industrial and Systems Engineering, Ohio State University. Funded by NIOSH, OHO26221-01 and 02.

Moore, B. (1994). *An evaluation of the effects of latex examination gloves on sensibility and manual dexterity of the hand.* Unpublished doctoral dissertation, University of Nebraska, Lincoln, NE.

National Institute for Occupational Safety and Health. (1994). *Workplace use of back belts—Review and recommendations* (DHHS Publication No. 94–122). Cincinnati, OH: Education and Information Division.

National Institute for Occupational Safety and Health. (1995a). *Cumulative trauma disorders in the workplace* (DHHS Publication No. 95–119). Cincinnati, OH: Education and Information Division.

National Institute for Occupational Safety and Health. (1995b). *The international classification of diseases* (9th rev., 5th ed.). Cincinnati, OH: DHHS

Occupational Safety and Health Administration. (1991). *Ergonomics program management guidelines for meat-packing plants.* Washington, DC: Government Printing Office.

Occupational Safety and Health Administration. (1995). *Ergonomic protection standard* (Draft). Washington, DC: Government Printing Office.

Pelmear, P.L., Taylor, W., & Wasserman, D.E. (1992). *Hand-arm vibration, a comprehensive guide for occupational health professionals.* New York: Van Nostrand Reinhold.

Pentikis, J. (1995). *Handtool assessment checklist.* Aberdeen Proving Ground, MD: U.S. Army Center for Health Promotion and Preventive Medicine.

Putz-Anderson, V. (1992). *Cumulative trauma disorders, a manual for musculoskeletal diseases of the upper limbs.* London: Taylor & Francis.

Redfern, M., & Chaffin, D. (1988). The effects of floor types on standing tolerance in industry. In F. Aghazadeh (Ed.), *Trends in ergonomics/human factors V* (pp. 901–905). New York: Elsevier.

Sanders, M.S., & McCormick, E.J. (1993). *Human factors in engineering and design.* New York: McGraw-Hill.

Schneid, T. (1992). *The Americans with Disabilities Act.* New York: Van Nostrand Reinhold.

Schwartz, R.K. (1997). Outcome assessment of prevention programs. In M. Sanders (Ed.), *Management of cumulative trauma disorders.* Boston: Butterworth–Heinemann.

Smith, S.L. (1995, July). Why industry needs to watch its back. *Occupational Hazards,* 30–34.

Snook, S.H., & Ciriello, V.M. (1991). The design of manual handling tasks: Revised tables of maximum acceptable weights and forces. *Ergonomics, 34,* 1197–1213.

United Auto Workers–General Motors Joint Committee on Health & Safety. (1990). *Ergonomics process planning guide.* Warren, MI: UAW-GM Human Resource Center for Health and Safety.

Waters, T.R., Putz-Anderson, V., Garg, A., & Fine, L.J. (1993). Revised NIOSH equation for the design and evaluation of manual lifting tasks. *Ergonomics, 36,* 749–776.

Wells, R, Moore, A., Potvin, J., & Norman, R. (1994). Assessment of risk factors for development of work-related musculoskeletal disorders. *Applied Ergonomics, 25,* 157–164.

Appendix 10-1
Design: Developing Solutions

Basic Principles

Anthropometry

Designers use anthropometric data to ensure the workstation, reach distances, clearances, tools, and equipment fit the user population. The first step in applying anthropometric data involves defining the actual working population. Numerous anthropometric data sources provide information on the physical dimensions of workers by gender, age, and ethnic origin (Gordon et al., 1998; Kelly & Kroemer, 1990; National Aeronautics and Space Administration, 1978). Use the data source that best matches the working population.

The next step is identifying the body parts and dimensions of interest, which will be determined by the task performed. For example, the task may involve reaching, seated or standing operations, use of controls, tools, and containers. The designer then identifies the percentile and gender of interest (e.g., fifth percentile female and ninety-fifth percentile male), extracts the data from the anthropometric sources, and applies the information.

There are three design approaches to applying anthropometric data. The preferred approach is to design for the range. Workstations and equipment designed using the design-for-the-range approach usually fits the majority of workers, from the ninety-fifth percentile male to the fifth percentile female, thus accommodating approximately 90% of the working population. Design for the extreme involves designing for the smallest female or the largest male in the population. The smallest workers (fifth percentile) determine reach dimension (such as fire extinguisher placement) and visual clearances. The largest workers (ninety-fifth percentile) determine clearances (doorways, walkways). Finally—and this should be the last resort—some workplaces and equipment take the design-for-the-average approach. Although this approach is more economical, the equipment or workplace will *not* accommodate the majority of the workforce.

Neutral Posture

Neutral posture is the position the body naturally assumes in a weightless environment. It is the most comfortable, least stressful, strongest, and most efficient position for workers (Eastman Kodak, 1986; Huchingson, 1981). Ergonomists should design workstations, job tasks, tools, and equipment with the neutral posture in mind.

Workplace Design Principles

Four basic workplace design principles can be applied to improve workstation arrangement and work flow while reducing risk factors (Sanders & McCormick, 1993):

1. Importance principle. The important components of a job should be placed in convenient

locations. Importance refers to the criticality of the component in the achievement of the objectives of the system.

2. Frequency of use principle. The frequently used components should be located in convenient locations (the copy machine should be near the department secretary or whoever photocopies the most).

3. Function principle. Components should be grouped and arranged according to their function, such as the groupings of displays, controls, or machines that are functionally related in the operation of the system. (For example, direction indicators and direction controls should be located together.)

4. Sequence of use principle. In some operations, sequences or patterns of relationship frequently occur in performing a task. Components should be arranged to take advantage of the sequences or patterns. This principle should be followed wherever and whenever possible as it has the greatest positive effect on performance, productivity, and errors.

Space considerations are important when evaluating a work area. Spaces that should be assessed include the kick space, leg room, free floor space, work area depth, lateral workspace (vertical position of shelves and drawers), storage space, and handle locations.

Common Problems and Solutions

Workstation Design

The work surface is determined by the anthropometric dimensions of the worker and the type of work being performed. The visual angle required to perform the work usually decides the work-surface height and angle. Work surfaces that are either too high or too low force the worker into awkward and stressful postures, especially of the neck and back.

Slanted work surfaces can improve the neck and back posture but must be appropriate for the type of work performed. For example, such fine or detailed work as drafting or an inspection task requires the work to be closer to the eyes. The work surface must also allow sufficient leg clearance depending on the anthropometric dimensions of the workers, the nature of the work, and worker position (seated or standing).

Workstation Height Guidelines*

Working height must provide for the optimum visual distance for fine or precise manipulation.

Delicate work (e.g., drawing) is best performed when the elbow is supported to help reduce static loads in the muscles of the back. A good working height is about 2–4 in. above the elbow.

The best working height for **lighter work** while standing is 2–4 in. below the elbow.

When performing **manual work**, the worker often needs space for tools, materials, and containers of various kinds. A suitable height for these is 4–6 in. below the elbow.

Heavier work, involving much effort and use of the weight of the upper part of the body (e.g., woodworking or heavy assembly work), should be done at a lower working surface, from 6–16 in. below the height depending on the force required.

If the employer cannot provide adjustable workstations, working heights should be set for the tallest worker and accommodate shorter workers by giving them something to stand on.

The **maximum speed** of operation for manual jobs carried out in front of the body is achieved by keeping the elbows down at the sides and the arms bent at a right angle.

Standing

Workers required to stand for prolonged periods are at an increased risk for back injuries. Standing workstations should provide a sit-stand stool, prop seat, or foot railing to relieve some of the stress on the lower back. Antifatigue matting, with a minimum 0.5-in. thickness (Redfern & Chaffin, 1988), should also be provided to relieve lower extremity and back stress.

---

*This section was modified from E. Grandjean. (1988). *Fitting the task to the man* (4th ed.). New York: Taylor & Francis.

Seating

Seat design should meet the anthropometric dimensions of the worker population. A number of recommendations have been published regarding chair design. The ANSI (1988) standard on video display terminals is frequently referenced for office seating guidelines. A chair feature checklist is presented in Figure 10-5. The critical seat features include seat height, seatpan depth, width, and slope. The backrest dimensions of interest are the backrest height, horizontal adjustment, lumbar support location, width, shape, and contour. The important armrest features are the armrest height, length, width, and the width between the armrests.

Reach Distances

Shoulder fatigue develops quickly as the shoulder flexes forward. Overhead reaching and static holding activities increase the risk for back, shoulder, and upper extremity injuries. Overhead reach distances should be set for the shortest worker; this ensures the majority of the workers will be able to reach the shelf or object. Generally, it is not possible to place all of the objects within the shortest worker's reach distance, in which case two basic workstation design principles (importance principle and frequency of use principle) can be applied in designing the reach distances. The important and frequently used items, tools, and equipment should be placed to accommodate the shortest worker. Where possible, the *individual* worker's reach envelope should determine the placement of objects, equipment, and materials. Whenever possible, static holding activities should be eliminated, using jigs, fixtures, or counterbalances.

Video Display Terminal Work

The majority of problems seen in the office can be easily resolved by rearranging the workstation, providing appropriate equipment and seating, and modifying the work pattern, either by increasing the frequency of rest breaks or interspersing nonstressful tasks throughout the work day. Each of the office components and recommendations is discussed in turn below (ANSI, 1988; Eastman Kodak,

1986; Grandjean, 1987; Huchingson, 1981; Lopez, 1993; Sanders & McCormick, 1993).

1. Desk. The type of desk determines the ergonomist's design approach. An adjustable desk is optimal. The adjustable desk allows the monitor height, wrist position, elbow angle, and thigh clearance to be fit to the individual worker. If the desk is not adjustable or funds are limited, the chair must allow proper worker positioning for the fixed work surface. Occasionally, the work surface is too low for the worker: it is a simple matter to elevate the work surface with blocks or commercially produced devices.

2. Chair. The chair is the single most important piece of office equipment. Chair features were previously discussed. A good chair allows optimal positioning of the worker based on the type of work performed.

3. Footrest. Shorter workers often are forced to sit dangling their feet or without reaching the backrest of the chair. This situation can lead to lower extremity circulation problems and back pain. If the worker must be raised to a fixed work surface, a footrest must be included in the workstation arrangement.

4. Monitor. The monitor position should be adjusted to accommodate the individual worker's preferred viewing distance (usually 500 mm, or 20 in., or more) and viewing angle (between 0 and 60 degrees). The monitor should be placed as close as possible to the worker's medial plane but no more than 35 degrees from the medial plane. If the worker uses prescription glasses or contacts, the preferred viewing distance may vary depending on the type of visual limitations. If the worker uses bifocals or trifocals, the preferred viewing angle is generally lower.

5. Keyboard. The keyboard should be placed at a height that allows the worker to keep the elbows between 75 and 135 degrees of flexion. Shoulder angles should not exceed 10 degrees of flexion, extension, or abduction. The design of the traditional rectangular keyboard forces the worker to assume a position of ulnar deviation and wrist extension. There are many alternatively designed keyboards that improve the wrist position; however, these keyboards do not eliminate all of the risk factors in the office environment and can only be considered part of the overall solution. User acceptance is critical. Many of the alternate design keyboards are not well accepted by the users. The ergonomics

team should arrange user testing of these keyboards on a trial basis before purchase.

6. Document. The document should be positioned as close to the monitor as possible. This allows the worker to maintain a neutral head and neck position during typing.

7. Environment: Lighting. Eye strain is the most common complaint among office workers. Inadequate lighting and direct and indirect glare cause many of the vision-related problems seen in the office. Direct glare is caused by light sources in the field of view; whereas indirect glare is caused by light being reflected by a surface in the field of view. Solutions to common lighting problems are as follows:

- Position the monitor so that it is perpendicular to the light source (windows, overhead lights, task lighting).
- Reduce the source of glare by covering windows and baffling ceiling light fixtures, allowing light to be evenly dispersed.
- Use diffuse indirect lighting rather than direct lighting.
- Keep lighting levels within the recommended levels based on the type of work performed.
- Ensure task lighting does not create new glare sources.
- Ensure the luminance ratio for VDT work meets the recommended 1:3 ratio between the monitor screen and immediate surrounding area and 1:10 for remote areas.
- Avoid high luminance sources in the peripheral field of view.
- Move or tilt the screen so that reflections are not in the field of view.

Manual Materials Handling

Solutions to material handling problems involve changes to the workstation, job, or containers and tools. The design approaches listed below can reduce or eliminate many of the risk factors seen in materials handling tasks (Chaffin & Andersson, 1991; Eastman Kodak, 1986; Huchingson, 1981; Sanders & McCormick, 1993).

1. Workstation. The workstation design should optimize the horizontal and vertical position of the load, while considering the individual anthropometric dimensions of the workers (such as height and reach envelope). Suggestions for reducing or eliminating workstation design problems are listed below.

- Change the work area layout so that all material is provided at work level, rather than from the floor or overhead; this can involve a change in height of either the work surface or the worker level.
- Provide ways to adjust the height of materials to be handled so that less lifting and more sliding can be done (e.g., provide a spring-loaded cart that automatically raises the materials in the cart or scissors table to adjust the height of the load).
- Minimize the horizontal distance between the starting and ending points of a lift (minimize carrying and travel distance).
- Limit stacking heights to the shoulder height of operators.
- Keep heavy objects at knuckle height of the operators.
- Locate objects to be handled within the arm reach envelope of the operator.
- Avoid the use of deep shelves that require the operator to bend and reach to obtain objects toward the rear of the shelves.
- Design work areas to provide sufficient space for the entire body to turn.
- Provide space for in-process inventory in production line operations so time pressure does not drive the handler.
- Use gravity to move material wherever practical, such as gravity-fed conveyors.

2. Job. Reducing static work is important in reducing the worker's physiologic stress and risk of injury. Most tasks involve both static and dynamic work, but in many cases the static component is the limiting performance factor. Static work frequently results in local muscle fatigue even for short-duration activities. Acceptable limits for dynamic work range from minutes to hours, whereas acceptable limits for static work durations are measured in seconds and minutes. In the design of jobs, reducing the static component of any task can prevent local muscle fatigue from limiting productivity.

- Decrease the weight of the object being handled.
- Assign the handling to two or more persons.
- Change the type of manual materials handling activity—lifting, lowering, pushing, pulling, car-

rying, and holding are types of manual materials handling. It is preferable for a job to require lowering rather than lifting, pulling rather than carrying, and pushing rather than pulling.

- Maximize the time available to perform the job by reducing the frequency of lift, or by incorporating work-rest schedules or job rotation programs.
- Rotate people to a lighter job after 1–2 hours in a constant handling task.
- Automate production handling and storage functions when possible.

3. Containers and tools. The types and design of tools and equipment used for manual materials handling can also influence the risk factors a worker is exposed to. Suggestions for decreasing risk include the following:

- Reduce the size of the container.
- Reduce the container weight (e.g., use plastic drums rather than metal drums).
- Distribute the load into two or more containers.
- Change the shape of the object or the location of handholds to allow the object to be handled close to the body.
- Provide good handholds on containers or objects to be handled.
- Use mechanical aids (hoists, lift trucks, lift tables, cranes, elevating conveyors, gravity dumps, chutes).
- Use devices such as handles and grips to provide better control of the handled object.
- Balance the contents of containers.
- Provide rigid containers for increased operator control of the object.
- Avoid lifting excessively wide objects from the floor level.
- Provide carts, carrier bags, or handling aids to support the weight of objects that have to be carried for more than a minute or more than a few feet.
- Provide tools to help in hand-applied forces.
- Use jigs and fixtures to reduce the requirement for holding in assembly tasks.

Hand Tools

Hand tools, in one form or another, are used in many human occupations. Improperly designed tools can lead to injuries, accidents, and cumulative trauma disorders. Common problems seen with hand tools include awkward positions, mechanical compression, vibration, and forceful exertions. Hand-tool design shortcomings are generally easy to identify (a hand-tool assessment checklist is presented in Figure 10-3) and the majority of these problems can be resolved by applying some basic principles (Chaffin & Andersson, 1991; Greenberg & Chaffin, 1989; Pentikis, 1995; Sanders & McCormick, 1993).

- Use special purpose tools.
- Use lightweight, well-balanced or counter-balanced tools.
- Use a tool balancer, holder, or jig if prolonged use or holding is required.
- Design tools for use by both hands.
- Use power hand tools whenever possible.
- Use the best grip for the task, such as a "power grip" when high force is required.
- Ensure appropriate tool handle thickness, shape, and length.
- If the tool is used with gloves, design the handle thickness, shape, and material to allow safe and comfortable use with the gloves.
- Design tools with compressible and nonconductive handles, without sharp edges.
- Bend the tool handle (when appropriate), not the worker.
- Select tools that minimize stress on muscles and tendons.
- Ensure adequate finger clearance if trigger use is required.
- Provide a two-directional swivel for pneumatic-tool hose connections.
- Cover power tool handles with vibration dampening material.
- Ensure all tools are properly maintained and calibrated.

References

American National Standards Institute. (1988). *American national standard for human factors engineering of visual display terminals workstations* (ANSI/HFS Standard No. 100–1988). Santa Monica, CA: Human Factors Society.

Chaffin, D.B., & Andersson, G.B. (1991). *Occupational biomechanics* (2nd ed.). New York: Wiley & Sons.

Eastman Kodak Company, Human Factors Section. (1986). *Ergonomic design for people at work* (Vols. 1–2). New York: Van Nostrand Reinhold.

Grandjean, E. (1987). *Ergonomics in computerized offices.* New York: Taylor & Francis.

Greenberg, L., & Chaffin, D. (1989).*Workers and their tools.* Midland, MI: Pendell Publishing.

Huchingson, R.D. (1981). *New horizons for human factors in design.* New York: McGraw-Hill.

Lopez, M. (1993). An ergonomic evaluation of the design and performance of four keyboard models and their relevance to carpal tunnel syndrome. Unpublished doctoral dissertation, Texas A&M University, College Station, TX.

National Aeronautics and Space Administration. (1978). *Anthropometric source book—A handbook of anthropometric data* (NASA Report No. RP–1024). Springfield, VA: National Technical Information Service.

Pentikis, J. (1995). *Handtool assessment checklist.* Aberdeen Proving Ground, MD: U.S. Army Center for Health Promotion and Preventive Medicine.

Redfern, M., & Chaffin, D. (1988). The effects of floor types on standing tolerance in industry. In F. Aghazadeh (Ed.), *Trends in ergonomics/human factors V* (pp. 901–905). New York: Elsevier.

Sanders, M.S., & McCormick, E.J. (1993). *Human factors in engineering and design.* New York: McGraw-Hill.

Chapter 11

Physical Factors Case Study: Reducing Hazards During Highway Tunnel Construction

Bryan Buchholz and Victor Paquet

Learning Objectives

On completion of this chapter, the reader should be able to

- Perform a simple job analysis to identify and control exposures that are potential hazards for developing musculoskeletal disorders.

Key Words

Ergonomic job analysis
Construction
Musculoskeletal disorders
Intervention

Abstract

During many manual construction activities, workers are exposed to designs that are not ergonomically configured; that is, the designs do not fit the characteristics and capabilities of the workers. Thus, hazardous exposures exist that increase workers' risk for developing work-related musculoskeletal disorders. An evaluation of the job tasks involved in the ceiling-panel assembly operation in the third harbor tunnel of the Central Artery/Tunnel (CA/T) construction project in Boston was carried out to identify and reduce the hazards of the tasks involved. Each assembly operation employed 10 iron workers, each of whom performed one of four job tasks. The researchers divided each job task into activities and evaluated each activity for hazards using a systematic ergonomic job analysis. This analysis was used to identify the potentially hazardous activities and to list the work-related causes of the hazards (equipment or tool design, work organization). In the analysis, hazards were identified for the trunk, legs, shoulders, hands, wrists, and neck. These hazards included repetitive motions of the wrist and arms, forceful whole-body and hand exertions, awkward body postures, and localized contact stresses. The most frequently observed hazards were static, nonneutral body postures induced by low work heights, heavy pushing of ceiling panels on the assembly line, and forceful, repetitive hand movements with contact stresses during bolting activities.

Recommendations for the redesign of the assembly line to reduce the hazards were suggested. An operation was subsequently developed at a different location in the tunnel that was identical to the first, with the exception of having several of the recommended design changes. A follow-up evaluation on the redesigned operation found that approximately 43% of the previously identified hazards had been eliminated or reduced. This study demonstrates how hazards can be systematically evaluated and reduced with relatively simple and inexpensive interventions for the prevention of musculoskeletal injuries.

Introduction

Construction workers show elevated risks of developing work-related musculoskeletal disorders

(WRMDs) of the back and of the upper and lower extremities (Damlund et al., 1982; Burkhart et al., 1993; Holstrom et al., 1993). Although WRMDs are quite common in construction work, little has been done in the United States to systematically characterize the hazards for specific construction trades and operations (Schneider & Susi, 1994). Even less effort has been devoted to reducing these exposures.

The CA/T construction project in Boston is currently the largest public works project in the United States. The two main components of the project are (1) the building of a new underground highway, which runs beneath the city and connects freeways from the north and south, and (2) the construction of a third tunnel beneath Boston Harbor linking Logan Airport to downtown Boston.

The Construction Occupational Health Project (COHP) at the Department of Work Environment at the University of Massachusetts, Lowell, is funded by the National Institute for Occupational Safety and Health (NIOSH) through the Center to Protect Workers' Rights as part of a nationwide research effort to reduce WRMDs in the construction industry. The CA/T construction project has served as the site of the COHP's efforts to evaluate the hazards involved in large-scale highway construction projects. As part of this effort, the COHP has evaluated various finishing operations in the recently completed Ted Williams Tunnel, including wall plastering, wall tiling, ventilation duct panel installation, handrail installation, ceiling module assembly, and ceiling module installation. These operations are performed by a variety of union trades such as plasterers, tile mechanics and finishers, iron workers, and laborers.

The contractor responsible for the finishing operations in the tunnel recorded eight injuries on the Occupational Safety and Health Administration logs (OSHA-200 logs), over a 6-week period. Although this contractor employed many construction trades on this site, only iron workers had been injured during this period. Of the eight injuries, six were related to overexertion of the musculoskeletal system: two back strains, two shoulder strains, and two knee or ankle injuries. The contractor's site safety officer requested the COHP perform an analysis of the ceiling module assembly operation, which he considered to be hazardous. During this operation, iron workers assembled individual ceiling panels into 10-panel modules, which were later hung from the tunnel's ceiling.

Researchers conducted the evaluation to summarize some of the hazards found in the ceiling module assembly operation, and to provide recommendations for reducing the hazards and thus minimize the risk of future WRMDs. First, one assembly operation was evaluated and the resulting design recommendations to reduce hazards were given to the contractor. Later, the contractor developed a similar operation that included many of the design recommendations, and the hazards for the job tasks were re-evaluated with a similar analysis to determine which of the hazards had been eliminated or reduced.

Analysis

General Ergonomic Analysis Methods

The goal of an ergonomic job analysis is to identify the design aspects of a job that increase a worker's exposure to risk factors for WRMDs, in order to reduce these exposures. The commonly cited risk factors for WRMDs are

- Repetitive motions or prolonged activities
- Forceful exertions
- Awkward postures
- Localized contact stresses
- Temperature extremes
- Vibration

The analysis attempts to characterize the magnitude and duration of these exposures. An understanding of the entire work process is also important, so that interventions may be effectively targeted. Therefore, a systematic ergonomic job analysis similar to that described by Keyserling et al. (1991) is used in an ergonomic evaluation to identify the hazardous activities and list the work-related causes of these hazards (equipment or tool design, work organization). The steps involved in the ergonomic evaluation used in this study are listed in Table 11-1.

The initial steps in the ergonomic evaluation are used to describe the various levels of the overall work process. A taxonomy, or classification system, has been developed to aid in the description of the heavy highway construction process (Buchholz et al., 1996). The contents of this taxonomy are based on the "Standard Specifications for Highways and Bridges" used by the Massachusetts Highway

Table 11-1. Ergonomic Job Analysis Items

1. Describe the general process and construction stage.
   a. Identify the contractor for the construction site.
   b. Identify the operations being performed.
2. Describe the operation (number of workers, trades involved, locals, machinery, location on site).
   a. Provide a list of the workers (name, description, trade, level, years in trade, injury, symptoms, etc.).
   b. Describe work schedule (shift duration and scheduled breaks).
   c. Describe work pace for each job task (use interviews and observations).
   d. Describe job rotation (if any).
   e. Sketch layout of work area.
3. Describe each job task, break it into activities and identify ergonomic exposures.
   a. Identify ergonomic risk factors for each body region (back, arms, legs, and neck).
   b. Provide a list of tools and equipment, identifying factors influencing exposure level.
   c. Identify tasks/activities that need further evaluation.
4. Design and implement ergonomic interventions.
   a. List possible interventions for reducing hazards.
   b. Prioritize interventions based on anticipated effectiveness and feasibility.
   c. Implement appropriate interventions.
5. Re-evaluate the job tasks after interventions are made.
   a. Identify ergonomic risk factors for each activity of each job task.
   b. Identify tasks/activities that need further evaluation.
   c. List possible ideas for reducing hazards.

Department (1988). The taxonomy is organized hierarchically, with construction projects broken into a series of *stages* and, on a large construction project, different stages can be under way simultaneously along the length of the site. The primary stages in heavy highway construction are earthworks, drainage, paving, curbs and edging, fences and walls, and structures. Each stage may be composed of several *operations,* which are overseen by a foreman and other on-site supervisors and are completed by at least one crew of workers. Each operation consists of *job tasks* that are performed by an individual worker from a specific trade, which is usually defined jurisdictionally (i.e., construction trades negotiate for the right to perform specific job tasks). *Activities* are the fundamental acts required to complete a job task and are based on *work elements* (e.g., lift, carry, reach, grasp, and move) taken from the time-study methodology traditionally used by industrial engineers (Barnes, 1980). Because the taxonomy allows an analysis to be stratified by construction stage, operation, and task, as well as by the trades involved in each operation, it provides the means for achieving a task-based analysis. A comparable taxonomy could be developed for other industries to facilitate a similar task-based analysis.

The first step in the evaluation methodology then is to determine the stages and operations that are under way at the site. Workplace organization can have an important impact on the hazards, and therefore information about the operation's shift schedule, production demands, the physical layout, and material flow is obtained. This information is important for understanding the purpose of the operation of interest, how it is impacted by other operations and how it impacts other operations.

The operation to be studied is described in the second step using observationally collected information. To aid in this description, a narrative of the operation is obtained from engineers, supervisors, and workers on site. The gathered information includes a description of crew size and structure, a description of the work schedule and pace, and a sketch of the layout of the work area. The operation is then divided into job tasks performed by individual workers. Written documentation of the work (such as contract, engineering specifications or production schedules) may provide additional useful information.

In the third step, each job task is described and further divided into activities, listing the tools, equipment, and materials used. If possible, the work cycle is defined (i.e., a repeated set of activities are described in the order that they occur). This is usually difficult in the construction industry, because much of the work is noncyclical or the work cycles

Table 11-2. Important Ergonomic Risk Factors and the Guidelines Used to Identify Them

1. Repetitive motions
   a. Hand/wrist motions repeated once per second[1,2]
   b. Sustained static exertions[3]
2. Forceful exertions
   a. Whole body exertions >50 lb required to lift, push, or pull[4]
   b. Grip forces >10 lb[1]
3. Awkward (non-neutral) postures
   a. Trunk flexion >45 degrees[5]
   b. Trunk lateral bending or twist >20 degrees[5]
   c. Neck flexion or twist >30 degrees[6]
   d. Shoulder flexion or abduction >60 degrees[7]
   e. Wrist flexion/extension >45 degrees[2,8]
   f. Wrist radial/ulnar deviation >20 degrees[2,8]
   g. Pinch postures[2,8]
   h. Sustained kneeling or squatting[9,10]
4. Localized contract stresses[8]
5. Temperature extremes
   a. Heat[11]
   b. Cold[8]
6. Vibration
   a. Whole-body[12,13]
   b. Segmental (hand-arm)[14]

[1]Silverstein et al., 1986
[2]Armstrong et al., 1982
[3]Rohmert, 1973
[4]Waters et al., 1993
[5]Punnett et al., 1991
[6]Kilbom & Persson, 1987
[7]Bjelle et al., 1979[1]

[8]Armstrong, 1986
[9]Thun et al., 1987
[10]Felson et al., 1991
[11]Snook & Ciriello, 1974
[12]Wikstrom et al., 1994
[13]Seidel & Heide, 1986
[14]NIOSH, 1989

are long and irregular. However, in large heavy highway construction projects, workers usually perform the same daily job tasks for an operation, which takes weeks or months to complete, and some operations are even performed on temporary assembly lines.

Each job task is then analyzed for exposure to the risk factors for WRMDs. A checklist is usually used for this purpose. The advantages of a checklist are that it is fast, simple, and inexpensive to use. The primary disadvantage is that it gives no detail on the magnitude or duration of the exposure. Direct measurements using a force gauge, stop watch, tape measure, or goniometer can be used to add detail to the analysis. A systematic ergonomic job analysis similar to that described by Keyserling et al. (1991) is then used

to identify the potentially hazardous activities and list the work-related causes of the hazards (such as equipment or tool design, work organization). Hazards are identified for the trunk, neck, shoulders, hands, wrists, and legs. Some of the important ergonomic risk factors found in the literature and the guidelines used to identify them are shown in Table 11-2.

A number of methods are available, if a more detailed analysis is desired. More detail can improve intervention targeting and provide a better measure for evaluation. For example, estimates of the percent of time workers spend in awkward postures or the frequency of wrist posture deviations for activities and tasks can be estimated. Methods for detailed evaluation of posture and motion range from direct observations (Buchholz et al., 1996; Karhu et al., 1977) to methods using videotape (Armstrong et al., 1982; Keyserling, 1986) and to electrogoniometers, which are instruments for detailed posture and motion measurement (Marras et al., 1993). The level of detail in an ergonomic analysis is usually determined by logistical considerations, such as time and resources.

The fourth step in this process is to design and implement interventions to control the workers' exposure to the identified risk factors. Ideally, this should be a collaborative effort between the ergonomist, workers, management, and other stakeholders. The final step of the ergonomic method is to re-evaluate each of the job tasks for hazards using the same analysis that was used in the original evaluation, so that comparisons can be made between the pre- and post-intervention operations.

Specific Methods

In this study, three researchers observed the operation for approximately 4 hours on each of 4 days over a 2-week period. Each job task was carefully observed for five to ten work cycles. The cycle of activities was recorded and the time needed to complete a cycle (cycle time) was determined to provide estimates of the frequency of activities performed throughout the shift. The hazards for each activity were identified using a checklist-like approach. In some cases the hazards were quantified using direct measurements (frequency of repetitive hand motions, load weights or forces, exposure duration), but in most cases the hazards were only identified. Equipment or work area design problems thought to be the cause of the hazards were also noted. Still photographs were taken to document the hazards for each job task. Temperature extremes and vibration were not considered a problem because of the relatively mild climate inside the tunnel and only nonvibrating hand tools were used.

Recommendations to improve the design of the operation were given to the Site Safety Officer. Some of these recommendations were incorporated in another assembly line that was later constructed for this operation. One researcher observed the operation on the new assembly line for 2 hours on three occasions. Again, information about the work area layout and equipment used was collected. The operation was divided into job tasks and each job task was divided into activities. The hazards associated with each of the activities were then identified. The hazards were then compared to those of the original operation.

Results of the Initial Ergonomic Evaluation

Stage and Operation

The ceiling module assembly operation that was evaluated was part of the tunnel finishing stage of highway construction. Other operations in this stage include wall plastering, wall tiling, paving, guard rail installation, and ceiling module installation. Because attaching individual panels to the tunnel's ceiling would be difficult and time consuming, the contractor decided that it would be more efficient to first assemble groups of 10 panels together before installing them. Therefore, an assembly line that could accommodate a 10-panel module was constructed. An overhead monorail system was installed so that panels could be moved along the line. Pallets of panels and steel were delivered to the assembly line, and a large truck having a hydraulic flat bed was used to take the completed modules from the line and position the modules close to the ceiling for installation. The assembly line was located in one of the widest sections of the tunnel to minimize disrup-

tion of the other construction operations. When the assembly line was set up, little consideration was given to how well the characteristics of the line were suited for the workers assembling the ceiling modules.

The layout of the assembly line is shown in Figure 11-1. The work area was approximately 250 feet long and the assembly line was located 20 in. above floor level. Individual ceiling panels were 4×11.5 feet and weighed approximately 700 lb. The panels and steel connector beams were moved and lifted onto an assembly line with powered lifts. The lifts were activated with a four-button control and virtually eliminated manual lifting of the panels and connecting steel. However, panels and steel were manually adjusted (pushed or pulled across the rollers) after being placed on the assembly line. A crew of 10 iron workers (one woman and nine men) participated in the operation. The crew worked a standard 8-hour shift (7 AM to 3 PM). Job tasks were performed at a moderate, steady pace. The crew did not rotate among the various job tasks.

Job Tasks and Hazards

The operation was divided into four job tasks:

1. *Panel sorting.* Ceiling panels and beams required for assembly were sorted with one of the monorail's powered lifts.

2. *Panel preparation.* Rubber gaskets were glued onto the ceiling panels and the panels were delivered to the submodule assembly using the powered lift.

3. *Submodule assembly.* Sets of three to four panels were aligned and connected with steel l-beams and H-beams.

4. *Module assembly.* Submodules were bolted together into one 10-panel module.

Each assembled module was then connected to another of the monorail's lifts and loaded onto a truck having a hydraulic flat bed. In a separate operation, the module was later delivered to the installation location.

The cycle or sequence of activities for each job task was identified (Table 11-3). Cycle times for job tasks was variable, but the order in which workers performed the activities during a job task was relatively consistent. Each of the job tasks and the activities for which hazards were found are

TOP VIEW

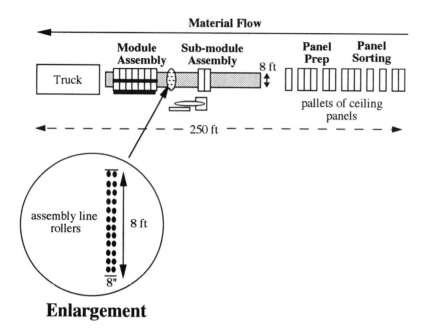

SIDE VIEW

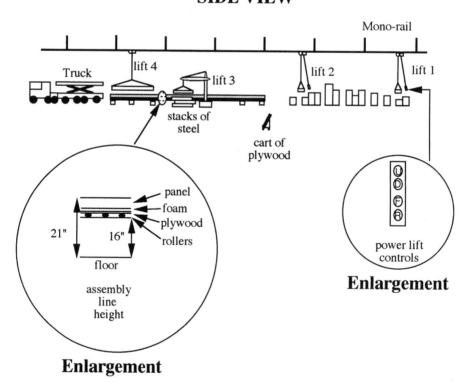

Figure 11-1. Ceiling module assembly operation.

Table 11-3. Job Tasks and Cycles of Activities During Ceiling Module Assembly

Number of Workers	Major Activities
Panel sorting and stacking (cycles ranged between 1 and 10 minutes)	
2	Wrap strap around ends of pallet and connect strap to lifting cable
1	Operate powered lifter
1	Guide load
2	Disconnect strap from cable and unwrap strap from ends of pallet
Panel preparation (cycles ranged between 6 and 25 minutes)	
1	Use powered air-hose to blow screw holes clean of debris
1	Screw hooks into four corner screw holes
1	Wipe edges of panel with rag
1	Retrieve bolts, gaskets, and glue bottles
2	Align gaskets along edges of panel
2	Brush glue along panel edges
2	Brush glue on gasket
2	Glue gaskets onto panels*
2	Cut excess gasket with scissors*
2	Operate powered lift, guide load, place panel onto rollers
2	Push panel down assembly line*
2	Take out corner hooks
1	Operate powered lift to pick up new ceiling panel
1	Perform miscellaneous clean-up (align boards, etc.)
1	Screw hooks into new panel
Submodule assembly (cycles ranged between 20 and 70 minutes)	
2	Align three or four panels on rollers*
2	Retrieve clamps
2	Clamp together submodule
2	Retrieve rubber gaskets and glue bottles
2	Align gaskets
1	Retrieve cart of wood, place wood in cart
2	Brush glue along submodule
1	Position washers, nuts, bolts near holes
1	Glue gasket onto submodule*
2	Hook lift to I-beam
2	Operate lift/guide load
1	Press gasket onto submodule
2	Push submodule under I-beam
2	Align I-beam with pins*
2	Bolt I-beam to panels*
1	Hook lift to H-beam, operate powered lift
1	Continue ratchet work
1	Align H-beam on pins*
1	Bolt H-beam to submodule*
1	Tighten bolts with 45 ft-lb ratchet*
2	Unhook clamps
Module assembly (cycles ranged between 60 and 200 minutes)	
1	Push submodule 1 down the assembly line*
1	Align submodule 1
1	Push submodule 2 down the assembly line*
1	Align submodule 2
3	Get ratchets, wrenches, and bolts
2	Put brackets and hardware on I-beams and H-beams

Table 11-3. *Continued*

Number of Workers	Major Activities
1	Push submodule 3 down the assembly line*
1	Align submodule 3
2	Bolt brackets to submodules 24 times*
2	Tighten down brackets with a 350 ft-lb calibrated torque wrench 8 times
1	Hook winch to assembled module
1	Operate powered winch to move module*

*Potential hazards.

described below. The hazards for each of the listed activities and related work area design problems are summarized in Table 11-4.

Panel Sorting. Two iron workers sorted the ceiling panels and connecting steel with one of the monorail's lifts (one worker operated the lift, the other guided the panel). The panels were sorted in the order in which they were to be assembled. Each ceiling panel had been tagged with an alphanumeric identification code. The activities in this job task were not considered particularly hazardous.

Panel Preparation. Two iron workers retrieved individual ceiling panels with another of the monorail's lifts, and stacked them near the assembly line. The iron workers glued rubber gaskets onto the ceiling panels and then delivered the panels to the assembly line using the powered lift. The panels were lowered onto plywood sheets, which protected the panels from being damaged by the rollers and were pushed manually on the rollers to the submodule assembly. Potential hazards were identified for three activities:

1. *Gluing the gasket onto the panel.* The gaskets were carefully aligned and pressed against the glued submodules. The work height was at or below waist level (depending on where the panel was located during the sorting job task) for more than half of the work cycles observed. When the work height was low the workers flexed their trunk more than 45 degrees (usually close to 90 degrees) or squatted when pressing the gasket onto the panel in order to view the gaskets. The workers assumed these postures for approximately 2–5 minutes each time they glued the gasket onto a panel that was at or below waist height.

2. *Cutting the excess gasket with scissors (Figure 11-2).* Cutting the excess gasket was also an activity requiring a high degree of precision and therefore the worker again kept the gasket near the eyes. The worker flexed the trunk or squatted while cutting the gasket, although such postures were usually maintained less than 1 minute.

3. *Pushing the panel down the assembly line.* This was the most physical activity during panel preparation. After each panel was placed on the assembly line of rollers it was manually pushed 10–30 feet down the assembly line. Because the height of the panel when on the assembly line was approximately 21 in., the workers were required to flex or twist their trunk over 45 degrees while pushing. Workers also mentioned that it was sometimes difficult to push the panels because the plywood did not roll easily on the rollers.

Submodule Assembly. Sets of three or four panels were aligned by one or two iron workers. Steel beams were aligned with a powered crane lift (not on the monorail) and bolted to the ceiling panels to form a submodule by two iron workers. Potential hazards were identified for five activities:

1. *Aligning the panels on rollers (Figure 11-3).* The workers were required to flex or twist their trunks over 45 degrees and usually twist their necks while aligning the panels. The weight of the panels placed high forces on the workers' backs and shoulders while pushing the panels.

2. *Gluing the gasket onto the submodule (Figure 11-4).* The workers were required to flex their trunks more than 45 degrees or squat when pressing the gasket onto the submodule. The workers assumed these postures for approximately 2–5 minutes for each gasket.

3. *Aligning the steel with the pins (Figure 11-5).* The steel I- and H-beams each weighed more than 200 lb and the workers were required to push or pull the

Table 11-4. Summary of the Potential Hazards Identified for Each Job Task

Activity	Body Area	Highly Repetitive Motions	High Forces	Static Non-Neutral Postures	Contact Stresses	Work Area Design Problems
Panel preparation						
Gluing gasket onto panel	Trunk			√		Low work surface
	Legs			√		
Cutting excess gasket with	Trunk			√		
scissors	Legs			√		Low work surface
Pushing panel down	Trunk		√	√		Winch not accessible
assembly line						or fast enough
Submodule assembly						
Aligning the panels on	Trunk		√	√		Manual alignment required
rollers	Neck		√	√		and work surface is low
	Shoulder					
Gluing the gaskets onto	Trunk			√		
the submodule	Neck			√		Low work surface
Aligning the steel with	Trunk		√	√		
the pin	Neck			√	√	Low work surface
	Legs					
Bolting the steel to the	Trunk		√	√		Low work surface and
panels	Shoulder	√	√		√	tighten bolts manually
	Hand/Wrist			√	√	
	Legs					
Tightening the bolts with	Trunk		√	√		Low work surface and
the 45 ft-lb ratchet	Shoulder	√	√		√	tighten bolts manually
	Hand/Wrist		√	√	√	
	Legs					
Module assembly						
Pushing submodule down	Trunk		√	√		Winch not accessible or
assembly line	Shoulder		√			fast enough
Tightening bolts	Trunk			√		Low work surface and
	Neck		√	√		tighten bolts manually
	Shoulder	√	√		√	
	Hand/Wrist			√	√	
	Legs					
Operating powered winch	Trunk			√		Winch low
	Legs			√		

beams manually to align them. While doing this, the workers had to flex their trunks over 45 degrees and assume squatting or kneeling postures and remain in these postures for as much as 3 or 4 minutes.

4. *Bolting the steel to the panels.* Two beams were each attached to a submodule with approximately 10 bolts. For each bolt, the workers usually had to flex their trunks greater than 45 degrees or squat or kneel for up to 1 minute. During this time, the workers flexed or extended their wrist at least 45 degrees approximately 60 times. Therefore, workers assembling submodules deviated their wrists approximately 300 times per submodule (two workers connected the 10 bolts).

5. *Tightening bolts with the 45 ft-lb ratchet.* One worker finished tightening each of the bolts with a ratchet calibrated to 45 ft-lb. This activity required the worker to jerk the ratchet toward his body during each turn of the bolt. This was done until the bolt was tightened the desired 45 ft-lb, at which time the ratchet released its resistance (slipped). The worker usually assumed a three-point crawling (knees and one hand on panel) or kneeling posture while using the ratchet.

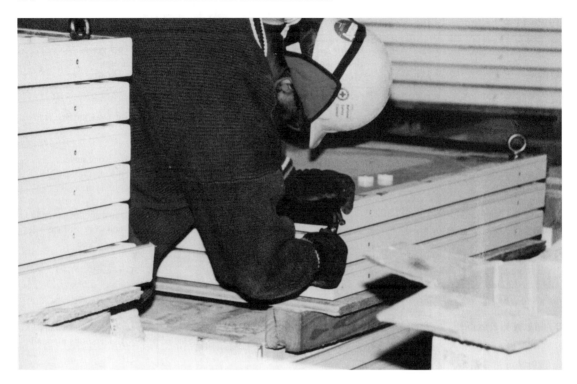

Figure 11-2. A low work height forced the worker to flex his trunk when cutting the excess gasket during panel preparation.

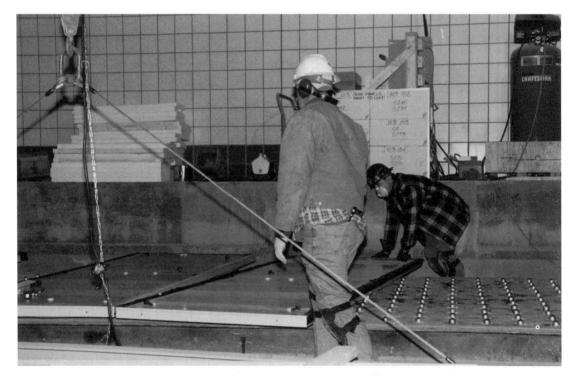

Figure 11-3. Workers aligned the panel on the rollers for the submodule assembly. The weight of the panel (approximately 700 lb) and the low height of the assembly line resulted in non-neutral postures of the trunk and neck and high forces on the shoulders and back.

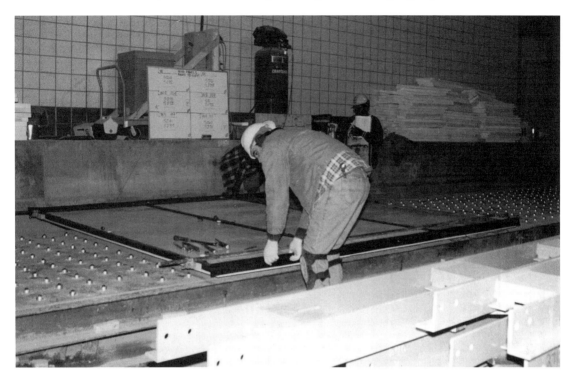

Figure 11-4. The worker flexed his trunk while gluing the gasket during submodule assembly because the assembly line height was below his knees.

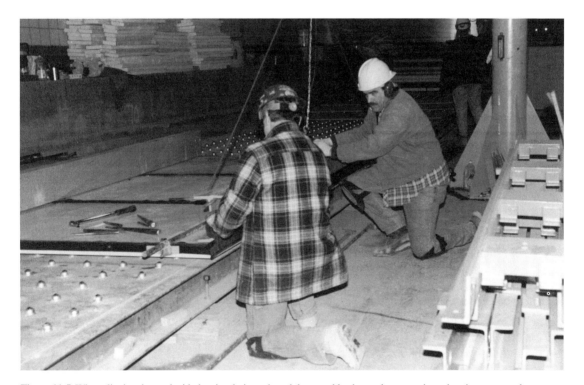

Figure 11-5. When aligning the steel with the pins during submodule assembly, the workers experienced static non-neutral postures of the legs and trunk and high forces on the back. The workers wore knee pads to reduce the contact stress placed on their knees.

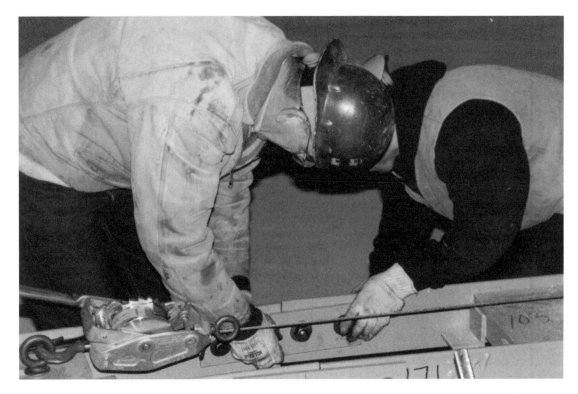

Figure 11-6. The low height of the assembly line required workers to flex their trunk while tightening the bolts that splice the submodules together into one module.

Module Assembly. Three to four iron workers manually pushed the submodules 20–60 ft. Two to four iron workers bolted groups of three submodules together into one assembled module. The iron worker foreman inspected the modules. The assembled panels were then connected to another of the monorail's lifts and positioned on the truck. Hazards were found for three activities:

1. *Pushing the submodule down the assembly line.* The three or four workers who manually pushed the submodule, weighing 2,500–3,200 lb, down the assembly line had to flex or twist their trunk greater than 45 degrees. This activity was considered to be the one that required the greatest overall exertion by the workers. This was done once every 20–70 minutes.

2. *Tightening bolts (Figure 11-6).* The workers were required to bend their trunk greater than 45 degrees while bolting the submodules together. Workers were observed with their neck flexed greater than 30 degrees during this activity. Twelve bolts were used to connect two submodules. While bolting, the workers flexed or extended their wrist at least 45 degrees approximately 60 times. Each bolt took up to 1 minute to tighten.

3. *Operating the powered winch.* The powered winch, used to move the assembled module beneath the monorail's third lift, was located below knee height. Therefore, the worker was required to assume awkward trunk and leg postures. This activity took approximately 1 minute to complete.

Summary of Potential Hazards

Some of the most stressful hazards included

1. Non-neutral trunk, neck, and leg postures caused by the low work-surface heights

2. Heavy loading and static non-neutral trunk

postures during the manual pushing of ceiling panels and submodules

3. Repetitive/forceful wrist deviations during bolting activities

Design Intervention

The researchers made several recommendations to improve the design of the assembly operation and increase worker awareness of the hazards. These recommendations were first communicated to the site safety representative verbally, and later were included in a brief report to the contractor. In the report, it was recommended that the workers be consulted before any of the interventions were implemented. It was thought that the workers should have control over which of the suggested interventions to accept, and that the workers would have the best understanding as to whether or not the recommendations would disrupt the operation. Most of the recommendations called for changes in the design of the workplace because engineering controls have been shown to be more effective than administrative controls or personal protective equipment for reducing hazards.

Recommendations for Ceiling Module Assembly

1. *Raise the height of the working surface for panel preparation.* Providing a work surface height of at least 40 in. (approximately waist height) for the panel gluing activity during panel preparation would reduce the frequency and duration of awkward trunk and leg postures during the panel preparation job task.

2. *Increase the height of the rollers and add stairs.* Increasing the height of the assembly line rollers to approximately 36 in. (slightly below waist height) would reduce the frequency and duration of non-neutral trunk and leg postures during the submodule and module assembly job tasks. Stairs would then need to be installed to allow workers to easily get on and off of the assembly line.

3. *Possible use of powered ratchets.* Using powered ratchets, calibrated to the 45 ft-lb of torque that is required in the bolting activities would reduce the frequency of wrist motions during the submodule and module assembly job tasks and reduce the duration in which workers are in non-neutral trunk postures.

4. *Improve the design of the powered winch.* The powered winch was not always used to move submodules for submodule assembly because the winch frequently malfunctioned, was not easy to use, or was not fast enough. The winch should be raised to approximately 36 in. from the floor. If feasible, the speed at which the winch pulls the submodules should be increased. A back-up winch should be purchased to replace the winch when it is not functioning properly.

5. *Provide ergonomics training.* Providing the workers with basic ergonomics training that explains the importance of maintaining neutral postures and minimizing heavy manual material handling should increase each worker's ability to recognize hazards and may help reduce the risk to musculoskeletal injury caused by hazardous work procedures.

New Design

A similar ceiling module assembly work area was later developed at a different location in the tunnel. Several improvements were made to this work area that reduced some of the hazards mentioned above. The improvements included

1. *Increased panel preparation work height (Figure 11-7).* Panels were raised with the powered lift to over 40 in. from the floor during panel preparation.

2. *Increased assembly line height (Figure 11-8).* The height of the assembly line was increased and slightly tilted downward from beginning to end so that gravity would assist the workers when pushing panels and submodules. The assembly line heights ranged from approximately 36 in. at the beginning to 18 in. at the end. This was done simply by installing sheets of wood of different heights beneath the assembly line. Stairs were installed so that workers could get on and off of the assembly line easily.

3. *Fork truck replaced powered winch.* A fork truck replaced the powered winch eliminating the awkward static trunk and leg postures when the winch was operated.

4. *Ergonomics training.* The workers in this operation received a basic 20-minute training session about body mechanics and lifting techniques for reducing stress on the lower back during manual material handling.

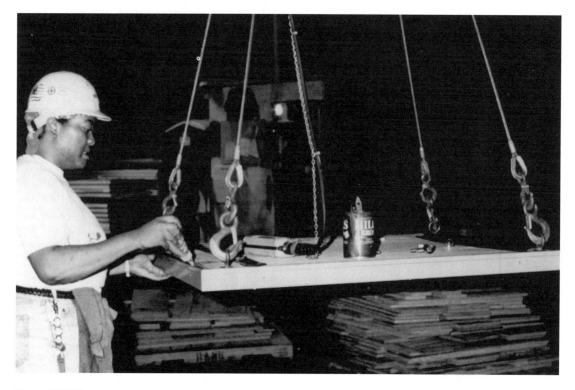

Figure 11-7. The panels were raised to a more suitable working height to reduce static non-neutral trunk and leg postures during panel preparation.

Test and Evaluation

The effectiveness of an ergonomic intervention may be evaluated by measuring the change in morbidity data (such as musculoskeletal injuries rates, absenteeism due to musculoskeletal injuries, prevalence of musculoskeletal symptoms) or the change in hazards that follows the intervention. Sometimes, morbidity or exposure data can be compared to that of a similar group of workers that are not introduced to the intervention (a control group).

It is important to understand some of the logistical difficulties that arise when evaluating an intervention. There are a variety of factors that may confound the effect of an intervention. For example, changes in production demands and economic considerations may affect absenteeism, willingness to report symptoms, and job turnover. Additionally, when only a small group of workers are affected by an intervention, it may be difficult to show a positive change in morbidity or exposure with conventional scientific methods due to a lack of statistical power. Finally, reductions in injuries or symptoms

may not immediately follow an intervention. It is therefore important to select a time interval for the intervention that is short enough to minimize the potential possibility for external changes in the workplace and long enough for the true benefit of the intervention to be observed (such as reduction in morbidity or exposure).

In this study, injury data specific to the assembly operations could not be obtained from the contractor (only trade-specific information was available). Therefore, a reassessment of the exposure to poor ergonomic design (i.e., hazards) for each of the tasks was chosen to evaluate the new assembly line. Because of the small number of workers and generally crude measures of exposure, no formal statistical tests were performed. Two important assumptions for this type of analysis are that change in exposure can be identified reliably and that the exposure is a true predictor of the musculoskeletal health outcome of concern.

The work area layout, job tasks, and number of workers performing each job task on the new assembly line were almost identical to those of the original

Figure 11-8. Wood was inserted beneath the rollers to increase the height of the assembly line. This helped reduce static non-neutral trunk and neck postures during the submodule assembly.

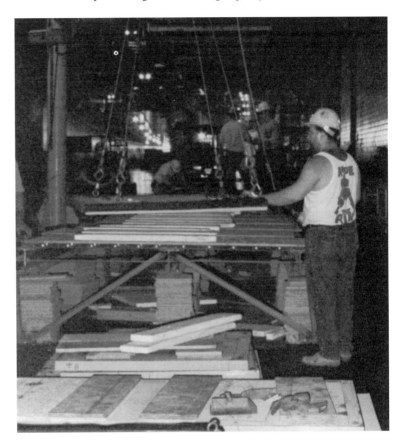

assembly line with the exception of the improvements mentioned above. The sequence of activities within each cycle as well as cycle times was also similar to the initial operation. The cost of the improvements was limited to the cost of labor and materials (wood) used to raise the height of the line. The training was provided by the researchers as a free service. (The only cost to the contractor was wages for 20 minutes for the 10 iron workers.) Slightly more than 43% of the hazards identified during the earlier operation were eliminated or reduced (Table 11-5). Static non-neutral trunk and leg postures during panel preparation were eliminated with the increased work height. The higher assembly line reduced static non-neutral trunk and leg postures during the manual handling of panels. The tilted assembly line helped reduce forces on the trunk and shoulders during manual pushing of the panels.

Non-neutral static trunk and leg postures for several activities during submodule assembly were affected very little, because workers had to work on top of the panels when aligning and bolting steel. The forceful and repetitive hand motions also remained unchanged during bolting activities. Workers had explained that powered ratchets could not be used because construction design specifications required manual bolting to obtain the desired torque.

Conclusion

Although not all hazards were eliminated with the new ceiling module assembly operation, this case study demonstrates how hazards can be systematically evaluated and how relatively simple interventions can be used to reduce hazards and help prevent musculoskeletal injuries from occurring in the future. Interventions such as assembly work heights at or above waist height, locating controls

Table 11-5. Summary of the Potential Hazards for Each Job Task with the Improved Design

Activity	Body Area	Highly Repetitive Motions	High Forces	Static Non-Neutral Postures	Contact Stresses	Work Area Design Improvements
Panel preparation						
Gluing gasket onto panel	Trunk			E/R		Height of work surface
	Legs			E/R		increased
Cutting excess gasket with scissors	Trunk					
	Legs			E/R		Height of work surface
				E/R		increased
Pushing panel down assembly line	Trunk		E/R	E/R		Assembly line height increased and tilted
Submodule assembly						
Aligning the panels on rollers	Trunk		E/R	E/R		Assembly line height
	Neck		E/R	E/R		increased
	Shoulder					
Gluing the gaskets onto the submodule	Trunk			E/R		Assembly line height
	Neck			E/R		increased
Aligning the steel with the pin	Trunk		√	√		
	Neck			√	√	
	Legs					
Bolting the steel to the panels	Trunk		√	√		
	Shoulder	√	√		√	
	Hand/wrist			√	√	
	Legs					
Tightening the bolts with the 45 ft-lb ratchet	Trunk		√	√		
	Shoulder	√	√		√	
	Hand/wrist		√	√	√	
	Legs					
Module assembly						
Pushing submodule down assembly line	Trunk		E/R	E/R		Assembly line height
	Shoulder		E/R			increased and tilted
Tightening bolts	Trunk			E/R		Assembly line height
	Neck		√	E/R		increased and tilted
	Shoulder	√	√		√	
	Hand/wrist			√	√	
	Legs					
Operating powered winch	Trunk			E/R		Winch not used
	Legs			E/R		

E/R denotes a hazard that was eliminated or reduced in the improved design.

at or above waist height, and ergonomics training may be applicable to a variety of assembly operations, including those not on construction sites.

Acknowledgments

This research was supported by the Center to Protect Workers' Rights with a grant from the National Institute for Occupational Safety and Health (NIOSH grant No. U02/CCU308771-02). The authors acknowledge Michael Grasso and William Rodwell for their assistance with data collection. The authors appreciate the active participation and cooperation of Michael Joel, Site Safety Officer for Walsh Construction Company, and members of the International Association of Bridge Structural and

Ornamental Iron Workers (Local 7), without whom this study would not have been possible.

References

Armstrong, T.J. (1986). Ergonomics and cumulative trauma disorders. *Hand Clinics, 2,* 553–565.

Armstrong, T.J., Foulke, J.A., Joseph, B.S., & Goldstein, S.A. (1982). Investigation of cumulative trauma disorders in a poultry processing plant. *American Industrial Hygiene Association Journal, 43,* 103–116.

Barnes, R. (1980). *Motion and time study: Design and measurement of work* (7th ed.) (pp. 116–128). New York: Wiley & Sons.

Bjelle, A., Hagberg, M., & Michaelsson, G. (1979). Clinical and ergonomic factors in prolonged shoulder pain among industrial workers. *Scandinavian Journal of Work Environment and Health, 5,* 205–210.

Buchholz, B., Paquet, V., Punnett, L., et al. (1996). PATH: A work sampling–based approach to ergonomic job analysis for construction work and other nonrepetitive work. *Applied Ergonomics, 26,* 177–187.

Burkhart, G., Schulte, P., Robinson, C., et al. (1993). Job tasks, potential exposures, and health risks of laborers employed in the construction industry. *American Journal of Industrial Medicine, 24,* 413–425.

Damlund, M., Goth, S., Hasle, P., & Munk, K. (1982). Low back pain and early retirement among Danish semiskilled construction workers. *Scandinavian Journal of Work, Environment & Health, 8,* 100–104.

Felson, D., Hannan, M., Naimark, A., et al. (1991). Occupational physical demands, knee bending, and knee osteoarthritis: Results from the Framingham Study. *Journal of Rheumatology, 18,* 1587–1592.

Holstrom, E., Lindell, J., & Moritz, U. (1993). Healthy lower backs in the construction industry in Sweden. *Work and Stress, 7,* 259–271.

Karhu, O., Hansi, P., & Huorinka, I. (1977). Correcting working postures in industry; a practical method for analysis. *Applied Ergonomics, 8,* 199–201.

Keyserling, W.M. (1986). Postural analysis of the trunk and shoulders in simulated real time. *Ergonomics, 29,* 569–583.

Keyserling, W.M., Armstrong, T.J., & Punnett, L. (1991). Ergonomic job analysis: A structured approach for identifying risk factors associated with overexertion injuries and disorders. *Applied Occupational and Environmental Hygiene, 6,* 352–363.

Kilbom, A., & Persson, J. (1987). Work technique and its consequences for musculoskeletal disorders. *Ergonomics, 30,* 273–279.

Marras, W.S., Lavender, S.A., Leurgans, S.E., et al. (1993). The role of dynamic three-dimensional trunk motion in occupationally related low back disorders. The effect of workplace factors, trunk position, and trunk motion characteristics on risk of injury. *Spine, 18,* 617–628.

Massachusetts Highway Department. (1988). *Standard specifications for highways and bridges.* Boston: Author.

National Institute for Occupational Safety and Health. (1989). *Criteria for a recommended standard: Occupational exposure to hand-arm vibration.* (DHHS [NIOSH] Publication No. 89–106). Cincinnati, OH: Author.

Punnett, L., Fine, L., Keyserling, W., et al. (1991). Back disorders and nonneutral trunk postures of automobile assembly workers. *Scandinavian Journal of Work Environment and Health, 17,* 337–346.

Rohmert, W. (1973). Problems in determining rest allowances. Part 1: Use of modern methods to evaluate stress and strain in static muscular work. *Applied Ergonomics, 4,* 91–95.

Schneider, S., & Susi, P. (1994). Ergonomics and construction: A review of the potential hazards in new construction. *American Industrial Hygiene Association Journal, 55,* 635–649.

Seidel, H., & Heide, R. (1986). Long-term effects of whole-body vibration: A critical survey of the literature. *International Archives of Occupational and Environmental Health, 58,* 1–26.

Silverstein, B., Fine, L., & Armstrong, T. (1986). Hand-wrist cumulative trauma disorders in industry. *British Journal of Industrial Medicine, 43,* 779–784.

Snook, S., & Ciriello, V. (1974). The effects of heat stress on manual handling tasks. *American Industrial Hygiene Association Journal, 35,* 681–685.

Thun, M., Tanaka, S., Smith, A., et al. (1987). Morbidity from repetitive knee trauma in carpet and floor layers. *British Journal of Industrial Medicine, 44,* 611–620.

Waters, T.R., Putz-Anderson, V., Garg, A., & Fine, L.J. (1993). Revised NIOSH equation for the design and evaluation of manual lifting tasks. *Ergonomics, 36,* 749–776.

Wikstrom, B-O., Kjellberg, A., & Landstrom, U. (1994). Health effects of long-term occupational exposure to whole-body vibration: A review. *International Journal of Industrial Ergonomics, 14,* 273–292.

Suggested Reading

Chaffin, D., & Andersson, G. (1991). Methods of classifying and evaluating manual work. In *Occupational biomechanics* (2nd ed.) (pp. 264–301). New York: John Wiley & Sons.

Kiser, D., & Rodgers, S. (1986). Evaluation of job demands (Part III). In Eastman Kodak Company, *Ergonomic design for people at work,* Vol. 2 (pp. 95–121). New York: Van Nostrand Reinhold.

Putz-Anderson, V. (1988). *Cumulative trauma disorders: A manual for musculoskeletal diseases of the upper limb.* London: Taylor & Francis.

Chapter 12

Psychosocial Factors Case Study: Work Organization and Work-Related Musculoskeletal Disorders

Marla C. Haims and Pascale Carayon

Learning Objectives

On completion of this chapter, the reader should be able to

- Understand the importance of using a systems approach when considering work-related musculoskeletal disorders (WRMDs).
- Apply a systems approach to interventions in the work place for reducing or preventing WRMDs.
- Define a variety of techniques (data collection methods) for extracting important information from the work system.
- Define some principles for implementing participatory WRMD interventions.

Key Words

Work-related musculoskeletal disorders
Work organization
Psychosocial work factors
Participatory ergonomics
Process of intervention

Abstract

A potential link between job stress and WRMDs has been indicated by recent studies (NIOSH, 1992; Smith et al., 1992; Sauter & Moon, 1996), and theories on these links have been proposed (Sauter & Swanson, 1996; Smith & Carayon, 1996). WRMDs are found in many occupations, particularly in those with well-known psychosocial stressors, such as high workload, work pressure, job future ambiguity, low job control, and low supervisory support (Cooper & Marshall, 1976; Smith, 1987). Therefore, it is possible that job stress and psychosocial work factors have an influence on WRMDs. Several models have been proposed to explain the potential links between WRMDs and work organization, psychosocial work factors, and job stress (Smith & Carayon, 1996). There is also some empirical evidence of the relationship between work organization, psychosocial work factors, and WRMDs among workers (Houtman et al., 1994), in particular among office workers and computer users (Carayon, 1995a, b; Levoska & Keinänen-Kiukaanniemi, 1994; Lim & Carayon, 1995; Linton & Kamwendo, 1989; NIOSH, 1992; Smith et al., 1992). We believe that to fully understand the etiology of WRMDs and to prevent or control WRMDs, it is important to examine both ergonomic and psychosocial work organization factors and to adopt a systems approach. A longitudinal case study for examining WRMDs and the effectiveness of work organization interventions for reducing or preventing WRMDs is presented. The case study provides an example of how to use a systems approach when attempting to understand and control WRMDs in a practical work setting.

Introduction

WRMDs are increasingly becoming a concern to occupational health and safety professionals, ergonomists, engineers, employers, unions, and workers. WRMDs represent a collection of health problems that have three characteristics: (1) cumulative disorders (i.e., injuries that develop over a long period as a result of repeated, continuous exposure of a particular body part to stressors); (2) trauma of tissues and joints that develops as the result of repeated, continuous exposure to stressors; and (3) physical ailments or abnormal conditions (Putz-Anderson, 1988). There has been a recognition that a link may exist between WRMDs and stress (Armstrong et al., 1993; Bongers, de Winter, Kompier, & Hildebrandt, 1993; Cox & Ferguson, 1994; Hagberg et al., 1995; Sauter & Swanson, 1996; Smith & Carayon, 1996). We propose that work organization has a determinant role in the development and experience of WRMDs.

Importance of Work Organization

The importance of examining overall work organization and psychosocial work factors in the development and experience of WRMDs has been emphasized by many researchers (e.g., Bongers et al., 1993; Carayon & Smith, 1994; Smith & Carayon, 1996). Research studies of offices and workers using video display terminals have shown that psychosocial work factors, such as lack of job control, cognitive workload, and monotonous tasks, are related to WRMDs (Lim, 1994; NIOSH, 1990, 1992; Smith et al., 1992).

Work organization is defined as the way work is structured, distributed, processed, and supervised (Hagberg et al., 1995). As such, it is an *objective* characteristic of the work environment and depends on many factors, including management style, type of product or service, characteristics of the workforce, level and type of technology, and market conditions. Examples of work organization factors include job content and responsibility, individual versus team work, methods of time management, management style, and organizational design. Psychosocial work factors are *perceived* characteristics of the work environment that have an emotional connotation for workers and managers and can result in stress and strain (Hagberg et al., 1995). Examples of psychosocial work factors include work overload, work pressure, lack of control, social support, and job future ambiguity. Psychosocial work factors result from the interplay between the work organization and the individual.

Smith and Carayon (1996) have defined two types of mechanisms by which work organization and psychosocial work factors can influence WRMDs. First, work organization factors, which can cause psychological stress, may influence or be related to ergonomic stressors, such as force, posture, and repetitiveness. Work organization defines the nature of the work activities (variety or repetition), the exposure to loads, the number and duration of actions, and other ergonomic considerations such as workstation design, tool and equipment design, and environmental features. These factors interact as a system to produce an overall load on the person that can lead to WRMDs. Second, work organization can contribute to WRMDs through physiologic, psychological, and behavioral stress reactions to various work factors. There are psychobiological mechanisms that make a connection between stress and WRMDs plausible and likely. Stress can lead to an increased physiologic susceptibility to WRMDs by affecting hormonal responses and circulatory responses that exacerbate the influences of traditional ergonomic risk factors (i.e., force, repetition, and posture). Stress may also increase the sensitivity to and reporting of pain, by increasing negative psychological affect and mood. In addition, stress can affect employee attitude, motivation, and behavior, which in turn can lead to actions that increase the risk of WRMDs. Work organization and psychosocial work factors have been shown to be related to stress (Cooper & Marshall, 1976; Smith, 1987) and therefore could, in turn, influence musculoskeletal disorders. Figure 12-1 is a conceptual model that presents the proposed relationships linking work organization to WRMDs. Mediating this relationship are ergonomic risk factors (posture, force), psychosocial work factors, the stress loads produced by both, as well as the interactions between them.

Balance Theory

The balance theory of job design for stress reduction proposed by Smith and Carayon-Sainfort (1989) is a theoretical framework that can tie together work organization with ergonomic and psychosocial factors, and can conceptualize work factors that influence stress and WRMDs. The theory asserts that the

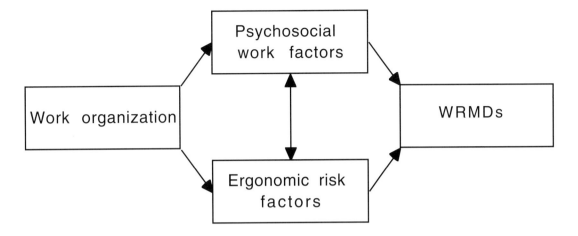

Figure 12-1. Research model of work organization and work-related musculoskeletal disorders (WRMDs).

work system has five elements (i.e., job tasks, organizational factors, tools and technologies, the work environment, and the individual) that influence each other and interact with one another to define a "stress load" that can then lead to various types of strain reactions and health disorders.

According to Smith and Carayon-Sainfort (1989), stress results from an imbalance between the various elements of the work system. This imbalance produces a "stress load" on the human response mechanisms that can produce adverse psychological and physiologic reactions. The human response mechanisms, which include behavior, physiologic reactions, and cognition, act to bring control over the environmental factors that are creating an imbalance. These efforts, coupled with an inability to achieve balance, produce an overload of the response mechanisms that leads to mental and physical fatigue. Prolonged exposure and fatigue lead to strain and disease. The model emphasizes the definition of sources of occupational stress (stressors) that can then be manipulated to produce proper balance in the work system. These stressors can be categorized into one of the following elements of the work system: (1) the task, (2) the organizational context, (3) the tools and technologies used, (4) the physical and social environment, and (5) the individual.

The balance theory model is useful to determine and design work-based interventions for dealing with WRMDs. The essence of the balance theory is to reduce the stress load and associated negative health consequences by balancing the various elements of the work system. Proper work design can be achieved by designing into each element of the work system those characteristics that meet recognized criteria for physical and mental loads, work cycles, and job content. However, the ideal work design—which would eliminate all sources of stress—often cannot be achieved. Therefore, the proposed approach emphasizes the use of positive job elements to compensate for poor job elements. Whenever possible, the poor job elements of the work system should be eliminated or reduced. But when this is not possible, the balance theory recommends the use of positive elements to balance the poor job elements. The stress load created by the poor job elements can be compensated by the moderating effect of positive job elements. For example, it has been shown that repetitiveness of tasks can be both physically (Putz-Anderson, 1988) and psychologically stressful (Cox, 1985). Therefore, repetitiveness in any job should be eliminated or reduced to a minimum. However, this is not always possible because of economic and technical constraints. When repetitiveness cannot be reduced, its negative impact on stress and WRMDs may be moderated by, for instance, appropriate rest breaks. In this example, a work organization factor (rest breaks) is used to balance the negative effect of a task characteristic (repetitiveness).

A major advantage of the balance theory is that it does not highlight any one job factor, such as frequency of motions, or any small set of factors, such as workload and posture. Rather, it examines the design of work from a systems perspective. It emphasizes the potential positive job elements that can be used to overcome the negative job elements in a job. Thus, all aspects of the work system (the individual, the nature of the tasks performed, the organizational context, the tools and technologies used, and the physical and social environment) and the interactions among them are considered in developing a proper design.

The remainder of this chapter is dedicated to the description of a longitudinal case study conducted to further advance our knowledge on the etiology of WRMDs and effective intervention strategies. It uses a systems approach to consider work organization and its influences on psychosocial and ergonomic risk factors in the development of WRMDs. As the balance theory asserts, many elements of the work system and a multitude of interactions between these elements must be taken into account in studying the development of WRMDs. It is hoped that the presentation of this case study sheds some light on strategies, methods, and techniques that can be used in the complex tasks of understanding, reducing, and preventing WRMDs in the working population.

A Longitudinal Case Study in a Public Service Agency

A longitudinal office automation study was initiated in 1991 at a public service agency in the Midwest. The agency requested that our university research team conduct an assessment of the ergonomic and health considerations associated with the use of computers in specified areas within their organization. The work areas initially identified for study consisted of jobs in data and word processing and data entry. The jobs demanded an average of 7.2 hours of computer use per day, and approximately 85% of the 200 job positions were occupied by female employees.

An agreement was reached between the employer, employee representatives, and research team to conduct a study for assessing office operations, submitting and implementing recommendations for enhancing the productive use of office automation, improving the ergonomic aspects of office working conditions, and collecting research data concerning the relationship between office ergonomics, organi-

zational conditions, and employee health and well-being. The agency had an interest in determining the most effective application of ergonomics to their office automation for enhanced productivity and worker health; the researchers had a related interest in determining the specific effectiveness of particular work interventions for the reduction and prevention of occupational stress and WRMDs.

Analysis

Overall Methodology

The overall methodologic design of the case study reflects a systems approach using a longitudinal and action research paradigm. Action research is a methodologic approach that involves researchers and organizational members in a combined process aimed at meeting research and client (intervention) goals (Argyris, 1993). It is an iterative process that includes diagnosis, planning, action, intervention, evaluation, and learning among all participants (Israel, 1991).

The systems or macro-ergonomic approach requires a recognition and understanding of the interrelationships among various aspects of the work system (Hendrick, 1991; Smith & Carayon-Sainfort, 1989). It is important to understand that solving ergonomic problems encompasses improvements not only in the physical environment and job tasks, but also in the structuring of work organization, the supervision of work activities, and the development of organizational policies and procedures. To best understand the various levels of an organization's functioning for effective ergonomic interventions, it is important that researchers develop a long-term relationship with the organization and its employees. An action research study design allows for this relationship to develop over time.

The keyword of the methodology is *multiple*. To gain an adequate understanding of the entire work system—for implementing appropriate preventive measures against occupational stress and WRMDs—multiple elements of the work systems must be considered. Table 12-1 provides the important characteristics of a study design that uses a systems approach to the prevention of stress and WRMDs. Action research, time, and multiple actors, methods, and study variables are global methodologic elements; participatory ergonomics and the train-the-

Table 12-1. Characteristics of the Study Design

Design Elements	Objective
Global elements	
Action research: planning, action, intervention, and learning among both researchers and organizational members	To meet both research and intervention goals through the combined knowledge and action of researchers and organizational members
Time: longitudinal study, multiple data points	To study the effects of change/interventions over time
Actors: multiple participants at different levels/units in the organization	To ensure representativeness of and input from concerned parties
Methods: multiple data collection methods	To obtain valid and reliable data
Study variables: multiple stressors and outcomes	To have a systemic overview of problems and solutions
Specific elements	
Participatory ergonomics: employee participation in identifying ergonomic risk factors and developing and implementing ergonomic solutions	To identify "hidden" risk factors, enhance employee knowledge of ergonomics, and allow for participation in the work environment
Train-the-trainer: employee group trained by research team to train other employee groups	To quickly disseminate ergonomic information throughout the organization, involve employees, and enrich their jobs

trainer (TTT) approach are specific to this particular case study. A description of the methodology and its application in other case studies of office automation can be found in Carayon (1994a, b).

Action Research. The methodology relies on action research to ensure research and intervention goals are met. Action research involves participation (in that employees serving on an action research project team are involved in both the research and the intervention), a balance between research and practical action, a joint relationship between researchers and employees, continuous feedback, learning among all involved, employee empowerment, and system development (Argyris, 1993; Hugentobler, Israel, & Schurman, 1992; Israel, Schurman, & Hugentobler, 1992). It is a powerful method for dissemination of information, training, application of appropriate interventions, and employee acceptance of these interventions for the goal of decreasing occupational stress and enhancing health. The action research process might itself be health enhancing, because participation and its increases in job control, learning, and social support have been shown to be linked to stress reduction and enhanced health conditions (Johnson, Hall, & Theorell, 1989; Karasek & Theorell, 1990; Sauter, Hurrell, & Cooper, 1989).

Time. The methodology involves collecting data at multiple data points to study the effect of change or interventions over time. For instance, comparison of

data before and after the implementation of an intervention provides information on the effectiveness of the intervention. Baseline data are collected as the first step of the process. These baseline data used to make a diagnosis of the work system and to design interventions to reduce physical and psychological stress and prevent or reduce WRMDs. Data are then collected on a regular basis to examine how physical and psychological stress evolves over time, and to assess the effectiveness of interventions.

Actors. Multiple actors are involved in the study, as the project is built to encourage cooperation and joint learning between the research team and the organization. For example, a study agreement between the research team, top management, and the union is developed as a cooperative effort. It specifies the objectives and content of the study as well as roles of the diverse parties involved. Data are collected from multiple actors within the organization (e.g., office workers, supervisors, technical staff, and top management), and different employees are involved in the study at different points in time and in different forms.

Methods. Multiple data collection methods are used to collect a large variety of data. Questionnaire surveys, ergonomic evaluations, interviews, videotaping or observation, and the examination of company records are used to assess the work environment, develop recommendations for change, and evaluate specific interventions. Other, more qualitative methods, such as the evaluation of the researcher's study diary, in-depth interviews with the action research project team, and continuous feedback evaluation forms from this group, are used to assess specific effects of the action research on the project team. Further description of data collection tools and their uses is provided in the next section.

Study Variables. Based on the theoretical systems framework presented earlier in this chapter, multiple stressors and multiple outcomes are examined. In addition, relationships and interactions among the study variables are examined. In our systems approach, relationships between physical and psychological aspects of the work system are important. For instance, the role of work organization, ergonomic factors, psychosocial factors, and psychological stress are all important contributors in the development and report of musculoskeletal disorders (Bongers et al., 1993; Carayon & Smith, 1994; Lim, 1994; Lim & Carayon, 1994, 1995; NIOSH, 1992; Smith & Carayon, 1996). These aspects are usually central to the identification of problems and the development of systemic recommendations.

Participatory Ergonomics. Participatory ergonomics is one specific methodologic component of the case study design, used as a tool for implementing ergonomic changes, reducing stress, and improving health. Noro and Imada (1991) describe participatory ergonomics as a method in which end-users of ergonomics (workers) take an active role in the identification and analysis of ergonomic risk factors as well as the design and implementation of ergonomic solutions. It includes ergonomic training of the workforce, information exchange between ergonomic experts and individual employees, employee participation in decision making about ergonomics and ergonomic design changes, and participation in the implementation and evaluation of these changes (Smith, 1994; Wilson, 1991). The participatory ergonomic approach and its employee involvement can be health enhancing in itself and is particularly important with respect to WRMDs, as some risk factors may be difficult to identify, quantify, or change.

Train-the-Trainer. The objective of the TTT approach is for the research team (or other ergonomic experts) to train an initial group of employee partici-

pants (referred to as *ergonomic coordinators* [ECs] in this case study) in basic ergonomic knowledge and for this group to provide ergonomic training for other employees in the organization. The rationale of the TTT approach is that people can be trained to train others, allowing knowledge to be transferred throughout an organization at an exponential rate (Hajnal & Carayon, 1994; Silverstein, 1991). Advantages of the TTT approach are efficiency, employee involvement, job enrichment, and increased problem-solving skills; drawbacks of the approach include loss of information in the transfer and the difficulty of employees becoming true ergonomic experts (Hagberg et al., 1995; Silverstein, 1991).

Data Collection Methods

Table 12-2 presents a comprehensive list and brief description of the data collection methods used throughout the course of the case study. The use of multiple sources of evidence and the combination of both qualitative and quantitative methods serves to add scope, breadth, confidence, and validity to case study findings. Different methods with different types of data were used at different stages of the study, as appropriate for the specific questions to be answered. For example, the questionnaire survey provides quantitative data for assessing aspects of the work environment, physical discomfort, psychological stress, and health status. Interviews are a qualitative method for obtaining more in-depth information that may serve to expand on or clarify questionnaire survey results. It should be noted that both the type and timing of measurement techniques were dictated by both the research study and the action research team's goals. (Refer to the timeline in Figure 12-6 for the use of these methods over time.) Several methods and examples of their measurement instrument content are described in detail below.

Questionnaire. A standardized questionnaire survey developed by the research team was used to collect information from employees at the beginning of the study and then after the implementation of each intervention put into place over the course of the study. This survey is a comprehensive instrument that examines employee perceptions of (1) working conditions, (2) job satisfaction, (3) job content, (4) supervision, (5) social relations, (6) psychological stress, (7) health status, and (8) demographic characteristics. The sur-

Table 12-2. Data Collection Methods Used Throughout the Course of the Study

Data Collection Method	Description and Use
Questionnaire survey	Measures various study variables. Data collected at the beginning of the study and then about every year during the study
Ergonomic evaluations	Examines computer characteristics, workstation design, and characteristics of the physical environment and is performed by trained ergonomists
Videotaping/observation	Provides information for job analysis, including tasks, postures, and pace
Interviews	Individual interviews verify results from other data collection methods and tap individual participant's perceptions
Evaluation of company records	Worker's compensation claims, performance data, etc. examined pre- and post-intervention to assess needs and intervention effectiveness
Feedback evaluation forms	Provides a means for continuous feedback on the reactions, outcomes, and impact of the participatory process
Diary	Provides a record for the researcher of study timeline, activities, interventions, and organizational reactions, outcomes, and impact

vey takes approximately 30–40 minutes to complete. It includes many questions that have been used in previous studies, especially studies conducted by NIOSH (Smith et al., 1981). Several rounds of survey data allow for exploring potential relationships between ergonomic risk factors, psychosocial factors, musculoskeletal discomfort, psychological stress, and health status over time. The survey is also used to assess the impact of various interventions on the physical and psychological health of employees within the organization. Table 12-3 outlines the major sections of the questionnaire survey and Figure 12-2 provides the specific questions that constitute the two scales—musculoskeletal discomfort and postural stressors.

Ergonomic Evaluations. A specially designed ergonomic evaluation form is used to assess ergonomic and postural characteristics of importance to the health of computer users. The form was developed and used by researchers at the University of Wisconsin-Madison, and its reliability and validity have been tested in previous studies of office automation (Carayon et al., 1987). The evaluation examines basic workstation characteristics and general environmental features, such as dimensional characteristics, adjustability, control, functional features, accessory positioning, ventilation, lighting, glare, and noise. Measuring devices such as rulers, meter sticks, goniometers, inclinometers, and spot photometers are used to make measurements at each workstation. The evaluation of physical characteristics of the workstation is performed in the absence of the employee at the workstation; the

Table 12-3. Content of Questionnaire Survey

Section A: Job information
Section B: Characteristics of work environment
Section C: Job satisfaction
Section D: Health information
Section E: Physical environment at your workstation
Section F: Mood scale
Section G: Musculoskeletal discomfort
Section H: Demographics

employee's presence is necessary for examining postural characteristics and the fit between the workstation and the individual employee. Such measures include visual distance to the screen, knee clearance under the work surface, and wrist deviation while keying. Table 12-4 outlines the content of the ergonomic evaluation form and Figure 12-3 displays the section for evaluating the chair at the workstation.

Observation and Videotaping. Observation of jobs familiarizes the researcher with the tasks, scheduling, and physical and psychosocial aspects of the work. In this case study, evaluation of ergonomic stressors was of primary importance during baseline measurements, and thus became the focus of data collection in observations and video analysis. Each workstation is observed for 20 minutes, during which postural stressors and their corresponding job activities are recorded. Each workstation is also videotaped for 20 minutes to further quantify the ergonomic stressors. Figure 12-4 is a blank observation and videotape

MUSCULOSKELETAL DISCOMFORT SCALE (15 questions)

The following questions concern your body and the way you and it function. Please try to answer each question by circling a number to indicate how often you have experienced each of the following items within the past year in general.

Hand/Arm Discomfort	Never	Occasionally	Frequently	Constantly
1. Pain down your arms	1	2	3	4
2. Loss of feeling in the fingers or wrist	1	2	3	4
3. Cramps in hands/fingers relieved only when not working	1	2	3	4
4. Loss of strength in arms or hands	1	2	3	4
5. Stiff or sore wrists	1	2	3	4

Leg Discomfort	Never	Occasionally	Frequently	Constantly
6. Leg cramps	1	2	3	4
7. Difficulty with feet and legs when standing for long periods	1	2	3	4

Upper Body Discomfort	Never	Occasionally	Frequently	Constantly
8. Back pain	1	2	3	4
9. Pain or stiffness in your neck and shoulders	1	2	3	4
10. Feeling of pressure in the neck	1	2	3	4
11. Shoulder soreness	1	2	3	4
12. Neck pain that radiates into shoulder, arm, or hand	1	2	3	4

General Discomfort	Never	Occasionally	Frequently	Constantly
13. Swollen or painful muscles and joints	1	2	3	4
14. Pain or stiffness in your arms or legs	1	2	3	4
15. Persistent numbness or tingling in any part of your body	1	2	3	4

Figure 12-2. Musculoskeletal discomfort and postural stressor scales from questionnaire survey.

POSTURAL STRESSORS SCALE (7 questions)

	Never	Occasionally	Frequently	Constantly
1. How often does your job require you to leave your desk and move around the office?	1	2	3	4
2. How often does your job require you to work in uncomfortable positions?	1	2	3	4
3. How often does your job require you to use awkward work motions?	1	2	3	4
4. How often do you have to stretch or twist to reach necessary working materials throughout the day?	1	2	3	4
5. How often do you hold your arms in one position for long periods of time when performing your job?	1	2	3	4
6. How often does you job allow you to change positions and sit or stand when you want?	1	2	3	4
7. How often do you sit or stand in the same position for several hours?	1	2	3	4

analysis form. The 20-second time intervals for recording postures across the top of the form are used only during video analysis. It should be noted that obtaining valid postural data from videotaping can be difficult (insufficient camera angles, sampling problems) and analysis of videotape is time-consuming. Videotaping can be useful, however, for quantifying frequency of postures, confirming results obtained using other methods, and reviewing the job tasks off-site.

Interviews. Interviews with employees, supervisors, and other personnel are conducted to supplement the data from the questionnaire, ergonomic evaluations, observations, and videotape. Specific questions are asked regarding employees' perceptions of the work environment and their levels of physical comfort at work. Table 12-5 is an example of one such interview form. Interviews with various members of the organization have been conducted for different reasons throughout the course of the study. For instance, the research team interviewed all EC members (members of the action research team) to assess the reactions, outcomes, and impact of the EC program on its participants and to help develop guidelines for the successful implementation of participatory programs (see Figure 12-6). One-on-one interviews, in many instances, reveal underlying causes and individual perceptions. Further, the interview context provides an opportunity for members at various levels of the organization to contribute their input and ideas to study project goals.

Evaluation of Company Records. Evaluation of company records provides important, rich information on the status of physical and psychological stress

Table 12-4. Content of Ergonomic
Evaluation Form

  I. Work area
     A. Describe type of office
     B. Draw diagram of the work space, indicating
        dimensions of workstation, position of equipment
        and furniture, placement of luminaries, and flow
        of traffic (an indicator of privacy)
 II. Video display terminal (VDT)
     A. Keyboard
     B. Mouse
     C. Display
     D. VDT characteristics (i.e., glare, visual distortion,
        adjustments)
III. Workstation design
     A. Workstation
     B. Working surface
     C. Chair
     D. Document holders, footrest, wrist, and arm rests
     E. Accessories
 IV. Environment
     A. Lighting
     B. Noise
     C. HVAC (heating, ventilation, and air conditioning)

---

within the organization. Worker's compensation claim data, performance data, absenteeism and turnover rates, and injury or accident rates provide the researcher with an overview of the state of affairs within the organization at the outset of the project. These data aid the researcher in defining priority areas within the organization in need of immediate attention and intervention. Showing improvements in any of these data types, following the implementation of interventions, is strong support of intervention effectiveness and is well received by management. It is important to understand, however, that such results are not expected to be realized early, especially in instances of WRMDs. In addition to the period of adaptation needed to adjust to the intervention, WRMDs generally develop over long periods and cannot be reversed (at least immediately) through any implementation initiative. Interventions are intended to help reduce symptoms in those with WRMDs and prevent development of new WRMDs. The longitudinal nature of the study design is crucial for discovering improvements in company performance and accident-related data.

Research Diary. A research diary is kept of all project activity, involvement, and progress. Diary entries allow for a continual, unobtrusive method of data collection, the identification of temporal relationships, and the recording of details and occurrences experienced and perceived by the researcher. Continuous updating of the diary forces the researcher into an ongoing data analysis of sorts. It fosters reflection on reactions to and outcomes of the program and helps the researcher make appropriate adjustments to program design.

Feedback Evaluation Forms. Feedback evaluation forms are used as a method for the research team to gather information on the EC group's reactions to the project, and their perceptions of its outcomes and potential impact on the organization as a whole. Forms are distributed to the group at 2-month intervals and returned to the researchers. The research team summarizes results and presents the summary to the EC group at the following meeting. Questions include instruction-oriented questions (effectiveness of instruction or training), participant-oriented questions (quality of communication between group members), and process-oriented questions (level of control in the EC program and the comfort associated with it). Some questions vary over time, according to current EC activities and areas of interest. Figure 12-5 is an example of one feedback evaluation form used with the EC group.

Intervention Design and Process

An overall intervention strategy was developed to accomplish the goals that had been laid out by the researchers (discerning the relationship between psychosocial factors and WRMDs, determining the effectiveness of specific interventions) and the organization (remediating ergonomic risk factors, enhancing productivity and employee health). This strategy followed an iterative process over time. The iterative intervention process was designed in a methodical way: there was evaluation, intervention, reassessment, another intervention, reassessment, and so on; however, it was flexible enough to continually meet the changing needs of researchers and the organization as a whole. For instance, intervention strategies changed over time, according to the changing immediate needs of the organization and the level of effectiveness of previous interventions. In addition, the use of data collection methods

Chair

Model: _____

Seatpan height: _____ cm

Range of pan height: low _____ cm; high _____ cm

Seatpan compression: _____ cm   Seatpan depth: _____ cm

Seatpan width: _____ cm   Top of backrest/pan distance: _____ cm

Backrest angle: resting: _____ fully reclined: _____

	Yes	No
Split backrest?	❑	❑
Seatpan: backrest tilt linked?	❑	❑

If yes, describe tilt link mechanism: _____

Armrests provided?   ❑   ❑

If yes, height of armrest from seat pan: _____ cm

If yes, distance between armrests (inner to inner at center): _____ cm

Ease of adjustments (circle one): (1 = can be done from seated position, 2 = average,
   3 = hard to do, 4 = no adjustment, 5 = tools required, 6 = NA)

Seatpan height	1	2	3	4	5	6
circle one:	*pneumatic*	*manual*				
Back angle	1	2	3	4	5	6
Seatpan angle	1	2	3	4	5	6
Armrest height	1	2	3	4	5	6
Backrest tension	1	2	3	4	5	6
Backrest height	1	2	3	4	5	6

	Yes	No	NA
Is the lumbar support adequate (10–20 cm above seat level, slight protrusion of <5 cm)?	❑	❑	❑
Do armrests interfere with movement?	❑	❑	❑
Do the armrests fit under the work surface?	❑	❑	❑
Does the seatpan have a rounded front edge?	❑	❑	❑
Does the seatpan tilt forward?	❑	❑	❑
Does the seatpan tilt backward?	❑	❑	❑
Is the seat surface appropriately padded?	❑	❑	❑
Does the chair have a five-leg base?	❑	❑	❑
Do the shape of the seatpan and backrest allow for free movement?	❑	❑	❑
Does the backrest interfere with movement?	❑	❑	❑
Does this operator use cushions/pads in the chair?	❑	❑	❑

If yes, describe and specify if for seatpan or back support: _____

Figure 12-3. Ergonomic evaluation form: chair assessment.

	0 secs	20 secs	40 secs	1 min	1 min 20 secs	1 min 40 secs	2 mins	2 mins 20 secs	2 mins 40 secs	3 mins	3 mins 20 secs	3 mins 40 secs	4 mins	4 mins 20 secs	4 mins 40 secs	5 mins
Back																
1. Straight																
2. Leaning back																
3. Leaning forward																
4. Leaning sideways																
5. Twisted or twisting																
Neck																
1. Neutral position																
2. Bent forward																
3. Bent to one side																
4. Bent backward																
5. Twisted																
Legs																
1. Sitting																
2. Standing																
3. Walking																
Arms/shoulders																
1. Arms in neutral position, close to body																
2. One or both arms flexed >30 degrees and <90 degrees																
3. One or both arms at or above shoulder level																
4. One or both upper arms abducted																
Wrists																
1. Flexion																
2. Extension																
3. Ulnar deviation																
4. Radial deviation																
5. Resting on edge																
Activity:																

Figure 12-4. Observation or videotape analysis form.

Table 12-5. Sample Interview Questions to Supplement Results of Questionnaires, Ergonomic Evaluation Forms, Observations, and Videotaping

Environment
What do you think about the lighting?
What do you think about the temperature?
What do you think about the humidity level?
What do you think about the air quality?
Is the noise level a source of distraction to you? Why? What is the source?
Do you think you need more privacy to conduct your work? Why? How would you like that to be done?

Comfort
What furniture, equipment, and accessories (if any) do you find uncomfortable to use at your workstation?
What do you think about the layout of your workstation? About the amount of space you have to work there?
Which tasks (if any) in your job contribute to your feeling of discomfort?
In general, are you comfortable at work? If no, why?
Do you have any health complaints that you feel may be connected to your work or working conditions?

Conclusions
Is there anything that you would like to change in your office? What would you like to change first? Next?
General comments:

changed over time. Some methods presented in the previous section were used during the initial evaluation of the identified work areas (questionnaires, ergonomic evaluations), whereas others were developed along the way to meet specific needs of reassessment after the introduction of various interventions. In the following section, a description of the progress of the case study is provided as an example of putting the research methodology and the data collection methods described in the previous sections to use in the field. It follows the iterative process over an extended period to ensure research and organizational goals are met.

*Description of the Office Automation
Study Over Time*

Figure 12-6 is a timeline of the longitudinal office automation study, its data collection phases, and its interventions. Data collection methods are provided in bold typeface, whereas intervention efforts are presented in italic typeface.

Baseline data in the form of questionnaire surveys and ergonomic evaluations of workstations were collected from a total of 171 office employee study participants in (85% response rate) two separate waves of data collection during 1991 and 1992. The data served as a systemic needs assessment of the work areas. Results demonstrated fair ergonomic conditions, high levels of musculoskeletal health

problems, high levels of visual discomfort, and high levels of psychological stress.

The organization's primary interest was the improvement of physical ergonomic conditions in their automated offices. Recommendations in the form of physical workstation adjustments were communicated to employees and management; several recommendations were implemented, reflecting a physical ergonomic intervention. It was also determined that ergonomic training for employees, supervisors, and managers was warranted. Through the course of several feedback sessions with management and employees, it was decided that the TTT approach would be used to develop an office ergonomics program for employees throughout the organization. The goal was to create and develop an ergonomics program within the organization that would continue to improve poor ergonomic conditions, reduce or prevent musculoskeletal discomfort, enhance general well-being, and increase productivity over time. The researchers hoped that establishing an independent, internal, participatory ergonomics program would ensure sustained interest within the organization for addressing ergonomic and health issues, and that it would serve as an ongoing problem-prevention program.

In late 1992, 14 employees were identified or volunteered to participate in a 2-day ergonomics training session provided by the research team (Hajnal & Carayon, 1994). Topics covered in the session

1. What do you think about the current ergonomic coordinator program?

	No, not at all			Yes, definitely	
In general, is the program useful to you?	1	2	3	4	5

	Poor			Excellent	
How would you rate the program overall?	1	2	3	4	5

2. What do you think about the material presented and discussed during the meetings?

	No, not at all			Yes, definitely	
Did the program content meet your expectations?	1	2	3	4	5
Are the skills learned and information emphasized useful and applicable to your workplace environment?	1	2	3	4	5
Is the material presented too technical?	1	2	3	4	5
Is the material presented clearly explained?	1	2	3	4	5

3. Do you feel confident in your ability to use   1   2   3   4   5
   the evaluation equipment?
   What, if anything, do you feel uncomfortable using? _____

   _____

   _____

4. Have you been using the evaluation equipment and doing evaluation   Yes   No
   activities within your work area?
   Why or why not? _____

   _____

5. Are you using the library facility?   Yes   No
   Why or why not? _____

6. Do you communicate with other members of the program   Yes   No
   concerning issues relevant to the program during the time between
   monthly meetings?
   Please comment: _____

   _____

7. Do you feel free/comfortable to participate in the ergonomic   Yes   No
   coordinator meeting discussions?
   More so or less so than previously? _____

8. Do you feel free/comfortable to participate in the activities related   Yes   No
   to the ergonomic coordinator program within your section?
   More so or less so than previously? _____

9. Do you feel you have enough "say" in the content and direction   Yes   No
   of the program?
   Please comment: _____

   _____

10. Do you have any suggestions for improvement?   Yes   No
    Please comment: _____

    _____

Figure 12-5. Example of a feedback evaluation form used to obtain information from the ergonomic coordinator group on an intermittent basis.

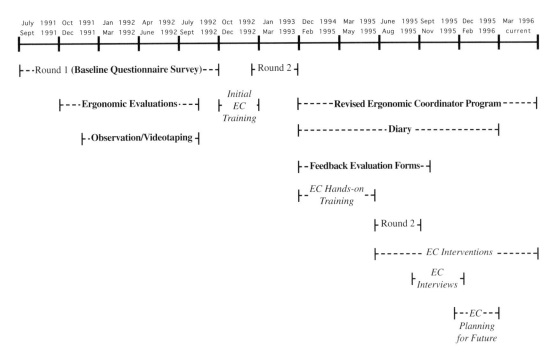

Figure 12-6. Timeline of longitudinal office automation study, its data collection phases, and interventions. Data collection methods are provided in bold typeface; intervention efforts are presented in italic typeface.

included an overview of ergonomics, aspects of the physical work environment, musculoskeletal problems in computerized offices, and specific workstation design and work practice changes that could be implemented in the local work environment. Lecture and group exercise formats were used to present the material. The overall concept was for these employees (the EC group) to be trained in ergonomic principles, become resource people for other employees, train additional employees (TTT approach), identify problems in the work environment, and bring identified problems to the attention of the organization.

A second round of questionnaire data was collected at the beginning of 1993, shortly after the initial training of the EC group. A total of 129 employees participated in this second round (64% response rate), 113 of which had also participated in the first round of questionnaire data collection in 1991 and 1992. Although results indicated an increase in employee awareness of workstation adjustments, levels of musculoskeletal discomfort and visual problems generally had increased from the first round of data collection, and reports of awkward and uncomfortable postures remained high. The lack of improvement in ergonomic risk factors and musculoskeletal discomfort in round

2 data was not discouraging, however, as the impact of the EC intervention was not expected to have taken effect in such a short time.

A follow-up session with the trained EC group was held a year and a half after the initial 2-day training session. An update on the research findings was presented to the EC group by the research team, and feedback was solicited from the group as to their progress and their perceived needs. At this meeting, the EC group expressed a need for a more developed ergonomics program, regular meetings, and more practical information and training for enhanced communication capabilities. EC program activity and effectiveness had been limited due to minimal follow-up by the research team, the non-continuous nature of the training, lack of available resources within the organization, and minimal support of the program from management. The research team was informed, however, that there was an interest in reconstructing the EC group.

Toward the end of 1994, members of the original EC group were contacted by researchers and solicited for their ideas for program redesign. A revised EC program was developed using an action research and participatory ergonomics paradigm

(Haims, 1995). Both the EC group and the research team recognized that a more in-depth, dedicated approach to training, resource development, program structuring, and planning was required to build a long-term ergonomics program within the organization. The revised program placed particular emphasis on ongoing training and learning among EC members for development of an internally regulated or in-house participatory ergonomics program. The aim was still physical ergonomic redesign (i.e., redesign of the physical environment, such as workstation components) and job redesign for reducing stress and improving health, but there was a more cognizant effort among the research team for establishing a self-sustaining ergonomics program within the organization and using an intervention process that would more directly influence and improve negative psychosocial factors existing in the work environment.

Regular meetings were established between researchers and the EC group, hands-on ergonomic training conducted, continued feedback solicited, and planning for the future emphasized. Meeting and training topics included workstation ergonomics, job design, WRMDs, and group dynamic skills. Later in the program, there was a focus on management, planning, and design skills for EC maintenance of the ergonomics program once university researchers left the site. The revised EC program included 13 regularly attending members (a combination of university researchers, risk and safety management, production employees, and supervisors) and three part-time members (other researchers and members of the organization's management), who represent approximately 450 office employees within the organization.

Several new methods of data collection were developed to evaluate the revised EC program intervention—a research diary to record the process and content of program implementation, in-depth interviews with EC members, and regular feedback evaluation forms from EC members (Haims, 1995). These methods were used to assess EC reactions, outcomes of program initiatives, and perceived impact of the intervention on a continuous basis for the purpose of program evaluation and continuous improvement (Goldstein, 1993).

The revived EC program has been in place for approximately 33 months (15 months with university researchers and 18 months since university withdrawal) and is very active within the organization. In the summer of 1995, EC members collected a third round of questionnaire data. Based on preliminary findings, they have been conducting ergonomic evaluations in problem areas, spending time educating and training those employees with the most severe problems, and collaboratively developing recommendations and implementing ergonomic changes. Since the university withdrawal from the organization in February 1996, the EC group has also broadened its program to target employees not previously identified for study and to ensure program sustainability. Related activities have included the planning and staffing of an ergonomics booth at the organization's safety fair, the dissemination of ergonomic information through presentations and regular publications in the organization's newsletter, the development of procedures (for employees and themselves) to be used as guidelines in various instances of ergonomic problems, and the creation of a "chair lab," through which employees seeking a new chair for their workstations can loan, test, and purchase a variety of ergonomically designed chairs. All of these recent activities have been initiated by the EC group, with little input from university researchers. Through increased levels of ergonomic activity, continuous training, feedback, and enhanced job control and decision-making opportunities over time, the EC group has developed the skills, capabilities, and motivation to control the content, direction, and administration of the ergonomics program (Haims, 1995).

Summary of Design and Process for Interventions

Aside from the research components of the case study (examination of the relationships between work organization, ergonomic factors, psychosocial factors, and WRMDs; examination of the effectiveness of various interventions), there were two other related, practical goals of the study: (1) a short-term goal of presenting findings and recommendations to the organization to begin making ergonomic improvements; and (2) a long-term goal of building an internal ergonomics program to continue making improvements over time. Over the course of the case study, the project has included (1) the collection of baseline data about many aspects of work to be able to determine the benefits of improvements; (2) the assessment of current workplace and workstation design characteristics; (3) the establishment of a priority system, based on the data collected, for undertaking interventions in a phased process with the most critical needs being addressed first; (4) the development of general guidelines for purchasing ergonomic furniture and for making improvements in environmental conditions; (5) the testing of innovative approaches in office ergonomics to examine their effectiveness in addressing specific worker performance and health/safety issues; and (6) the education and training of the office workforce in office ergonomics, job design, and various interventions.

The content of specific interventions throughout the study period has mainly focused on assessing and improving physical ergonomic conditions. This focus reflects the practical desires of management within the organization. The approach or processes used by the research team to implement such interventions (action research, participatory ergonomics, TTT), however, address psychosocial factors and work organizational issues. Through the implementation processes in the study, employees are given opportunities for learning and skill enhancement, enhanced participation in decision making, increased levels of job control, and enhanced networks for social support, all of which have been identified as important considerations for the reduction of occupational stress (Cooper & Marshall, 1976; Jackson, 1983; Karasek, 1979; Smith, 1987). The research approach used recognizes and addresses physical factors, psychological stress factors, and the relationship between the two within the work system. The content of intervention, such as workstation redesign, targets physical ergonomic risk factors, whereas the process of implementation through education and participation serves to improve various psychosocial factors of the work environment. As suggested in Figure 12-1, this double-edged approach is believed to be effective for the prevention and reduction of WRMDs.

Test and Evaluation Results

There are two different types of results from this longitudinal case study: (1) the reactions to, outcomes from, and impact on stress levels and health from various intervention efforts over time, and (2) the identification of some preliminary guidelines or principles for designing and implementing successful participatory interventions in the field for the reduction of WRMDs. Although there is academic research and theory rationalizing the use of participation in the workplace for the reduction and prevention of WRMDs (Bammer, 1993; Bongers et al., 1993; Carayon & Smith, 1994) and several research studies advocating this approach (Karasek, 1992; Westlander, Viitasara, Johansson, & Shahnavaz, 1995), there is a weak, if not nonexistent, framework addressing the process of implementing participatory practices. Thus, the question "how is participation effectively implemented within organizations?" was of primary interest in conducting this case study.

The results presented below focus on the implementation of the revised EC program in December 1994 (see Figure 12-6). The effectiveness of this particular intervention is of prime importance, as it is the final intervention in the case study, represents the accumulation of knowledge over the course of the study (both in the development of occupational stress and health and in the needs and desires within the organization) being put into practice, is a program internal to the organization to remain in operation in the future, and represents a first step in the identification of principles for designing successful work organization interventions to reduce WRMDs. Summary results from the research diary, feedback evaluation forms, EC interviews, and questionnaire surveys are presented. The diary, feedback evaluation forms, and interview methods of data collection serve as a means for evaluating EC participant reactions to and outcomes of the specific program. The three rounds of questionnaire surveys are used to assess the impact of the participatory ergonomics program on all members of the organization throughout the course of the study.

Diary Results

Diary entries were recorded regularly throughout the entire revised EC program, allowing for a continual method of data collection, the identification of temporal relationships, and the recording of details and occurrences as experienced and perceived by the researcher. These aspects of the diary provided for a richer understanding of the developmental process for the implementation of a participatory ergonomics program and the principles, strategies, and techniques that should or should not be used for progression within this process. Below is a summary of the major themes and corresponding findings that arose from the diary analysis (Haims, 1995).

Communication and Feedback. Communication within the EC group grew stronger over time, leading to increased effectiveness in action initiatives and a greater sense of group cohesiveness and trust. Frequency of EC meetings increased over time and were scheduled as members of the group saw fit. As time went on, communication links were extended beyond group meetings to include telephone conversations, e-mail correspondence, and separate meetings among various individuals to solve specific problems. As the ECs began performing ergonomic evaluations and making recommendations, they also began to consult each other and the university for advice, support, input, and solution targeting. Open communication between the EC group and the university researchers only developed, however, after the EC group was sufficiently convinced the research group had its best interests at heart, the researchers were committed to working with them for a long time, there was a clear purpose of the group, and there was an advantage to having access to university resources and expertise.

Feedback existed in the forms of communication between the EC group, researchers and organizational members, the use of feedback evaluation forms, direct interaction and action within the work environment, and interviews of individual ECs by the researchers. Feedback was an essential tool used throughout the project. It served to tap into the EC group's reactions to the program, to detect necessary changes in the program contents or structure, and to foster learning among the EC group.

Learning Over Time. There was continual learning for the EC group (including researchers) over the course of the project, and there was a continuous desire for further expansion of knowledge and learning as levels of participation in the program grew and greater action was taken. Content of learning changed over time, from purely ergonomic skills at the beginning of the program to skills for managing and implementing change at later points in time (such as development of tools for identifying workers with ergonomic needs and wanting to learn how to use statistical software for evaluation of the impact of the program). The EC group became increasingly innovative and resourceful over time, and as the

focus of education and training for the EC group began to shift from technical ergonomics to a broader scope, the EC group began to play the role of educators themselves (a reflection of the TTT approach).

Transfer of Control from Researchers to the Ergonomic Coordinator Group. Initially, the university group had almost complete control over the design process of the participatory EC program and did the bulk of the work to get the program off the ground. The EC group, however, gained increasingly higher levels of control in the design, content, and direction of the program as learning was enhanced over time. For example, ECs began to make decisions regarding what material should be covered in meetings, what tasks should be accomplished between meeting times, the types of questions to add to the round 3 questionnaire survey, and plans for the future.

Flexibility of a Dynamic Process. The EC project was designed by the university group to be structured, yet flexible enough to meet the changing needs of the organization, the changing needs of all individuals involved, and to allow for transfer of control over the program to organizational members over time. It was important that researchers took on different roles (e.g., designer/planner, expert, facilitator, educator, trainer, resource, advocate, project manager, analyst) called for by various situations over time and were eager, rather than reluctant, to give up control over the participatory program as EC group members became more self-confident and competent. Flexibility was planned into the structure of the program from the start, and thus input from EC members, affected employees, and management became a strength of the program rather than a source of frustration or inhibitor of attaining original goals. The dynamic, flexible nature of the program saved the program from disintegrating at several points during circumstances of unexpected organizational change.

Feedback Evaluation Forms

Feedback evaluation forms were completed, summarized, and returned to the EC group in the second, fourth, sixth, and ninth months of the revised EC project as a means of obtaining reactions to and outcomes of the program among members. Below are some general results from both the quantitative

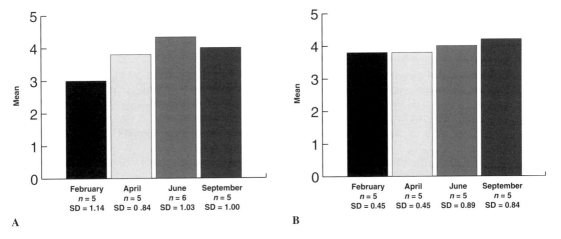

Figure 12-7. A. Feedback evaluation form results: overall usefulness of the ergonomic coordinator (EC) program. **B.** Feedback evaluation form results: overall usefulness of skills learned in the program.

and qualitative aspects of the feedback evaluation forms (Haims, 1995).

Quantitative Results. Figure 12-7 shows the overall usefulness of the EC program and the usefulness of skills learned in the program as reported by EC members. Responses were recorded on a Likert scale from 1 (No, not at all useful) to 5 (Yes, definitely useful). In general, usefulness increases over time.

Qualitative Results. The importance of the relationship between the university and the organization was emphasized by EC members. ECs also reported development through training and projects, an increased sense of direction and purpose over time, and the benefits of long-term learning and growth.

Ergonomic Coordinator Interviews. Table 12-6 presents a summary of the EC interview responses pertaining to communication and feedback, learning over time, the transfer of control from researchers to the EC group, and barriers to success encountered over the course of the program. Overall, EC members report increased communication and learning over the course of the program, the potential for the attainment of enhanced control, and a variety of barriers to success (Haims, 1995).

Questionnaire Survey

Survey results from rounds 1, 2, and 3 of data collection can be compared for evaluating the impact of interventions over the entire study period. Although there is currently a lack of data to represent the entire organization at all three measurement times and it is early in the revised EC program implementation to expect considerable organizational impact, some interesting findings are reported here (Haims, 1995). In Figures 12-8 and 12-9, data from one work section, targeted as a priority area for intervention at the beginning of the study, are presented. Data concerning upper body discomfort and hand/arm discomfort have been chosen as an example because they are considered surrogate measures for WRMDs. The percentages reported represent overall incidence, which indicates the percentage of employees who complain of the health problem at least occasionally.

Within this work area, back pain and pain or stiffness in the neck and shoulders are the most frequent upper body health problems; stiff and sore wrists are the most frequently reported hand/arm health complaint. Overall, there is a general trend of upper body and hand/arm discomfort increasing between rounds 1 and 2 and then decreasing between rounds 2 and 3. For example, large increases in the incidence of both pain or stiffness in the neck and shoulders and loss

Table 12-6. Summary of Interview Results Pertaining to Communication and Feedback, Learning, the Transfer of Control, and Barriers to Success

Interview Question	Summary of Responses
Is there a perception of an increased and/or improved communication network between group members? Between members of the organization as a whole? Between the organization and the researchers?	Increased quantity and quality of communication among EC members, among EC members and other employees in their respective work areas, and between researchers and the EC group over time Self-formation of subgroups among EC members for solving specific problems
Has being involved in the EC program and being a part of the participatory process contributed at all to your level of learning and knowledge? (1) in ergonomics? (2) in general? (3) relative to how the organization functions? (4) in your ability to make decisions and implement changes? and (5) Will the learning period continue in the future?	Increased learning in ergonomics and physical aspects of the work environment Increased skill in group dynamics and communication Increased understanding of the organizational structure and functioning Enhanced confidence in ability to influence organizational decisions and to make changes in the physical work environment Expression of need for training in the process of making changes Expression of desire and need to continue learning
Do you feel you had enough say or control in the process? Too much control/responsibility?	Researchers had most control at beginning of the program EC members had adequate input into program contents EC members always had the freedom to take more control
What have been the barriers (if any) to optimal success of the program?	Lack of general management support Conflicts between job and EC duties Lack of formal means for providing input to decision making at the organizational level Budget and time constraints Organizational changes Resistance to change among organizational members

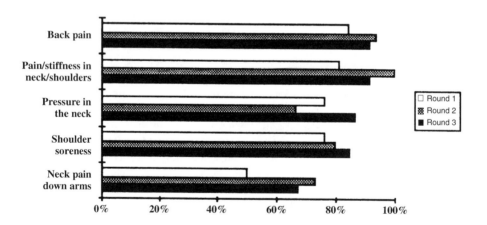

Figure 12-8. Percentage of employees in one work section reporting upper body discomfort for the three rounds of questionnaire data. Round 1 (1991–1992), $n = 20$; round 2 (1993), $n = 16$; round 3 (1995), $n = 46$.

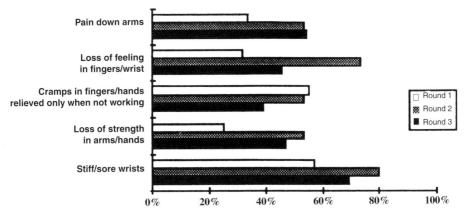

Figure 12-9. Percentage of employees in one work section reporting hand/arm discomfort for the three rounds of questionnaire data. Round 1 (1991–1992), $n = 20$; round 2 (1993), $n = 16$; round 3 (1995), $n = 46$.

of feeling in fingers and wrists were found between rounds 1 and 2, with a reduction in round 3. This trend did not, however, hold for experiences of pressure in the neck, shoulder soreness, or pain down the arms. Round 2 of data collection was done immediately following the initial TTT program for ECs, and round 3 surveys were distributed at the beginning of the revised EC participatory program. Thus, the effect of these particular interventions on results is probably minimal. The general trend for reduction in complaints of musculoskeletal discomfort at round 3 is, however, encouraging (Haims, 1995). It suggests a potential positive impact of the EC program, along with the overall longitudinal study and its ergonomic interventions, on the physical well-being of employees within this work area. The researchers and some organizational members are presently assessing the potential for collecting a fourth round of survey data to evaluate the long-term impact of the revised EC program on physical health and stress throughout the entire organization.

Resulting Principles for Implementing Participatory WRMD Interventions

There is increasing empiric evidence of the relationship between work organization, psychosocial work factors, and WRMDs among workers (Houtman et al., 1994), and NIOSH has recently initiated and funded a series of field studies for examining work organization interventions for the reduction and prevention of WRMDs. As these efforts con-

tinue, it is becoming increasingly important to develop a framework for the implementation of work organization interventions to ensure their effectiveness. Although there is academic research and theory rationalizing the use of participation as an effective work organization intervention strategy (Karasek, 1992), there has been little research aimed at the identification of guidelines or principles for designing and implementing effective participatory interventions. Developing a set of principles that can be used as a guide for designing work organization interventions is an avenue of research with some practical implications for the work place. This study represents a first step in identifying principles for the design of successful work organization interventions to reduce WRMDs. The design implications discussed in this section are not intended to be all inclusive, but rather to highlight the most important principles and strategies that came out of this case study (Haims, 1995).

Preliminary findings show the important role of control, feedback, and learning in designing the implementation of a participatory intervention (Haims & Carayon, 1995). Action within an environment that allows for control and continuous feedback promotes learning (Smith & Smith, 1988; Goldstein, 1975), and thus progression in the ability of participants within the organization to retain and continue to develop the participatory program on their own over time. Learning occurs through the coupling of action and feedback in the work environment and through more formal means of training. Some of the findings related to training in this study reflect those asserted by Goldstein (1975). These include the importance of maximum and immediate feedback, the recognition that problem solving potential increases with enhanced learning (i.e., learning to learn), the value of spaced versus massed practice, the importance of matching tasks with an individual's capabilities, and the importance of training in stages of increasingly higher levels of difficulty.

An additional training principle recognized in this case study was that training content must meet the current needs of the organization. This statement is basic common sense, but points to the importance of recognizing that priorities and needs within organizations are in constant flux. Thus, intervention programs must strike a balance between having both structure and flexibility. Programs must have stated purposes and goals, but must also be capable of adjusting to changes in organizational policy, structure, and procedure. This point is emphasized by Westlander and colleagues (1995) in their evaluation of two participatory interventions with data-entry work in Sweden. A participatory intervention must also be adaptive and dynamic to account for its continual internal development, through the enhanced knowledge, abilities, and control of its participants over time.

Along these same lines, the role of the researcher (or other intervention expert) must also be dynamic and flexible. The researcher must be willing and able to take on many different roles throughout the implementation process. For instance, at the beginning of the program the researcher may play the role of project leader and facilitator, but as learning and control are enhanced among participants, the role changes to one of supporter and external resource. This changing role has been observed in other intervention studies (Israel et al, 1992; Westlander et al., 1995).

Another important implication for design reflects the macro-ergonomic concept that organizational design and management factors are inherently connected to making changes at the micro-ergonomic level (Hendrick, 1991). Support for the participatory program and its ergonomic changes is required from the strategic decision makers of the organization for the program to be effective. For example, management in the organization must provide participant employees with time, access, and opportunities to exercise their gained knowledge and expertise for improving ergonomic work conditions.

It is not only management, however, that is required to commit to such an endeavor. The implementation of a participatory program for the reduction of WRMDs is not a quick and simple process, and commitment must be secured from all parties involved—management, supervisors, employee representatives, employees, researchers, and technical and safety staff. A great deal of time and effort must be committed for developing a trusting relationship among the action research project team, training and skill development among the project team, implementing changes within the organization, and developing the program as part of the organization's overall structure. Furthermore, the nature of WRMDs and their multifactorial etiology suggest that these disorders develop over time and will not disappear rapidly. The implementation of a participatory intervention is a proactive, rather than a reactive, approach for addressing WRMDs, and results, such as reduction in worker's compensation claims, should be expected to take some time to evolve.

Conclusion

The research model in Figure 12-1 demonstrates the importance of addressing both physical ergonomic risk factors and psychosocial work factors when developing work organization interventions for the reduction and prevention of WRMDs. This case study represents a model for addressing both issues by using a systems or macro-ergonomic approach. Multiple methods, actors, and study variables are examined over time to assess the various needs of the organization and its members and to define the necessary content of the intervention program. Action research, participatory ergonomics, and the TTT technique are approaches for developing or designing a process for the implementation of such intervention programs. When attempting to prevent or reduce WRMDs, it is not only important to decide what to change, but also how to change it. Both the content of the intervention and the process for implementing it are important for obtaining the best possible outcomes (Carayon, 1995b; Westlander et al., 1995).

It is becoming increasingly clear that there is a multiplicity of work-related risk factors for WRMDs (Hagberg et al., 1995). Therefore, it is necessary to adopt a systems approach for preventing or reducing WRMDs. In this vein, macro-ergonomic techniques, such as participatory ergonomics and action research, are important to take into account. Understanding the organizational context in which the intervention is occurring is also useful for ensuring the long-term success of an intervention. Each organization has its unique characteristics (e.g., history, organizational climate and culture, labor-management relations, technology, experience with organizational change), and it is important to take these into account when developing strategies for the reduction of WRMDs. Designing a set of principles that can be used as a guide for designing and implementing work organization interventions is an avenue of research that has important practical implications. We need to attempt to close the gap that exists between what Argyris (1993) calls *scholarly research* and *salable knowledge* for the reduction and prevention of WRMDs.

References

Armstrong, T.J., Buckle, P., Fine, L.J., et al. (1993). A conceptual model for work-related neck and upper limb musculoskeletal disorders. *Scandinavian Journal of Work Environment and Health, 19,* 73–84.

Argyris, C. (1993). *Knowledge for action: A guide to overcoming barriers to organizational change.* San Francisco: Jossey-Bass.

Bammer, G. (1993). Work-related neck and upper limb disorders—social, organisational, biomechanical and medical aspects. In A. Gontijo, & J. de Souza (Eds.), *Secundo Congresso Latino-Americano e Sexto Seminario Brasileiro de Ergonmia* (pp. 23–38). Florianopolis, Brazil: Ministerio de Trabalho.

Bongers, P.M., de Winter, C.R., Kompier, M.A.J., & Hildebrandt, V.H. (1993). Psychosocial factors at work and musculoskeletal disease. *Scandinavian Journal of Work Environment and Health, 19,* 297–312.

Carayon, P. (1994a). A systems approach to reducing physical and psychological stress: Application in automated offices. In G.E. Bradley, & H.W. Hendrick (Eds.), *Human factors in organizational design and management—IV* (pp. 733–738). Amsterdam: Elsevier.

Carayon, P. (1994b). Research on prevention strategies in automated offices. In G.E. Bradley, & H.W. Hendrick (Eds.), *Human factors in organizational design and management —IV* (pp. 707–712). Amsterdam: Elsevier.

Carayon, P. (1995a). Work pressure as a determinant of job stress and cumulative trauma disorders in automated offices. *Second International Scientific Conference on Prevention of Work-Related Musculoskeletal Disorders: PREMUS 95* (pp. 172–174). Montreal.

Carayon, P. (1995b). *Cumulative trauma disorders and work organization: The balance theory as a theoretical and practical framework.* Paper presented at the conference Work and Well-Being: An Agenda for Europe. Nottingham, UK.

Carayon, P., & Smith, M.J. (1994). Work organization factors and musculoskeletal disorders in offices. *Proceedings of the International Conference on Occupational Disorders of the Upper Extremities,* December 1–2, 1994. San Francisco.

Carayon, P., Swanson, N., & Smith, M.J. (1987). Objective and subjective ergonomic evaluations of automated offices. In J.M. Flach (Ed.), *Proceedings of the Fourth Midcentral Ergonomics/Human Factors Conference* (pp. 358–66). Urbana, IL: University of Illinois.

Cooper, C.L., & Marshall, J. (1976). Occupational sources of stress: A review of the literature relating to coronary heart disease and mental ill health. *Journal of Occupational Psychology, 49,* 11–28.

Cox, T. (1985). Repetitive work: Occupational stress and health. In C.L. Cooper, & M.J. Smith (Eds.), *Job stress and blue collar work* (pp. 85–112). New York: Wiley & Sons.

Cox, T., & Ferguson, E. (1994). Measurement of the subjective work environment. *Work and Stress, 8(2),* 98–109.

Goldstein, I.L. (1975). Training. In B.L. Margolis, & W.H. Kroes (Eds.), *The human side of accident prevention* (pp. 92–113). Springfield, IL: Charles C. Thomas.

Goldstein, I.L. (1993). *Training in organizations: Needs assessment, development and evaluation* (3rd ed.). Pacific Grove, CA: Brooks/Cole Publishing.

Hagberg, M., Silverstein, B., Wells, R., et al. (1995). *Work-related musculoskeletal disorders (WRMDs): A reference book for prevention.* London: Taylor & Francis.

Hajnal, C., & Carayon, P. (1994). Reflection of a research paradigm: The development and implementation of an ergonomic intervention. In *Proceedings of the 12th Triennial Congress of the International Ergonomics Association* (Vol. 6, pp. 135–137). Toronto: Human Factors Association of Canada.

Haims, M.C. (1995). Theory and practice for the implementation of a participatory program: A case study in a public service organization. Master's thesis, University of Wisconsin-Madison.

Haims, M.C., & Carayon, P. (1995, September). *Participatory ergonomics: A tool for reducing stress and improving health.* Paper presented at the conference Work, Stress and Health '95: Creating Healthier Workplaces, Washington, DC.

Hendrick, H.W. (1991). Ergonomics in organizational design and management. *Ergonomics, 34,* 743–56.

Houtman, I.L.D., Bongers, P.M., Smulders, P.G.W., & Kompier, M.A.J. (1994). Psychosocial stressors at work and musculoskeletal problems. *Scandinavian Journal of Work Environment and Health, 20,* 139–145.

Hugentobler, M.K., Israel, B.A., & Schurman, S.J. (1992). An action research approach to workplace health: Integrating methods. *Health Education Quarterly, 19(1),* 55–76.

Israel, B.A. (1991). A participatory action research approach to occupational stress and health. In *Conference Program of Healthy Work Environments / Healthy People: Partici-*

patory Approaches to Improving Workplace Health (pp. 158–162). Ann Arbor, MI: University of Michigan.

Israel, B.A., Schurman, S.J., & Hugentobler, M.K. (1992). Conducting action research: Relationships between organization members and researchers. *Journal of Applied Behavioral Science, 38,* 74–101.

Jackson, S.E. (1983). Participation in decision making as a strategy for reducing job-related strain. *Journal of Applied Psychology, 68,* 3–19.

Johnson, J.V., Hall, E.M., & Theorell, T. (1989). Combined effects of job strain and social isolation on cardiovascular disease morbidity and mortality in a random sample of the Swedish male working population. *Scandinavian Journal of Work, Environment and Health, 15,* 271–279.

Karasek, R. (1979). Job demands, job decision latitude, and mental strain: Implications for job redesign. *Administrative Science Quarterly, 24,* 285–308.

Karasek, R. (1992). Stress prevention through work reorganization: A summary of 19 international case studies. *Conditions of Work Digest, 11(2),* 23–41.

Karasek, R., & Theorell, T. (1990). *Healthy work: Stress, productivity and the reconstruction of working life.* New York: Basic Books.

Levoska, S., & Keinänen-Kiukaanniemi, S. (1994). Psychosocial stress and job satisfaction. *Work and Stress, 8,* 255–262.

Lim, S.-Y. (1994). An integrated approach to upper extremity musculoskeletal discomfort in the office environment: The role of psychosocial factors, psychological stress, and ergonomic risk factors. Unpublished doctoral dissertation, University of Wisconsin-Madison.

Lim, S.-Y., & Carayon, P. (1994). Relationship between physical and psychological work factors and upper extremity symptoms in a group of office workers. *Proceedings of the 12th Triennial Congress of the International Ergonomics Association* (Vol. 6, pp. 132–134). Human Factors Association of Canada.

Lim, S.-Y., & Carayon, P. (1995, September). Psychosocial and work stress perspectives on musculoskeletal discomfort. *Second International Scientific Conference on Prevention of Work-Related Musculoskeletal Disorders: PREMUS 95* (pp. 175–177). Montreal.

Lim, S.-Y., & Carayon, P. (1995). Psychosocial work factors and upper extremity musculoskeletal discomfort among office workers. In A. Grieco, G. Molteni, B. Piccoli, & E. Occhipinti (Eds.), *Work with display units 94* (pp. 57–62). Amsterdam: Elsevier Science.

Linton, S.J., & Kamwendo, K. (1989). Risk factors in the psychosocial work environment for neck and shoulder pain in secretaries. *Journal of Occupational Medicine, 31,* 609–613.

NIOSH. (1990). *Health Hazard Evaluation Report—HETA 89-250-2046—Newsday, Inc.* Washington, DC: U.S. Department of Health and Human Services.

NIOSH. (1992). *Health Hazard Evaluation Report: HETA 89–299–2230—US West Communications.* Washington, DC: U.S. Department of Health and Human Services.

Noro, K., & Imada, A.S. (Eds.). (1991). *Participatory ergonomics.* London: Taylor & Francis.

Putz-Anderson, V. (Ed.). (1988). *Cumulative trauma disorders: A manual for musculoskeletal diseases of the upper limbs.* London: Taylor & Francis.

Sauter, S.L., & Moon, S.D. (Eds.). (1996). *Beyond biomechanics: Psychosocial aspects of musculoskeletal disorders in office work.* London: Taylor & Francis.

Sauter, S.L., & Swanson, N. (1996). An ecological model of musculoskeletal disorders in office work. In S.D. Moon, & S.L. Sauter (Eds.), *Beyond biomechanics: Psychosocial aspects of musculoskeletal disorders in office work* (pp. 3–21). London: Taylor & Francis.

Sauter, S.L., Hurrell, J.J. Jr., & Cooper, C.L. (Eds.). (1989). *Job control and worker health.* New York: Wiley & Sons.

Silverstein, B.A. (1991). Developing shop-floor ergonomic expertise using a train-the-trainer approach. In *Conference Program of Healthy Work Environments / Healthy People: Participatory Approaches to Improving Workplace Health.* (pp. 74–78). Ann Arbor, MI: University of Michigan.

Smith, M.J. (1987). Occupational stress. In G. Salvendy (Ed.), *Handbook of ergonomics/human factors* (pp. 844–860). New York: John Wiley & Sons.

Smith, M.J. (1994). A case study of a participatory ergonomics and safety program in a meat processing plant. In *Proceedings of the 12th Triennial Congress of the International Ergonomics Association* (Vol. 6, pp. 114–116). Toronto: Human Factors Association of Canada.

Smith, M.J., & Carayon-Sainfort, P. (1989). A balance theory of job design for stress reduction. *International Journal of Industrial Ergonomics, 4,* 67–79.

Smith, M.J., & Carayon, P. (1996). Work organization, stress, and cumulative trauma disorders. In S.D. Moon, & S.L. Sauter (Eds.), *Beyond biomechanics: Psychosocial aspects of musculoskeletal disorders in office work* (pp. 23–42). London: Taylor & Francis.

Smith, M.J., Carayon, P., Sanders, K.J., et al. (1992). Electronic performance monitoring, job design and worker stress. *Applied Ergonomics, 23(1),* 17–27.

Smith, M.J., Cohen, B.G.F., Stammerjohn, L.W. Jr., & Happ, A. (1981). An investigation of health complaints and job stress in video display operators. *Human Factors, 23,* 387–400.

Smith, T.J., & Smith, K.U. (1988). The cybernetic basis of human behavior and performance. *Newsletter of Ideas in Behavioral Cybernetics,* p. 15.

Westlander, G., Viitasara, E., Johansson, A., & Shahnavaz, H. (1995). Evaluation of an ergonomics intervention program in VDT workplaces. *Applied Ergonomics, 26(2),* 83–92.

Wilson, J.R. (1991). Participation: A framework and a foundation for ergonomics? *Journal of Occupational Psychology, 64,* 67–80.

Section V

User-Centered Equipment Design

Chapter 13

An Introduction to Design, Evaluation, and Usability Testing

Marilyn Sue Bogner

Learning Objectives

On completion of this chapter, the reader should be able to

- Consider the diversity of the users of rehabilitative, assistive, and health care equipment.
- Understand the importance of addressing the impact of the context, the system, in which health care equipment is used on the performance of equipment users and maintainers.
- Appreciate the value of designing equipment, including procedures and instructions for its operation and maintenance, in such a way that the design compensates for potential deleterious effects of system factors on its use.
- Structure the evaluation criteria and usability testing of equipment to address real-world use and maintenance issues.

Key Words

User characteristics
Systems approach
Human error
User-driven design

Abstract

This chapter introduces the concept of user-centered design using an ergonomic systems approach. When designing health care, rehabilitative, and assistive equipment, the perspective of the user populations, the systems in which the equipment will be used, and the tasks to be performed all must be considered. Each of these elements is discussed in detail. Human error can result when user-centered design is not implemented and an example of such is presented. Finally, the methods considered integral to conducting user-centered design are presented.

Introduction

Know thy users, for they are not you.

—*Human Factors International*, 1995

People consider the world from their own perspective, projecting the way they understand it onto others. When engineers design and develop equipment solely from their perspective or their interpretation of users' needs, there is the potential to build in problems for the users. Without collaboration with actual users of equipment, the users' needs most likely will not be addressed. People who design equipment for others must be mindful that they, the designers, are not the typical users of the equipment. Equipment that is not designed for the actual users is likely to be difficult to use and induce error.

Error in using equipment in rehabilitation and health care can have dire consequences, ranging from not accomplishing the intended goal to causing injury and death. This chapter presents information that can be used to evaluate equipment to enhance ease of use and reduce the likelihood of error by (1) defining the user populations for health care and rehabilitation equipment, including assistive devices; (2) discussing user considerations in the design of health care equipment; (3) identifying user issues in evaluation and testing of equipment design; and (4) describing usability testing of rehabilitative, assistive, and health care equipment.* It is proposed that the context of use, real or simulated, be an integral part of operational usability testing.

User Populations

To provide an appreciation of the diversity of user populations, the equipment to be used is first described and defined. Consequently, the categories and characteristics of the users themselves are described.

Equipment

Rehabilitative equipment is used to change the functional status of a patient so that he or she can interact with the environment more easily or to improve a patient's overall health. Rehabilitative equipment is used during patient evaluations, such as functional assessment testing, strength testing, and perceptual tests. It also includes items used during the rehabilitation process, such as supportive slings to eliminate gravity while a patient relearns how to use his or her arms, as well as strengthening devices.

Assistive equipment aids a person in the performance of the activities of daily living, such as dressing (sock pullers), bathing, food preparation, and personal locomotion (wheelchairs, crutches). Assistive equipment is also used to perform job-related tasks. User-centered design of equipment is common in other domains such as aviation, nuclear power, and consumer products. The design of health care and rehabilitation assistive equipment is considered more complicated as both the diversity of the individual user characteristics as well as their specific health needs must be taken into account.

Health care equipment includes any device used in the diagnosis, treatment, and prevention of health problems as well as maintenance of people with chronic conditions. Drug delivery devices (e.g., infusion pumps that control the flow of therapeutic fluid into body tissue) are considered health care equipment, although the drugs themselves are not.

To adequately address issues affecting equipment design, it is necessary to know the characteristics of the user population and the context of use—the latter because factors in the environment impact on both the user and the operation of the equipment. Although not often considered, the equipment itself is a contextual factor, the design of which affects its use and maintenance. The human factors and ergonomics approach is to design and evaluate equipment through the application of user-designed criteria. The user-centered approach applies not only to equipment design, but also to the development of evaluation and testing criteria to ensure ease of use.

Categories of Users

Users of rehabilitative equipment and assistive devices typically are individuals with a physical condition caused by accident, illness, or genetic factors who require therapeutic activity to regain functionality. Other users are the health care professionals who work with the equipment to enable patients to regain functionality. These two categories of users have different characteristics, skills, and abilities, and the categories of users are expanding.

Rehabilitative and assistive devices are no longer associated only with severely disabled individuals. Immunizations and other preventive health care measures, improved nutrition, antibiotics, artificial joints, and sophisticated surgical techniques have reduced the incidence of incapacity and early death considerably. Thus, ours is an aging population. The infirmities of age, the debilitating illnesses often associated with age (e.g., cancer), and the new diseases (e.g., acquired immunodeficiency syndrome) have expanded the population that requires rehabilitative equipment beyond those previously known disabilities acquired from accidents, illness, and genetic causes. Most people tend to deny the possibility of a disabling accident or condition, so they consider the users of health care equipment as

---

*Because this chapter addresses the three devices, and rehabilitation and assistive devices can be considered a subset of health care as a whole, the term *health care equipment* is used to denote all three types of equipment, unless otherwise specified.

them rather than *us*. This attitude is beginning to change and will continue to change as the elderly population increases substantially.

Rehabilitative care is no longer primarily the purview of highly trained professionals. Shortened hospital stays and changes in hospitalization patterns brought on largely by fiscal constraints have caused an increase in home health care. As home care increases, a third category of user is becoming more evident: lay care providers. This category includes family members, significant others, friends, and marginally trained health care professionals. The impact of the diversity of user populations on the operation and maintenance of health care equipment is profound. Because more people need rehabilitation and more people are providing such care, the users of rehabilitative, assistive, and health care equipment rapidly are becoming *us*. For safe and effective use by such diverse populations, rehabilitative care equipment should be designed from the perspective of these populations and the viability of the design evaluated through testing such as usability testing. That necessitates a focus on designing to accommodate the characteristics of all categories of users.

Characteristics of Users

As previously stated, the three categories of health care equipment users are very diverse in skills, abilities, knowledge, and ability to care for others and to function in the environment. Members of these categories include (1) professional providers, such as nurses, physicians, therapists, and technicians; (2) the individuals receiving care, with their varying ages, characteristics, and health problems; and (3) nonprofessional lay providers, including friends, spouses, parents, children, and siblings who provide rehabilitative care. In contemporary society, there are very few extended families and few nuclear families in which the woman, the traditional care provider, is available to give care because the majority of women are employed outside the home. In many instances, the care provider (the person who operates and to some extent maintains the equipment) is likely to be a retired person in late middle age caring for an older relative. Sometimes, however, an older parent cares for a son or daughter in late middle age (Applegate, 1994).

Care providers may be sick or infirm themselves, may have manual dexterity impaired by disease (e.g., Parkinson's or arthritis), or may experience perceptual problems that affect their use of equipment, such as deafness or poor vision. They also can have decreased cognitive functioning due to disease or medication and lack of fluency in English. Care providers also may be young people who help by providing care at the end of the school day. These individuals may have characteristics that affect equipment use, such as small stature, limited upper body and hand strength, and lack of experience.

It is clear that age, ability, and health status of care providers vary greatly, as do the characteristics of the care recipients, nearly as much as the general population. To increase ease of operation and reduce the likelihood of error and the resulting adverse outcomes in using health care equipment, user characteristics must be considered in design.

User Considerations in Equipment Design

The once-daunting directive for military systems to be designed for the fifth-percentile woman to the ninety-fifth–percentile man (i.e., those of the age and physical fitness to serve in the military) is a source of envy for those who try to consider user characteristics in designing health care equipment. The users of this equipment are far more diverse than the military population. The issue of diversity underscores the importance of designing for the user through an ergonomic approach. Because the approach is to design from the perspective of the user, the diversity of users increases the challenges of design. (To reduce what may be redundancy in referring to human factors and ergonomics, only the term *ergonomics* is used.)

Automobile advertisements show that the application of ergonomics to design can enhance usability. An ergonomically designed car is presented as one in which the user is more comfortable, can see the dials on the dashboard readily, can adapt to driving with some degree of intuition, and can maintain more easily than cars without the benefit of such design. These performance components also apply to health care equipment design: Well-designed equipment is easier to use and maintain than equipment designed without such design considerations.

Despite the advantages, efforts to incorporate ergonomic considerations into the design of health care equipment have not been accepted as they have for products in the general consumer marketplace. The following discussion pursues this apparent inconsistency by addressing the evolving nature of the discipline of ergonomics, describing the incorporation of these considerations into user-centered design of health care equipment, and presenting an example of design-induced error.

Current Trends in Human Factors and Ergonomics

Traditionally, ergonomics professionals have focused their attention on the physical aspects of equipment, often referred to as *knobs and dials*. This focus is reflected in the *Human Factors Guidelines and Preferred Practices for the Design of Medical Devices* published by the Association for the Advancement of Medical Instrumentation (AAMI, 1993). The knobs-and-dials approach was appropriate when equipment was directly manipulable with straightforward procedures, a modicum of details that required attention, and obvious feedback. Although some health care equipment meets this description, technology has made the equipment far more complex. Currently, many health care devices are controlled indirectly through complex, often convoluted, programming of a computer chip with opaque (i.e., nonapparent) feedback as well as numerous activities and checks to be conducted.

Changes in the nature of health care equipment have expanded the scope of issues addressed by the practitioners of ergonomics. That expanded scope includes cognitive workload (i.e., the mental activity necessary to use a piece of equipment), individual differences among people who will use a piece of equipment, and the impact of the context of use on the person operating and maintaining equipment.

Cognitive Factors

There is a trend in research in aviation, a domain with a history of involvement with human factors, to address performance and human error issues, with a focus that includes the users' cognitive functioning (Wickens, 1995). That focus reflects the broadening of issues addressed in equipment design to consider the operator's cognitive as well as physical demands or workload. This expansion of ergonomic issues is relevant for the design of health care equipment for diverse user populations. To be used safely and effectively, equipment should impose minimal (if any) cognitive or physical demands on the most impeded user, such as an individual impaired by medication, stress, and language unfamiliarity, who operates the equipment in a crowded home environment with marginal resources. In other words, the equipment should be designed from the perspective of the worst-case operator and maintainer. This approach contrasts with the interpretation of many design engineers of what they are told about the needs of the users.

Users' Perspective

The importance of Wickens' (1995) focus on ergonomics is underscored by McNeese (1995), who notes that in traditional, knobs-and-dials human factors design, the user's knowledge, experiences, and needs were underappreciated. These factors were considered more from the ergonomist's perspective and not primarily from the perspective of the user. This is a fine, but very critical, distinction. In a sense, this is the distinction between objectivity and subjectivity (Muckler and Seven, 1992). What an engineer believes to be the knowledge, experience, and needs of the target user population, the objective view, may be very different from the subjective view of an actual end-user. This discrepancy can be corrected by involving actual, typical, if not worst-case, users in design discussions, and in ongoing testing during product development.

Human Factors Guidelines

Inclusion of users in the design process can be mandated for the categories or domains of equipment purchased or procured using Statements of Work (SOWs) to provide design specifications. Health care equipment, unlike domains that issue

SOWs, is designed and developed by industry, then submitted for premarket regulatory review, and ultimately marketed. It is a cottage industry that tends to develop its product without external specifications. Therefore, there has been no effective way to mandate human factor and ergonomic considerations in the design process. In an attempt to benefit from the experience of the military with standards for equipment design, the *Human Factors Engineering Guidelines* (AAMI, 1993) were developed for medical equipment based on the military human factors standard, MIL-STD-1472. The *Guidelines* have certain problems, as noted by Sind-Prunier (1995), among others.

Inspection of the *Guidelines* raises concerns about the appropriateness of much of its information for the development of health care equipment. Information of questionable value includes four pages of diagrams of hand-span, reach, and other anthropometric data for seated and standing operators. This may be questionable because few operators of health care equipment perform tasks in static positions. The *Guidelines* also include information about minimum separation distance between controls, including the J-handle on a mounting structure (five pages), but few, if any, pieces of health care equipment currently have such controls. Information is included on the body size of a 40-year-old Japanese male and female in the year 2000 (six pages). Although such data can be useful in designing health care equipment for people of a given size, such detail may not be necessary for most rehabilitative care equipment. Another example of information of questionable value from the *Guidelines* is control selection criteria (11 pages): Most health care equipment does not have the types of controls described.

The focus in the *Guidelines* on controls and anthropometric data does not address issues of contemporary equipment. Current ergonomic concerns in health care equipment include presenting information to enable the user to understand what the equipment is doing. This is of vital importance when the device can perform different functions or be in different modes by the flip of a switch or pressing a specific key—actions that can happen accidentally. To prevent mode error (believing the equipment is operating in one mode when in fact it is operating in another), it should

be obvious to the user in which mode the equipment is functioning. This important user issue is not addressed in the *Guidelines*. Indeed, the *Guidelines* address the central tenet of human factors and ergonomics, that of user-centered design, only in a gross sense. This is not sufficient for health care equipment. Guidance documents that appear to convey useful information must be considered critically.

User-Centered Design

User-centered design is design from the perspective of the user. It fits the capabilities, limitations, and performances of the user, as well as the context in which the item will be used. Because of the extensive use of health care equipment in home care and the wide variety of people who operate it, the characteristics of the user population approach those of the general population. Although some equipment is designed for a large population of care recipient users (e.g., wheelchairs), much rehabilitative and assistive equipment is developed for relatively small, specific populations with defined needs, often of a personal nature. For example, a sock puller designed for a young, strong paraplegic cannot be used by an elderly person with arthritic hands, so another puller for the elderly person is produced. This can be considered by some to be an unnecessary expenditure of increasingly constrained resources that might be reduced through universal design.

Universal Design

Universal design is reflected in equipment developed for a disability that is common to many people. Such equipment is adjustable for individual needs. Universal design uses of anthropometric data for groups of care recipients. With this approach to design, equipment can be designed for a diverse population without compromising its utility. Canes and crutches that can be adjusted for each individual are examples of universal design. In the sock puller example, a generic, universal design of that assistive device could be modified for use by people with a range of manual dexterity.

Research is needed on issues of universal design. Another area of research is how the separation of controls differs for people with different handicaps, so that controls can be designed to optimally aid each person in performing the task. Despite the cost and inventory advantages of quasi-generic, adjustable assistive equipment, there are conditions in which equipment may, if not must, be designed for one individual. Designing equipment for a given individual is referred to as *ergonomics-for-one.*

Ergonomics-for-One

Although the AAMI *Guidelines* (1993) may not be appropriate for designing most contemporary health care equipment, they can be useful in addressing some issues relevant to designing rehabilitative and assistive equipment for the workplace. Anthropometric data for seated and standing operators are important for people with disabilities who are in the work force; however, those data often must be tailored for a specific person. User-centered design is important not only for individuals with idiosyncratic needs; it is important for all users.

Importance of User-Centered Design

Equipment that is difficult to operate and maintain, and can contribute to or induce error, has been described in anecdotal reports and is in the folklore of many users and care providers. Although detailed, formal reports of error would be useful to provide information to identify problems to be addressed and reduce the likelihood of error, these reports are difficult to obtain. That difficulty is due in large part to our litigious society and the nearly immediate assumption that when an error occurs, the person associated with the error is responsible for it. Without information, it is difficult to learn from the experiences of users who operate and maintain the equipment, so problems that lead to error will be perpetuated. This increases the importance of developing user-centered evaluation criteria and conducting usability testing that is close to the actual context of use.

Human Error Versus Equipment Error

The design of health care equipment is technology-driven rather than user-centered. When an error is reported, typically it is presumed that the user is the problem and the equipment is blameless. The pervasive assumption that guides the development of health care equipment is that the user should accommodate the equipment rather than the equipment accommodating the user. That assumption directs error-reducing efforts to changing the user through training or punishment and not to assessing whether the equipment contributed to the error. Observation and analysis of an individual using health care equipment, as well as the lack of success in training, leads to the conclusion that a blame-the-user approach to error is not productive. Efforts should be made to assess how the error might have been induced by factors other than the user. One such factor is the equipment; other error-inducing factors can occur in the context of use. Contextual factors can interact with characteristics of the users; for example, a user with poor vision has to change a setting on equipment in dim light. To determine the role of contextual factors in the use of equipment, they must be included in the evaluation criteria.

Error and Context Evaluation Criteria

Error is a flag for a problem in the context or the system in which the person functions. Such a contextual or system problem impacts on the user to induce error (Bogner, 1994; Leape, 1994; Moray, 1994; Woods et al., 1994). Without consideration of the context of use, it is impossible to identify factors, including equipment design, that may contribute to error. Attempts to correct an error by addressing only the individual associated with the error probably will not reduce the likelihood of the error recurring. It is as if the scenario that induces error is a script: Changing the players results in only slight variations but does not appreciably change performance. Although error is but one aspect of performance, it can indicate use and maintenance problems and lead to adverse events.

Error in health care is not a rare occurrence. It has been estimated, based on data from a major study, that 100,000 people per year (twice the annual highway death rate) die in the United States from preventable adverse events that occurred when they were hospitalized (Leape, 1994). In addition to the cost implications of malpractice and product liability litigation, error in health care incurs patient-related dollar costs.

Adverse events in hospitalized patients that resulted in extended hospital stays, further medical treatment, incapacity, and death have been estimated to cost $25 billion per year (Bogner, 1994). Given that many adverse events occur that do not result in death or debilitating injury and that many errors occur outside a hospital, the extent and costs of error in health care are profound. Although the evidence is not definitive because data were obtained through retrospective chart review (Leape et al., 1991), many of those adverse events are associated directly or indirectly with the use and maintenance of health care equipment.

A valid assumption when considering error in the use of equipment, particularly health care equipment, is that people do not intend to make an error; people want to operate the equipment to achieve the intended result. This desire to make equipment work is evidenced by users' elaborate modifications to equipment and to operational and maintenance procedures that users develop to accommodate design problems. Design that necessitates workarounds (i.e., user modifications of the equipment) indicates of a concern for error as well as of problems in using the equipment.

Given that people do not intend to make errors and indeed work hard to prevent them and that errors nevertheless occur, other aspects of the error-inducing situation, the system or context of use, should be examined for factors that affect the user and lead to error. Once potential error-inducing factors are identified, they should be integrated into evaluation criteria that are a part of usability testing. For example, excessive workload is a system factor that causes stress.

Stress

Stress is a pervasive factor in nearly all contexts in which health care is provided, and often contributes to error. Many factors can induce stress for health care professionals in a hospital setting, including organizationally determined workload as well as changes in shifts that counter the body's circadian rhythm (Kreuger, 1994). Home health care givers experience stress from the responsibilities of providing care and the concomitant psychological and physical fatigue. Because stress is so pervasive, it is an important user issue in the design of health care equipment.

Stress is an important design issue because it reduces a person's cognitive functioning. Such reduction in functioning affects a person in many ways, including the impairment of a person's ability to remember the many details required to operate complex health care equipment. When a person is stressed, details can be omitted and lead to errors. Design that considers the impact of factors caused by context of use, such as stress, result in reduced complexity (e.g., simple, intuitive design with few details).

Simple design, however, is not particularly marketable in our technology-driven society. The assumption that more technology is better has been manifest in no part of our society more than in health care, despite the impact on the user. To encourage the consideration of the user in health care equipment design, user issues should be integral to its evaluation criteria. This provides a basis for identifying problems in the use and maintenance of equipment through usability testing. Problems so identified can point to user issues not addressed in design that may be corrected and incorporated into future designs.

The following example of design-induced error underscores the importance of user-centered evaluation criteria, which can lead to design changes. The equipment in the example is not used by any specific clinical community, but its use problems illustrate several important issues indicative of design that is not user centered.

An Example of Design-Induced Error

Don Norman (1992, p. 170) has said, "Blaming the person [is] a way to avoid the real issues." An example of the blame-the-person approach is provided by blood glucose meters (BGMs). BGMs are computer chip–based, portable devices designed to measure the blood sugar level of a person with diabetes. The diabetic puts a drop of blood from a finger on a strip and inserts the strip into the meter, which calculates the sugar level and presents numbers indicating that level on a display. On the basis of that information, the diabetic regulates his or her exercise, diet, and insulin. People with advanced disease may be required to test their sugar level as often as five times a day. The meters are used in institutional settings, in the home, at sporting events, and in any setting in which diabetics find themselves when it is time to test their blood.

Death and serious injury have occurred because people gave themselves insulin or adjusted their exercise or diet inappropriately based on readings from the meter. Typically, this is interpreted as a clear case of user error: Incorrect operation of the BGMs gave inaccurate blood sugar readings. Because the problem is presumed to reside in the user, efforts are made to change the users' behavior by training. Training, however, does not significantly reduce the problem. This has led to the presumption that users are hopeless, which is far from the case. Those who develop criteria to evaluate the problem need to understand that the user is only one part of the equation. The equipment also should be scrutinized and considered from the perspective of the user, which can be done from evaluation criteria developed from that perspective.

When the design of certain BGMs is analyzed, not from the perspectives of the design engineer, the institutional risk manager, or the data analyst, but from the user's perspective, it becomes evident that the design of the meter contributes to if not induces error. The design of BGMs, although developed for people with diabetes, does not consider the effects of the disease on the user. For example, one of the physical conditions caused by the disease, diabetic retinopathy, impairs the diabetic's vision. Many BGMs are very small; some as small as pens and credit cards. The display on these BGMs is too small for the person with impaired vision to read accurately.

The markings are also small and difficult to read on a related piece of equipment, the insulin syringe. To compensate for that problem, an entrepreneur developed a plastic magnifying cylinder to place over the syringe so that numbers can be seen more easily. As Norman (1992) notes, such aids are signals of inappropriate design. The likelihood of error and associated adverse events could have been reduced by identifying the problem of size of displays and marking through user-centered evaluation criteria.

Another set of problems with BGMs is that people with diabetes experience impaired manual dexterity. This makes the insertion of a small test strip into a small opening very difficult, particularly on the credit card–size meters, and can lead to misinserted strips and resulting misreadings. It also makes cleaning a meter by disassembling and reassembling very difficult.

With respect to the impact of the context of use on BGMs, effects of stress can be manifest in many ways. Many BGM models require that a test strip with a drop of blood on it be inserted into the meter to be read. After repeated use, a residue of blood forms in the meter. To reduce the likelihood of inaccurate readings due to the residue, the meter must be cleaned. Time and workload stress make this a difficult task, particularly if the disassembly procedure is not intuitive and the instructions are difficult to understand, assuming that the location of the instruction manual is known. These factors, coupled with the stress related to the users' disease-related impaired manual dexterity, can result in the meter not being cleaned as often as it should be, which can lead to inaccurate readings. This indicates not so much user error as design error. If cleaning the meter is important to its accuracy, and the user is the maintainer, then it is incumbent on the manufacturer to design a meter that is easy for the user to clean.

It is an oft-stated maxim that user needs should be considered in designing not only the equipment but also the procedures for operating and maintaining it, the packaging, and any accompanying written material. All these are user issues for evaluation criteria, not those of the design engineer alone. In the BGM example, considering the vision problems of the diabetic users, written instructions should be of an easily read font size, and considering the millions of Americans who have diabetes, the instructions should be written in a way that the worst-case user can comprehend, perhaps presented graphically. In addition to accommodating the problems caused by the disease, the design should include a display large enough to be read by a user with diabetes-impaired vision, a large opening for the strip with internal guides, and simple cleaning procedures. Opportunities for error can be reduced by user-centered design, design that acknowledges and compensates for the perceptual and physical problems resulting from the medical condition for which the equipment is used. The viability of user-centered design can be assessed by testing the usability of the equipment against user-centered evaluation criteria.

User-Centered Issues in Evaluation Criteria

For the purpose of this discussion, *evaluation* is considered the assessment of equipment against a set of criteria. *Usability testing* is considered a dynamic assessment involving the execution of a procedure to determine ease of use as well as accuracy of performance. Before usability testing, user issues must be identified to be incorporated into evaluation criteria.

Evaluation Criteria Tools

Development of equipment primarily from the ergonomist's perspective can result in awkward interfaces or even design failure (McNeese, 1995). Although the ergonomist may have the knowledge and education necessary for usability testing, he or she may also base the design on personal experience, rather than involving the user. This happens particularly often in the design of health care equipment. Unlike automobiles or other equipment the ergonomists themselves may have used (for which they can project some user experience into the design), ergonomists are not likely to have had experience using health care equipment. Tools exist, however, that can assist them.

Domestic and international standards, guidelines, and recommended practices related to aspects of health care equipment can be incorporated into evaluation criteria, albeit often to a limited extent. Those documents are too extensive to enumerate here; information can be obtained by contacting standards development organizations. (Information, including addresses and phone numbers, about such organizations can be found in Irons, 1996.)

Although standards and guidelines can be useful in developing evaluation criteria and guiding design, they are often anecdotally rather than empirically based and address aspects of the overall design that may be indirectly related, if at all, to use issues. Over reliance on standards and guidelines without the active involvement of users can result in neglect of user-centered considerations in evaluation criteria. Such neglect can lead to equipment that induces errors and adverse outcomes.

Context of Use

The importance of context in equipment design is noted by McNeese (1995): He proposes that failure of knowledge engineers (individuals who specialize in the technological aspects of presenting information) "to consider the influences of socio-organizational and contextual factors" (p. 2) leads to equipment that can contribute to error. An approach to design that considers the context of use is important for understanding the impact of factors in the experiential-physical-social-cultural environment on the use of health care equipment. This is a systems approach (defined below), which can assist in designing equipment and developing criteria for the evaluation of the usability of health care equipment.

Systems Approach

Moray (1994) has proposed a systems approach to the problem of error in health care. He described the aspects of the system in which people give and receive health care that induce error as the "design of objects, activities, procedures, and patterns of behavior" (p. 67). A systems approach requires that the ergonomist examine all elements of a system including personnel, equipment, task, and environment. Therefore, when using a systems approach in examining error in health care, the contextual factors such as workload, stress, personal experience levels, and the physical, political, and psychosocial environments should all be considered. This all-encompassing approach is used to identify aspects of the system that are the primary culprits impacting people's behavior to contribute to or induce adverse events. Once identified, efforts can begin to rectify these problematic aspects directly or indirectly.

Palmer et al. (1985) found that tasks targeted for improvement in providing quality care were not improved when the tasks were associated with a need for delivery system changes that were beyond the control of the health care provider. Following Moray's systems approach, such targets for improvement may include reducing stress and fatigue that contribute to error by changing work schedules, behavior patterns, and attitudes of health care professionals. This could involve changing the policy of professional organizations and local, state, and even national policy. It is not a short-term approach:

Change in organizations and policy involves many people and can be a slow process. Legislation can expedite such change, but the ramifications of legislated change can cause other, often profound problems, and legislation itself does not happen quickly. Systems issues are central to evaluation. Using a systems approach to set evaluation criteria, conduct usability testing, and thereby guide equipment design should ensure that all variables are considered.

The expanded human factors and ergonomics approach, with its appreciation of context, not only supports the systems approach—it embodies that approach. The impact of the context is from the perspective of the user.

Consumer Involvement in Product Modification

A user-centered approach is vital to reducing the likelihood of error in the use of rehabilitative, assistive, and health care equipment. In developing general consumer products, evaluation criteria developed from the users themselves are often used in usability testing, thus increasing the "reality" of testing. The process used in developing a consumer product can be applied to the development of health care equipment. Because of the dearth of information on applying user-centered criteria to health care products, an example of consumer involvement in modification of a general product, lunch boxes, will be used. It illustrates how two types of users and user-centered criteria were used in design and evaluation.

In a project to redesign children's lunch boxes (Mitchell, 1995), user-based criteria were developed from the first phase of the project. That phase consisted of field research to identify the reactions of two categories of users, children and parents, to existing lunch boxes. The research included on-site observations of children using lunch boxes and children's sketches of an ideal lunch box. This information was refined and used to develop lunch box concept models. Before production, the models were taken to schools, and the children's use of them was observed and recorded. The models also were given to parents, and their reactions to packing the lunch boxes were assessed. Thus, the criteria for design of the equipment essentially started with user groups. Those who eat from them and those who pack and maintain them provided valuable information during the initial design phase, pro-vided evaluation criteria, and were included in testing and evaluation of the final product.

If that much concern was shown for user acceptance of lunch boxes, it seems reasonable that similar concern is merited for health care equipment. More particularly, health care equipment should be both developed and evaluated from the users' perspective, that is, by user-based criteria.

User-Based Criteria

User-based criteria for evaluating all assistive equipment was developed by Batavia and Hammer (1990). Although they identified factors that could be used in such evaluations, the authors consider their findings preliminary. This is due to several methodologic concerns, such as how representative the sample is of the long-term user populations. Their concern points to a problem with universal criteria: Not all assistive equipment is used by the same population. Batavia and Hammer noted that an analysis of the functional goals of the equipment, the context in which it is used, and the populations that will use it may indicate that a single, all-purpose list of criteria is not practical. They felt that the focus of their research, that of developing criteria for evaluating assistive devices in general, may have been too broad. The diversity in devices and users might be better served by developing the essentials of a universal design for assistive devices, with added criteria for specific modifications for particular end users.

Batavia and Hammer's work supports the case for user-based evaluation criteria for a refined definition of users. That refined definition appreciates the perspective of users who share common needs for special features of equipment for that particular subgroup of users. As criteria for various types of equipment are determined, they can be compared for commonalities, and perhaps an empirically based core criteria can be developed. Without this empiric basis, general criteria could be like a one-size-fits-all shirt that fits no one.

User Issues in Equipment Testing

To be user-centered, it is important that the evaluation of health equipment actively include criteria from a systems perspective of a range of contextual factors. These factors can be as specific as inadequate lighting or as general as the culture of a profession, for example, the "can-do" attitude of nurses (nurses' belief that they should be able to solve whatever problem may confront them, including equipment that is difficult to operate and maintain).

As with equipment design, there are two perspectives for user issues in evaluation: the engineer's assessment and the user's assessment. The following discussion of an infusion pump gives examples of each perspective. Evaluations from each perspective are shown in reports of problems with a specific model of an infusion pump. As with the BGM example, although the pump is not used by a specific clinical community, this case illustrates several ergonomic issues that pertain to all equipment.

An Example of Two-User Perspective: Infusion Pump

An infusion pump mechanically monitors the delivery of fluid into a vein or tissue. It is shaped like a box with a key pad and a display. It is placed on the pole from which the bag of fluid is hung. A tube carrying fluid from the bag is pressed into a channel in the pump, which is accessible when the door to the pump is opened. The channel contains small "fingers" that move in a peristaltic manner to pass the fluid through the tubing. Typically, the tubing is pressed into the channel from the top of the pump to the bottom of the pump, from which it continues until it is attached to a needle that delivers the fluid to the recipient's tissue or vein.

A model of an infusion pump was designed so that the tubing is installed inside the pump from the bottom up. During loading of this model, the pump door is open and the tubing that comes from the bottom of the bag and hangs in front of the channel is pressed into the channel from the bottom of the channel, which is at the bottom of the pump until it reaches the end of the channel at the top of the pump.

After the bottom-up pump was marketed, there were a number of incidents in which the tubing was installed in the pump but no fluid was infused. Also, in some instances, the bottom-up installation was interpreted to entail looping the tubing so that the pumping mechanism was reversed, and blood from the patient was found in the tubing. These problems allegedly happened because of user error in installing the tubing from the top down instead of from the bottom up.

The design of the bottom-up pump included several alarm capabilities and fail-safe features to avoid free flow of the fluid. (Free flow had been found to occur when the door to the pump is open, which eliminates control of the fluid without first stopping the flow through the tubing.) The pump was evaluated using several engineering techniques, such as Failure Mode and Effects Analysis and safety hazard assessments (Stamatis, 1995). The engineering assessment indicated that the pump was safe to use. Despite this finding, problems occurred that resulted in injury and death, and these problems were readily identifiable by the users.

The subjective experience of users, based on their clinical experience with infusion pumps, is that tubing is usually installed from the top of the channel to the bottom. To install tubing from the bottom up requires conscious effort. The system in which the pump is used reinforces the top-down manner of tubing installation in several ways. Users know that the often near-chaotic conditions of the context of use (e.g., an intensive care unit in a hospital) are likely to make the necessary cognitive effort for the atypical installation difficult; hence, the familiar procedure for installing tubing likely would be followed.

Compared to other pumps in the context of use, users found no readily observable cues to remind them to install the tubing bottom up: The interior of the bottom-up pump is essentially the same as that of the top-down pump produced by the same manufacturer. A small diagram of the bottom-up tubing installation procedure appears on the inside of the door to the pump, but that can be overlooked because of its size and location. If users had unlimited time to install the tubing, they might search and find the small diagram, but that typically is not the case.

In short, in the context of use there are no attention-getting, obvious cues to remind the user of the atypical, bottom-up tubing installation. In addition, there is no fail-safe mechanism in the tubing or in the design of the pump to prevent its being loaded top down. The design engineers did not incorporate the user's perspective, nor did they include the impact of the system in which equipment is used and maintained in the engineering assessments of the pump. The manufacturer's effort to address the misinstallation of tubing was to provide additional training and a pocket-sized instruction sheet for installing the tubing. The problem persists. The manufacturer recommends further training.

The infusion pump example illustrates the propensity to address only one aspect of the system in which error occurs, the user. It also illustrates the lack of viability of a solution that addresses only that aspect of the system. User-centered evaluation criteria can confirm the implementation of user-driven design when it is applied in a testing environment, such as usability testing.

Usability Testing

Usability testing refers to the systematic evaluation of the "interaction between people and the products, equipment, environments, and services they use" (McClelland, 1990, p. 218). Usability testing evaluates how easy a product is to use and whether it is functional and acceptable. One assumption of usability testing is that equipment can be evaluated by collecting data on the operation of the equipment in a controlled setting, most often a laboratory and currently is popular among ergonomists. To engender an understanding of its value and applicability for health care equipment, the history of usability testing is briefly discussed, issues regarding laboratory versus real-world testing are described, and laboratory versus simulation testing is addressed.

The computer industry developed usability testing to determine ease of learning software products, and once a specific software product is learned, how easy that product is to use (Mack & Nielsen, 1994). Errors in product use as well as factors that enhance performance are considered part of the usability of a product. In addition to identifying problems, a purpose of usability testing is to provide design-related resolution of problems.

The context for computer usability testing is often a laboratory with one-way windows, through which the participant can be observed interacting with the product. Video equipment typically is used to record the user's behavior and comments. A laboratory is not a requirement for usability testing, but it may be preferred. When people use a computer, they typically interact primarily, if not solely, with it and have little immediate interaction with other aspects of the physical or social environment, so the conditions of a usability laboratory are quite similar to the context of use for computers and software.

Testing Noncomputer Equipment

The conditions that are appropriate to test the usability of computers and software are not necessarily appropriate to test noncomputer equipment, such as health care equipment. A response by the software may not have been what was expected or desired by the user, but the range of software responses are limited, and the action that elicited the response most likely did not harm the software. The range of responses by the computer constrains the reactions of the user elicited by those responses. The range of responses from the interaction of health care equipment and the recipient of care, however, is wide and often unpredictable.

Workload for computer users does not change precipitously as a result of the computer's condition unlike the sudden workload change for a clinician should a patient's condition suddenly improve or worsen. Typically, people working with computers are not bombarded by the need to attend to other pieces of equipment being used for other, related purposes, as are users of health care equipment. Nor are the responses of a user to computer software comparable to the responses of a user of health care equipment, which can result in responses from the recipient of care that range from rapid improvement to death with significant impact on workload. Undoubtedly, there is stress in computer use as in air traffic control, but those stressful conditions differ significantly from the types of stress and workload changes experienced in health care settings. Therefore, usability testing must be performed under stressful conditions similar to those in actual use accurately identify user issues.

The importance of considering workload issues in health care technology assessment has been underscored by Sind-Prunier (1995). She proposes that to adequately assess how well the design of health care equipment accommodates the workload of the user, it is important to evaluate the design against the worst-case workload scenario experienced by actual users.

Many who develop health care equipment may protest that worst-case evaluation is not practical for their products. Indeed, some manufacturers believe that it is enough to conduct tests in the laboratories in which the equipment was developed, using as subjects those who developed the equipment or other people from the same organization. Others feel that such testing provides no objectivity or realism in the evaluation. A laboratory setting does have advantages, such as control of confounding factors. Confounding factors are part of the worst-case scenario in the use of health care equipment and should be considered in the evaluation of its usability.

Laboratory Versus Real-World Testing

The goal of having a controlled laboratory setting in which to test a product is seductive because it is a clean, uncomplicated way to collect data. A laboratory may not be an appropriate setting for testing of some products, but testing some aspects of equipment in a usability laboratory can identify problems and is often the first step in usability testing. However, an aspect of a device that is difficult to use in a laboratory setting could be impossible to use in the chaos of an actual health care setting. Given Mitchell's (1995) comment that there may be only one chance to test the equipment, which acknowledges the ergonomist's very limited opportunity for testing, it is imperative that any test provide as much information as possible about the characteristics of the equipment that are relevant to its actual use.

Ecologic Validity

Jordan and Thomas (1994) raised the issue of ecologic validity of a usability laboratory, that is, how closely the test environment resembles the actual environment in which the product will be used. They found that potential supporters of usability testing who were not ergonomists expressed the attitude that ecologic validity is central to usability evaluation. The ergonomists they interviewed did not share this opinion. The ergonomists expressed the attitude that if a high level of ecologic validity were important, the testing should be conducted in the field. They felt that one of the most valuable aspects of the usability laboratory was propaganda, that is, projecting the image of the ergonomists' work.

Much of what ergonomists do is work on paper or manipulate a piece of equipment, which, although quite valuable, does not appear scientific and is difficult to appreciate. Looking through a one-way window at a person working with a piece of equipment while that activity is being videotaped in a usability laboratory has much more of an aura of science and, as such, affords the ergonomists the trappings of science. Generalizability of findings from such testing, however, may apply only to people using the particular piece of equipment in a comparable setting. The importance of ecologic validity can vary according to the extent to which the product being tested is affected by factors in the context of its use. For products such as health care equipment, which are subject to myriad factors in actual use, ecologic validity is essential in obtaining findings that apply to the typical use of that equipment.

Although there are ethical issues in using prototype equipment in an actual health care setting, an actual setting can provide information about problems in using existing health care equipment. This is evidenced in videotapes of actual emergency room cases in research on decision making under stress by Mackenzie and his colleagues (1996). Although it was not the focus of the research, the videotapes provide serendipitous data on product problems, such as packaging that is difficult to remove and a monitor on which the user cannot retrieve information about the patient's vital signs.

Applicability of Laboratory Usability Testing Across Products

A technique such as laboratory usability testing is appealing and is sometimes adopted with enthusiasm without considering the degree to which the technique is appropriate to the problem under consideration. The worst-case scenario should be considered in equipment design and in its evaluation and usability testing. The laboratory setting for testing computer software, a setting very similar to the actual context of use, does not approximate the actual context of use for health care equipment and as such may not be an appropriate venue for testing its usability. The applicability of findings from such testing to actual users in the context of use is questionable.

Usability testing developed by and for computer and software products may be appropriate for products that are used in settings similar to computers, such as telephones and computer-based information-providing equipment, that are not subject to impact by environmental factors. As Scerbo (1995) notes, there is concern that findings from usability testing may lead to unrealistic expectations for a product. He also notes that some professionals express concern about the potential for subject and procedural bias as well as the reliability and validity of data from usability testing. Thus, usability laboratory testing of products such as health care equipment whose operation is affected by contextual factors in a usability laboratory could provide spurious findings.

Use of a health care device occurs in a complex environment with several dynamic factors that affect the user, including the physical and emotional state of the care recipient. Stressors affecting the use of health care equipment that occur in the context of use, such as those in the BGM example, most likely are not evident in the usability testing laboratory because of the lack of time pressure and the often-overlooked Hawthorne effect, in which the subject works especially hard to complete the task because she is being observed.

Karat (1994) emphasizes the importance of testing a product with techniques appropriate to the characteristics of that product and the context of its intended use. She states that although several usability assessment methods exist, they cannot be used indiscriminately. The objectives of a specific computer-related project, such as interface issues (the subject of her evaluations), must be carefully considered in selecting a method for use in a particular situation. If care is important in selecting methodologies for a specific class of products (e.g., computers), care should also be exercised in subjecting a broad class of products (e.g., health care equipment) to a testing situation appropriate to the testing objectives of that class of products.

Dumas and Redish (1993, p. 26) stated that "usability testing works for all types of products." The caveat is that the testing methods and process must be tailored to the system in which the product is used. It might be said that the only way to tell if usability testing really works is to examine the number of changes in the product identified as a result of the testing. It also may be said that only when no changes are indicated as a result of the testing is it demonstrated that the testing efforts were not effective. This raises two issues. One is that repeated testing occurs, which may not be possible, as Mitchell (1995) states. The second reiterates the question of the validity of laboratory findings for actual context of use. The competing demands of other equipment,

other health care providers, and the recipients of care and the variables they introduce are not represented in the laboratory. Findings from a laboratory setting may not "work" in reducing problems in using and maintaining health care equipment in actual use. For equipment minimally affected by interaction with dynamic entities in its context of use, laboratory-based usability testing is appropriate.

The enthusiasm for usability testing for all types of products, with the implication that such testing occurs in a laboratory setting, has evoked negative reactions (Scerbo, 1995). It would be a pity if the baby of rigor of usability testing were tossed out with the bath water of the laboratory setting. Unfortunately, those who extolled the virtues of laboratory usability testing eclipsed the important comment by Dumas and Redish (1993) that any means of observing a person using a product and recording his or her actions and comments can be the basis for a usability test—making simulation testing a viable alternative. This is evidenced in Rice's (1995) elegant, formal, hypothetical usability test of a walker. The real-world problem of maneuvering around a file cabinet using the assistive device was appropriately tested in a controlled setting, which approximated simulation testing. This takes usability testing out of the laboratory to be conducted in a realistic context of use with systematic recording of equipment use and comment, known as *operational usability testing*.

Laboratory Versus Operational Testing

For the purpose of this discussion, testing that has many of the features of usability testing but considers factors in the actual context of use for the product being tested is referred to as *operational usability testing*.

The operational aspect of testing, that of testing under conditions as near to those of actual operation of the equipment, has been used successfully in some domains. The military has a history of conducting operational tests of its weapon systems. This testing typically occurs in a physical setting like that of a possible battle (forested terrain, desert), using prototypes of the weapon system and nonexplosive ammunition, operated and maintained by the personnel who will use the system when it is fielded. Operational testing follows the scenario of the performance specifications of the system: a period of continuous operation of the system of a specified duration. Often, the activities of the crew are videotaped to determine problems of use. Findings from operational tests can lead to design modifications before the system is produced.

A variation of operational testing is conducted by the U.S. Consumer Product Safety Commission (CPSC). Consumer products with identified or potential safety hazards are subjected to tests emulating conditions of use, often extreme conditions to push the envelope of ease and safety in use. Although these tests do not necessarily involve actual users, the behavior that tests the products is comparable to that of a user, such as pulling at the buttonlike eyes of a stuffed animal or dropping a product from the height of a tall ladder.

Operational usability testing is in the spirit of the testing conducted by the military and the CPSC. It can occur in a laboratory or in locations other than a laboratory. Because health care products are used to provide care to vulnerable populations, aberrations in the operation of the products during testing could harm an actual health care recipient. This can be avoided by some form of simulation of either the situation or the patients, or both, simultaneously.

Simulation Tests

Simulation, a hybrid of usability laboratory and field testing, generally mimics real-world operation within a more controlled setting. It provides conditions for operational assessment of equipment during which no harm can occur. Applying evaluation criteria in simulated usability testing allows the preliminary determination of the appropriateness of the design for the workload conditions of use. Testing equipment by operating and maintaining it in a realistic simulated environment affords an opportunity to assess workload issues as well as issues pertaining to the actual ease of use of the equipment.

Simulations in operational environments used to address user-centered issues in rehabilitative care equipment builds on the strengths of usability testing, such as recording activity and comments, and avoids the weakness of questionable ecologic validity. Concern that the nature of health care devices may harm the patient is alleviated by providing a physiologically versatile manikin as the health care recipient. This allows

a simulated situation in which an actual health care setting is used to assess the ease of use of equipment. In that ecologically valid context, actual users function in an actual setting; only the recipient of care is not real. As shown in the widespread use of simulators in training aviation personnel, people can become very involved in a simulated operational situation.

A simulated patient (a manikin with certain computer-based physiologic characteristics) has been used to study the functioning of operating room (OR) personnel. In work by Gaba and DeAnda (1988), the manikin replaces an actual patient in an OR and can be programmed to react to the anesthesiologists' care in ways that challenge their skill. This videotaped activity provides an assessment of how an anesthesiologist responds and manages crisis situations. Helmreich and Davies (1996) also used a manikin as a patient in an actual OR and observed the cooperation of members of the OR team through videotaping. The functioning of each team member in response to programmed problems that occur during "surgery" on the manikin is assessed using information from the videotapes. In both instances, information from the actual context-based simulations has been used to improve team functioning.

The usability of health care equipment can be assessed in the context of use appropriate for the equipment being tested with actual users, people simulating care recipients, and programmable care recipient manikins. Equipment can be tested on a wide range of responses, including rare reactions, that can be programmed into the manikin. The context of use provides settings of unquestionable ecologic validity, and videotaping interactions with the equipment provides data for measurement.

The ultimate operational usability testing would be in an actual health care setting involving actual users, as was done by Mackenzie et al. (1996). In that research and, to a lesser degree, in simulation research, a problem arises with the magnitude of videotaped data. That problem underscores the importance of establishing evaluation criteria. To identify use issues with existing health care equipment, videotaping could be done in particular locations of interest, such as the physical therapy department, during specific time frames. Videotaping can be used to assess patients' use of equipment, such as ingress and egress from a vehicle with a particular wheelchair design or various types of breath control devices for powered wheelchairs. It also can be used to assess training manuals or training programs, such as teaching a patient to use and care for an artificial limb. Thus videotaping is useful for product improvements of existing equipment, for evaluation of prototypes, and for operational or simulation testing with manikins.

Conclusion

Operational usability testing of rehabilitative, assistive, and health care equipment brings the point of this chapter—the importance of user-centered design—full circle. To reduce the likelihood of error and optimize ease of use of equipment, a typical user must be involved in developing a device from its inception through testing, evaluation, and marketing. The user is not to be confused with a subject matter expert, who may or may not have current clinical experience with similar equipment.

The perspective of the user, not the engineers' interpretation of the needs of the user, forms the basis for user-centered design. This is not a new idea: In 1988, John Gould proposed that a user be a member of the design team. User-based criteria should be employed in evaluating equipment. To truly test the usability of equipment, it must be subjected to operational testing that assesses the importance of the context, actual or simulated, in which it will be used. Programmable manikins and videotaping afford the opportunity to conduct operational usability assessments, but it is an expensive way to test equipment. The spirit of systematic operational usability testing can be served much less expensively by using people as care recipient surrogates as much as possible.

Operational usability testing addresses the issues raised by Mitchell (1995). Because such testing simulates actual conditions, sufficient data can be obtained to avoid iterative design, for which there rarely is time or money. Findings from operational usability testing can be used to address the concerns of engineers and managers by convincing them of the value of ergonomic, user-centered activities.

The greatest value of using an ergonomic systems approach to conduct operational usability testing is to demonstrate that equipment developed from the perspective of the people who operate and maintain it, is easier to use, has a reduced likelihood of errors, as well as having fewer requests for user support, increased user satisfaction, and reduced product liability litigation. Operational usability testing will advance the discipline of human factors and ergonomics and improve the quality of life of those who use the equipment.

References

Applegate, M.H. (1994). Diagnosis related groups: Are patients in jeopardy? In M.S. Bogner (Ed.), *Human error in medicine* (pp. 349–372). Hillsdale, NJ: Lawrence Erlbaum.

Association for the Advancement of Medical Instrumentation. (1993). *Human factors engineering guidelines and preferred practices for the design of medical devices* (ANSI/AAMI HE48-1993). Alexandria, VA: AAMI.

Batavia, A.I., & Hammer, G.S. (1990). Toward the development of consumer-based criteria for the evaluation of assistive devices. *Journal of Rehabilitation Research and Development, 27*, 425–436.

Bogner, M.S. (1994). Human error in medicine: A frontier for change. In M.S. Bogner (Ed.), *Human error in medicine* (pp. 311–326). Hillsdale, NJ: Lawrence Erlbaum.

Dumas, J.S., & Redish, J.C. (1993). *A practical guide to usability testing.* Norwood, NJ: Ablex Publishing.

Gaba, D.M., & DeAnda, A. (1988). A comprehensive anesthesia simulating environment re-creating the operating room for research and training. *Anesthesiology, 69,* 387–394.

Gould, J.D. (1988). How to design usable systems. In M. Helander (Ed.), *Handbook of human-computer interactions* (pp. 557–789). Amsterdam: Elsevier.

Helmreich, R.L., & Davies, J.M. (1996). Human factors in the operating room: Interpersonal determinants of safety, efficiency, and morale. In A.R. Aitenhead (Ed.), *Bailliere's clinical anaesthesiology: Safety and risk management in anaesthesia.* London: Bailliere Tindall.

Irons, G.J. (1996). *Standards annual report.* Rockville, MD: U.S. Food and Drug Administration, Center for Devices and Radiological Health.

Jordan, P.W., & Thomas, D.B. (1994, October). Ecological validity in laboratory based usability evaluations. *Proceedings of the Human Factors and Ergonomics Society 38th Annual Meeting,* 128–130.

Karat, C. (1994). A comparison of user interface evaluation methods. In J. Nielson, & R.L. Mack (Eds.), *Usability inspection methods* (pp. 203–234). New York: John Wiley.

Kreuger, G.P. (1994). Fatigue, performance, and medical error. In M.S. Bogner (Ed.), *Human error in medicine* (pp. 311–326). Hillsdale, NJ: Lawrence Erlbaum.

Leape, L.L. (1994). The preventability of medical injury. In M.S. Bogner (Ed.), *Human error in medicine* (pp. 13–25). Hillsdale, NJ: Lawrence Erlbaum.

Leape, L.L., Brennan, T.A., Laird, N.M., et al. (1991). The nature of adverse events in hospitalized patients. Results of the Harvard Medical Practice Study II. *New England Journal of Medicine, 324,* 377–384.

Mack, R.L., & Nielson, J. (1994). Executive summary. In J. Nielson, & R.L. Mack (Eds.), *Usability inspection methods* (pp. 1–24). New York: John Wiley.

Mackenzie, C.F., Jefferies, N.J., Hunter, A., et al. (1996). Identifying systems problems in trauma patient anesthesia: An analysis of performance deficiencies in airway management as captured by video and self-reports. *Human Factors, 38,* 636–645.

McClelland, I. (1990). Product assessment and user trials. In J.R. Wilson, & E.M. Corlett (Eds.), *Evaluation of human work: A practical ergonomics methodology* (p. 218). New York: Taylor & Francis.

McNeese, M.D. (1995). Cognitive engineering: A different approach to human-machine systems. *Gateway, VI(5),* 1–4. Wright-Patterson AFB, OH: Crew System Ergonomics Information Analysis Center.

Mitchell, P.P. (1995). Consumer products techniques. In J. Weimer (Ed.), *Research techniques in human engineering* (pp. 246–267). Englewood Cliffs, NJ: Prentice Hall.

Moray, N. (1994). Error reduction as a systems problem. In M.S. Bogner (Ed.), *Human error in medicine* (pp. 67–91). Hillsdale, NJ: Lawrence Erlbaum.

Muckler, F.A., & S.A. Seven. (1992). Selecting performance measures: "Objective" versus "subjective" measurement. *Human Factors, 34,* 441–455.

Norman, D.A. (1992). Turn signals are the facial expressions of automobiles. Reading, MA: Addison-Wesley.

Palmer, R.H., Louis, T.A., Hsu, L.H., et al. (1985). A randomized controlled trial of quality assurance in sixteen ambulatory care practices. *Medical Care, 23,* 751–770.

Rice, V.J. (1995). Human factors in medical rehabilitation equipment: Product development and usability testing. In K. Jacobs, & C.M. Bettencourt (Eds.), *Ergonomics for therapists* (77–93). Boston: Butterworth–Heinemann.

Scerbo, M.W. (1995). Usability testing. In J. Weimer (Ed.), *Research techniques in human engineering* (pp. 72–110). Englewood Cliffs, NJ: Prentice Hall.

Sind-Prunier, P. (1995). Medical techniques. In J. Weimer (Ed.), *Research techniques in human engineering* (pp. 332–362). Englewood Cliffs, NJ: Prentice Hall.

Stamatis, D.H. (1995). Failure mode and effect analysis. Milwaukee, WI: ACQC Quality Press.

Wickens, C.D. (1995). Aerospace techniques. In J. Weimer (Ed.), *Research techniques in human engineering* (pp. 112–142). Englewood Cliffs, NJ: Prentice Hall.

Woods, D.D., Johannesen, L., Cook, R.I., & Sarter, N. (1994). *Behind human error: Cognitive systems, computers, and hindsight.* Wright-Patterson AFB, OH: Crew Systems Ergonomics Information Analysis Center.

Chapter 14

Medical and Rehabilitation Equipment Case Study: Design, Development, and Usability Testing of a Lift-Seat Wheelchair

Donald S. Bloswick, Ben Shirley, and Eric King

Learning Objectives

On completion of this chapter, the reader should be able to

- Understand methodologies for analysis and quantification of user needs and establish design criteria to meet these established needs.
- Recognize various criteria necessary for testing and evaluating wheelchair system design to include physiologic, mechanical, and performance-based criteria.
- Use laboratory and field studies to determine and quantify the comparative usability of wheelchair modifications and systems.

Key Words

Wheelchair
Stand
Assist

Abstract

Many people require assistance to move to a standing position from a seated position and vice versa. Those who must assist these individuals experience high back stresses. Currently available devices help the totally impaired to move to an upright position. These devices are complex and expensive, however, and are not suited for people requiring only partial assistance to stand. Two modified wheelchairs were designed to assist partially disabled users to move between seated and standing positions. Laboratory studies of leg electromyography (EMG) magnitude and field studies of usability indicate that the devices reduce the leg strength required to rise from a seated to standing position and vice versa and that they are a valuable assist to health care providers who must move people into and out of a wheelchair.

Historic Development of the Wheelchair

The first self-propelled wheelchairs were built by Johann Hautsch in Nuremberg during the 1640s. These wheelchairs were propelled by the occupant with two hand cranks and were used mostly by people with gout. During the 1700s, wheelchairs were self-propelled because one pair of wheels was large enough to be turned directly by the occupant of the chair. Wheelchair use in the United States dramatically increased during the late 1800s, mainly due to the significant number of disabled veterans from the Civil War. Most of these wheelchairs were constructed by attaching two large wooden spoked wheels to the front of a captain's chair. In almost all chairs, a single small wheel was placed in the rear underneath the seat. Wheelchairs with four wheels were very uncommon at this time. In the 1890s, wheelchair design took a step forward when Peter Gendron made wire-spoked wheels commercially available on wheelchairs. During the same period, rubber tires were applied to wheelchairs as well (Kamentz, 1969).

In the 1930s, Herbert A. Everest, a disabled mining engineer, and Harry C. Jennings, a mechanical engineer, founded the Everest and Jennings Company and in 1933 produced the first lightweight folding wheelchair (Crawford, 1985; Kamentz, 1969). This wheelchair was constructed mostly of metal, with some wooden components. The two large drive wheels were mounted on the rear of the frame, and two smaller wheels were mounted on the front corners of the frame to provide stability (Kamentz, 1969). This wheelchair design has become the standard used today by most wheelchair manufacturers.

Analysis

Problem Definition

Rising from a seated position and moving back into a seated position are common activities of daily living that are generally easily performed by young and physically strong individuals. Many people in long-term care facilities and other institutions, however, have difficulty rising out of chairs, and more than 2 million noninstitutionalized people age 65 and older face the same problems (Alexander, Schultz, & Warwick, 1991). Because many of these people can move around and function once they rise to a standing or semistanding position, the ability to rise and sit without assistance is important to maintaining an independent lifestyle. This ability also reduces the physiologic consequences of prolonged wheelchair confinement, such as poor circulation, bone degradation, and pressure sores. The ability to stand also helps to boost self-esteem, widen recreational activities, and allow face-to-face encounters (Bak, 1989). A related concern is that transferring patients from wheelchairs to beds and back again places those who assist with this activity at risk due to the high back stresses resulting from lifting heavy loads in awkward postures.

Many wheelchairs have been developed that assist individuals to move to and from the standing position. Joyce (1989) described a device known as Turbo, a battery-powered wheelchair for children with neuromuscular disease. It uses a standing frame that holds the user at the chest, hips, and knees. An article in *People Weekly* (1989) discussed another battery-powered wheelchair named Hi Rider, which allows paraplegics to stand and travel in the standing position while restrained at the lower chest and knees. Nash, Davy, and Orpwood (1990) described the wheelchair Mark II, which contains a foldout support frame that provides a standing function for midthoracic paraplegics. Another design, described by Bak (1989) as the Lifestand, raises disabled children with gas springs and four-bar linkage systems. All the designs reviewed were quite complicated and expensive, and most required motors. The stand-assist devices were designed primarily for the severely impaired and were not suitable or convenient for people requiring only partial assistance to stand.

Need for Lift-Seat Wheelchair

A research project was undertaken to design and evaluate simple and inexpensive wheelchairs with the capacity to assist partially disabled users to move between the seated and standing positions (Figure 14-1).

Design Criteria

Physiologic Design Criteria

Kelly and Kroemer (1990) indicate that two areas of concern for older persons are knee and grip strength and postural sway. They note that grip strength declines by 60% between ages 30 and 80, that knee strength of the elderly drops 56–78% relative to younger individuals, and that postural sway can be double that of younger individuals. The elderly also tend to use more hand force to compensate for reduced leg strength and greater body weight (Wheeler, Woodward, & Ucovich, 1985).

Two basic biomechanical requirements exist for rising from a chair. The first is to bring the body's center of mass over the area of foot support at the time of seat liftoff. The second is for the body posture to be such that the muscles can generate the joint moments required to lift the body. Alexander et al. (1991) suggest that the elderly place more importance on feet location to achieve postural stability than on reducing muscle exertion.

Figure 14-1. Use of tension spring wheelchair.

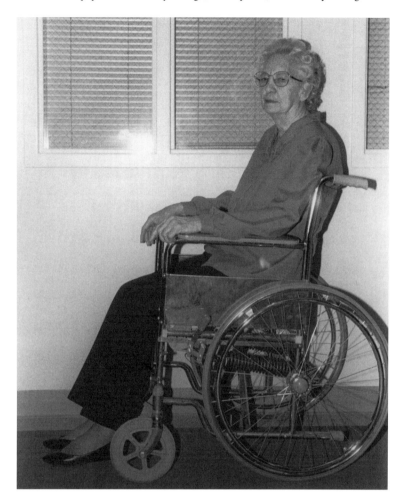

Mechanical Design Criteria

The following design criteria were established for this research:

1. A large initial force should be generated to start to lift the individual, which gradually decreases as the person's center of mass moves forward and upward during the standing process. The lower force in the "seat-up" position is needed to facilitate moving back into the chair.
2. A device to dampen the motion is imperative to allow the person to ascend and descend slowly. It is also very important for individual comfort and safety.
3. The chair should allow the lift seat to rise only when the wheels are prevented from rolling.
4. No outside power sources (other than gravity) are to be used.
5. All components are required to fit within the shape of the existing wheelchair.
6. The device must be adjustable for a variety of body weights.
7. The device must be simple to reduce breakdown potential and cost and to make the wheelchair more convenient to use.

Design and Intervention

Two wheelchairs were developed to fulfill the requirements listed in the previous section: the tension and torsion spring designs.

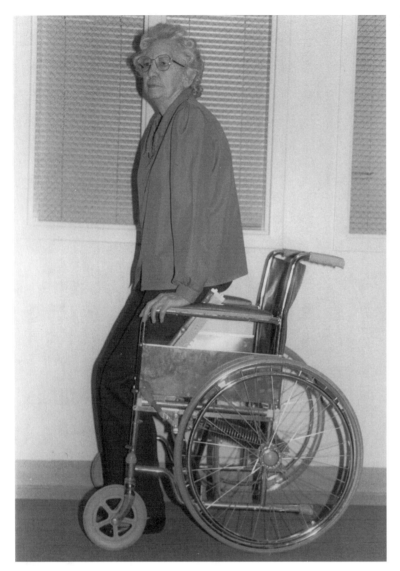

Figure 14-1. *continued*

Tension Spring Design

The primary components or characteristics of the tension spring design are the pivot seat (with lock), spring, cam, damper, and weight adjustability (Figure 14-2).

Pivot Seat

The standard wheelchair seat was replaced with a mechanism that used the original seat cover and

enabled the seat to pivot upward and forward. The pivot-seat device is constructed of aluminum and fits within the existing wheelchair frame. Press-fitted precision bearings are used in the side supports to allow smooth rotation. The seat can be locked down by means of a locking mechanism located at the back of the seat, which is connected to the wheelchair frame. When the release lever is pushed forward, it simultaneously applies the wheelchair wheel brake and releases the seat. The seat frame is a rigid piece that pre-

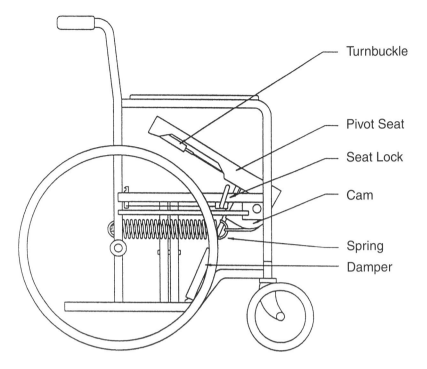

Turnbuckle

Pivot Seat

Seat Lock

Cam

Spring

Damper

A

Figure 14-2. Tension spring design (**A**) diagram; (**B**) photograph.

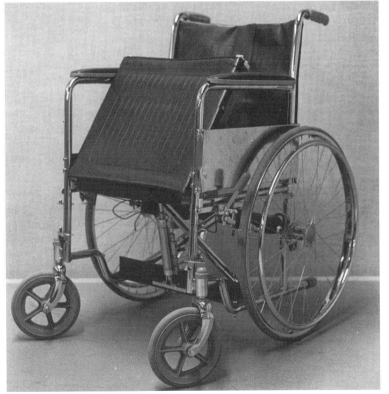

B

vents the wheelchair from collapsing; unfortunately, it also reduces portability.

Spring

Two 6-in. (15.24-cm) extension springs are attached to the back of the wheelchair frame, one on each side, and are connected to the pivot seat by wire ropes. The design parameters for the springs are as follows: (1) 3-in. (7.62-cm) displacement between the up and down positions, (2) approximately 1-in. (2.54-cm) extension at the maximum upright position (depending on body weight adjustment), (3) a spring constant of 70 lb per inch (31.5 kg per 2.54 cm), and (4) total extended length less than 12 in. (30.48 cm). The function of the springs is to lengthen, thereby storing the energy that is produced when the person sits down. This stored energy is then released to aid the person to later move to a standing position.

Cam

Two elliptical cams are attached to the bottom of the pivot-seat device. They are mounted so that the point of the cams is 1 in. (2.54 cm) in front of the axis of rotation. The wire rope passes through a groove over the cams and attaches to the pivot seat in such a way that the moment arm of the force generated by the spring decreases as the seat moves to the maximum upright position. This reduces the lift force when the seat is in the upright position.

Damper

A hydraulic cylinder is mounted between the frame and the pivot seat. The cylinder dampens and smooths the motion of the pivot seat by means of an adjustable pin valve, which controls the rate of flow of hydraulic fluid in a closed circuit. The lift force and pivot-seat movement velocity are independent. This function is important for comfort and safety during the sitting and standing process. The speed at which the pivot seat rises and lowers can be conveniently changed by adjusting the pin valve located on the hydraulic cylinder. When the valve is turned down, fluid flow is restricted, which slows the rate of seat movement.

Weight Adjustability

Adjustability for varying weight and user ability is achieved by incorporating one turnbuckle in series with each spring, which can be adjusted to increase or decrease the initial spring length. This increases or decreases the initial tension and therefore the spring force through the entire range of motion.

Width and Weight of Wheelchair

The seat width of the tension spring wheelchair is approximately 20 in. (50.8 cm); seat width for a comparable standard wheelchair without the lift seat is 18 in. (45.72 cm). The weight is 70 lb (31.5 kg); an unmodified wheelchair weighs 37 lb (16.65 kg). The footprint was unchanged. It should be noted that this was a prototype design, and most modifications were fabricated from metal. Any final production version will use lighter-weight parts.

Tension Spring Operation

To move from a seated to a standing position, the occupant engages the wheel brakes on the wheelchair and moves the seat release lever forward. The seat release lever is located next to the wheel brake on the right side of the wheelchair. The occupant then leans forward, which moves his or her center of mass over the seat pivot point, thus reducing the moment arm of the body weight resisting the lifting action. If the wheel brakes are not engaged, moving the seat release lever forward automatically locks the brake. This prevents the seat from being released without the brake being locked and the wheelchair rolling out from under the user. Moving the brake lever and seat release lever simultaneously requires approximately 6 lb (2.7 kg) of force.

To return to a sitting position, the operator simply sits in the seat. The pivot seat lowers and automatically locks into the "down" position when the seat is in the lowest position. The wheelchair brakes can then be released.

To adjust the speed with which the seat rises and lowers, the user must turn the flow valve knob (located on the hydraulic cylinder) clockwise for slower motion and counterclockwise for faster motion. As noted earlier, the lift force is independent of the seat movement speed.

Torsion Spring Design

The primary characteristics of the torsion spring design are the pivot seat, spring, damper, and weight adjustability (Figure 14-3).

Pivot Seat

The pivot seat for this design is essentially the same as the tension spring design except that the back support bracket is hinged, making it collapsible. Folding this support down allows the wheelchair to be folded. The general function of the seat is the same as in the tension spring design.

Spring

Two torsion springs are mounted on each side of the wheelchair frame. The springs were designed as follows: (1) produce approximately 448 lb-in. of torque (516 kg-cm) about its axis when the seat is in the down position, (2) made of carbon steel, (3) outside diameter of 4.5 in. (11.43 cm), (4) total length of 3 in. (7.62 cm), (5) eight total turns, and (6) maximum rotation of 150 degrees.

The general function of the springs is the same as in the tension spring design except that the longer spring provides a torsional moment by acting at the point of seat rotation instead of providing force along the longitudinal axis.

Dampers

Two hydraulic cylinders, one on each side, are mounted on the wheelchair frame and lift seat. The hydraulic lines are connected so that the fluid from the upper chamber of one cylinder flows to the lower chamber of the other cylinder. This means that the cylinder actuators cannot move independently, and a single control valve placed in the line controls both actuators. The seat locking mechanism consists of a ball valve mounted just below the left arm rest. This valve controls the cylinder actuators, which are connected to the pivot seat. This valve can be closed

at any time, allowing the seat to be locked in any position.

A flow valve conveniently mounted on the left cylinder controls the speed of the pivot seat's descent. The valve allows free flow in one direction and adjustable flow in the reverse direction. This means that the seat always ascends at a set (modest) speed but can be adjusted to descend at any rate.

Weight Adjustability

The lifting force of the seat is controlled by a pin locking mechanism, which increases or decreases the initial spring tension.

Width and Weight of Wheelchair

The seat width of the torsion spring wheelchair was approximately 17 in. (43.18 cm); seat width of a comparable standard wheelchair without the lift seat is 18 in. (45.72 cm). The weight was 42 lb (18.9 kg); an unmodified wheelchair weighs 37 lb (16.65 kg). The footprint was unchanged, but the torsion spring lift seat was approximately 8 in. (20.32 cm) wider at seat level due to the extension of the torsion spring out from the sides of the wheelchair. It should be noted that this was a prototype design, and most modifications were fabricated from metal. Any final production version will use lighter-weight parts. Also, the torsion springs themselves can easily be reduced in width by about 50%, which would reduce the 8-in. (20.32-cm) protrusion.

Torsion Spring Operation

To rise from a seated position, the user first locks the wheel brakes and then turns the seat lock control lever up to a horizontal position. This lever is located under the left armrest. The occupant then leans slowly forward and stands. To return to a seated position, the user sits into the seat, and the seat then lowers to the down position.

To lock the seat, the seat control lever must be turned to the down or vertical position. The seat can be locked at any point between the down and up positions. This is done by turning the control to the locked position when the seat is in the desired position. The movement of the seat control level requires minimum force (approximately 2 lb, or 0.9 kg).

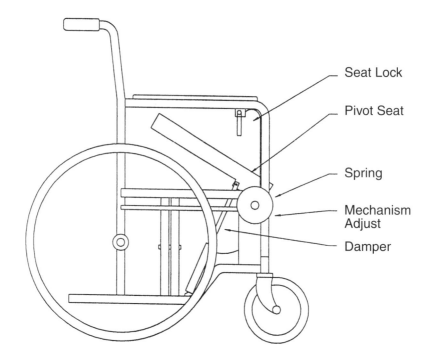

A

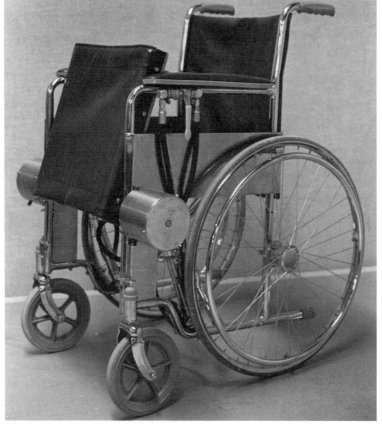

B

Figure 14-3. Torsion spring design (**A**) diagram; (**B**) photograph.

The rate at which the seat lowers is controlled in the same manner as in the tension spring design. The flow valve, however, is located on the left hydraulic cylinder. As for the tension spring design, the lift force is independent of the seat movement speed.

Test and Evaluation

Laboratory Electromyogram Test

The objective of this portion of the test was to compare the muscle exertion required to stand and sit from a conventional wheelchair to that of the modified wheelchairs. EMG data on the quadriceps muscle during the process of standing and sitting from a standard wheelchair and two modified wheelchairs was used to evaluate the assistance provided by modified wheelchairs. Institutional Review Board approval was received, and all subjects signed informed consent declarations. All subjects selected for this portion of the test were healthy college-age individuals.

Equipment

The test equipment consisted of a computer, EMG amplifier-filter box, EMG lead with preamplifier, EMG surface electrodes, and one conventional and two modified wheelchairs. The data acquisition system included an IBM-compatible 486 computer and a Data Translation model DT2801 analog-to-digital converter. Samples were collected at 60 Hz for 4 seconds using LabTech Notebook software, version 6.2 (Laboratory Technologies Corporation, Wilmington, MA). The EMG electrode signal voltage was amplified to ±10 V using an amplifier-filter box. The EMG leads between the surface electrodes and preamplifier were 3 ft long and made of double-shielded, data-audio, four-conductor coaxial cables. The surface electrodes (HP 1444SC) were nonirritating adhesive, disposable, monitoring electrodes made by Hewlett-Packard Medical Products Group (Andover, MA).

Procedure

Five subjects (one woman and four men) were tested using the following procedure:

1. The purpose of the experiment was explained to each subject, and informed consent forms were signed.

2. The purpose and operation of each wheelchair were explained and demonstrated to each subject.

3. Three button-type EMG patches were placed on the surface of the skin. Two active electrodes were placed on the quadriceps muscle along the muscle line of action 1 in. (2.54 cm) apart on centers, and one electrode (the ground) was placed just above the knee joint, where it was assumed that muscle activity would be very low.

4. The subjects were asked to sit in and rise from the chair a few times until they were comfortable with the chair operation. During the test, subjects were asked to stand and sit in a slow but normal fashion.

5. When collecting data, the subjects were asked to stand or sit five times using the same chair while data were collected. They were required to rest approximately 30 seconds each time they stood to reduce the effects of muscle fatigue. The data collection system was triggered manually just before the subject stood, and it recorded EMG data at 60 Hz for 4 seconds.

6. Step 5 was repeated until all chairs were used for both standing and sitting. The order of standing, sitting, and type of wheelchair was randomized.

The EMG data collected were not a direct measure, but an indication, of muscle activity. The data did not produce smooth curves when plotted but contained spikes and discontinuities due to random and 60-Hz "noise" and muscle twitches. To help reduce these fluctuations, a 10-point smoothing process was conducted on all data. Data were discarded when unusable due to an assignable cause, such as human or equipment error.

The smoothed data were plotted with voltage against time for each trial. The peak and the area under the curve were calculated and recorded for each trial. For each subject, the peak EMG activity and area under the curve were calculated and averaged for the five trials. The peak measure was assumed to be an indication of maximum muscle exertion during the trial, and the area measure was assumed to be an approximation of total energy.

To evaluate the statistical significance of the results, an analysis of variance between the wheelchairs and the subjects was performed. To facilitate analysis, the average for each wheelchair was calculated. The data collected during standard wheelchair use were established as 100% for each subject, and the peak and average forces required to rise from or move into the modified wheelchairs were then divided by the standard wheelchair forces for the same subject. This normalized all the data as a percentage of the EMG values for the standard wheelchair. The combined averages were then calculated across all subjects. The EMG data for one subject had peaks that were a factor of four higher than the other recorded data, and the smoothed curve contained very sporadic peaks that were inconsistent with other recorded data. This set of data was considered an anomaly due to equipment malfunction or EMG electrode attachment problem and was not included in the overall averages.

Electromyogram Test Results and Discussion

The purpose of the EMG test was to evaluate the difference in quadriceps muscle activity between the standard and modified wheelchairs. This was done by evaluating the maximum muscle exertion (peak on the EMG curve) and total muscle exertion (area under the EMG curve) required to sit and stand from each wheelchair and comparing their values to equivalent values for the standard chair.

Table 14-1 indicates the relative "total" and peak EMG values for each wheelchair compared to the standard wheelchair. In each case, the difference between modified wheelchair EMG values and the standard wheelchair values are significant at 0.01.

Overall, the EMG values for the torsion spring design were lower than those of the tension spring design. This may be because the torsion spring design provided lift support through a larger seat angle.

Field or Usability Test

The primary objective of this portion of the test was to evaluate the design of the two wheelchairs by testing them at a nursing home, St. Joseph Villa. Institutional Review Board approval was received, and all subjects (or guardians) signed informed consent declarations. All subjects selected for this portion of the test were residents of an extended care facility in the Salt Lake City area. Residents and

nurses, who use wheelchairs on a daily basis, were asked to evaluate the new wheelchairs.

Residents

The following information was collected from the residents:

1. Did you feel safe using the chairs?
2. Did the chairs help you sit down and rise more easily?
3. Did the chairs provide enough assistance in the lower and upper range of seat motion?
4. Did the seat locks work conveniently?
5. What did you like and dislike about each chair?
6. Which chair did you like the best?
7. Were the chairs generally convenient to use?
8. What recommendations do you have for future modifications?

Staff

The following information was collected from the staff (nurses and certified nursing aides):

1. Did you feel the chairs were safe?
2. Did the chairs help you transfer the patients?
3. Do the chairs provide enough assistance in the lower and upper range of the seat?
4. Did the seat locks work conveniently?
5. What did you like and dislike about each chair?
6. Which chair did you like the best?
7. Were the chairs convenient to use?
8. What recommendations do you have for future modifications?

Subject Selection Criteria

The residents had to be capable of using standard wheelchairs and be willing to cooperate in the test. Subjects of varying abilities were tested. Subjects included those who needed total assistance to be transferred, those who needed partial assistance, and those who were considered independent.

Procedure

The wheelchairs were taken to the St. Joseph Villa nursing home on several occasions. Nine residents and three nurses directly participated, using the following procedure:

Table 14-1. Normalized Quadriceps Electromyogram Analysis Results as a Percentage of Standard Wheelchair Effort to Use

Wheelchair	Total Expenditure (%)		Maximum Exertion (%)	
	Rising	Sitting	Rising	Sitting
Standard	100	100	100	100
Tension spring	78.13	71.56	74.14	57.85
Torsion spring	58.80	69.51	55.76	57.20

1. The purpose of the research was explained to each resident and nurse. Informed consent forms were then signed by the residents or their legal guardians, nurses, and witnesses. In some cases, the consent forms had been previously signed by appropriate guardians.
2. The purpose and operation of each wheelchair was explained and demonstrated to each subject.
3. The resident was transferred from a standard wheelchair to a modified wheelchair and then back again. This was repeated for the second modified wheelchair.
4. The use and operation were observed and documented by the researcher. Most of the transfers were videotaped for further evaluation.
5. The researcher asked the residents and nurses questions about the performance of the wheelchairs.

Several nurses and nursing aides observed the procedure, but neither signed consent forms nor participated directly. These staff members were asked the same type of questions as those directly participating.

Field or Usability Test Results and Discussion

Nine residents were tested. The comments listed below are from the residents who were best able to convey their opinions and do not reflect the total number of residents tested. The comments are keyed to the eight questions listed earlier.

1. None indicated that they felt unsafe or uncomfortable using either of the modified chairs.
2. Four of the residents said the chair helped them to get up and sit down easier, and two said it did not help.
3. Two indicated that the torsion spring helped them stand all the way up the easiest but felt the extension spring was better for sitting down because it had less force in the upper range. One liked the extension spring the best for all ranges and commented that it was the smoothest.
4. None liked the seat latch mechanism in the tension spring design, and all preferred the hydraulic seat lock on the torsion spring design.
5. Many were concerned with the comfort of the torsion spring chair, commenting that it was skinnier than conventional wheelchairs.
6. None would say they liked one chair more than the other because they liked different things about both chairs.
7. Three indicated that the tension spring chair would be convenient if it had the hydraulic lock. They felt the torsion spring design was too uncomfortable to sit in. This is likely due to the placement of a support piece at the rear of the seat for the torsion spring design that placed pressure on the buttocks.

Three nurses officially signed consent forms and participated in the study, but a total of eight other staff members watched, helped, and gave opinions. The comments are keyed to the eight questions listed earlier.

1. All felt that the modified chairs were safer than conventional wheelchairs. They thought that the modified chairs were safer for the residents and nurses due to the reduced physical exertion for the resident and reduced back stresses for staff members when transferring residents.
2. All believed that the modified chairs greatly helped in transferring patients and required

much less effort on their part, especially when helping a resident to move from a standing to a sitting position.

3. Six liked the torsion spring the best for all ranges because it helped the residents stand all the way up. The other five liked the lower force provided by the tension spring when the resident first started moving from the standing to the sitting position.

4. All believed that the hydraulic lock was the best because it would lock even if the seat was not completely down, as opposed to the latch lock on the tension spring design.

5. There were concerns over the comfort of the torsion spring chair, and some had difficulties getting the seat to start going down.

6. Overall preferences were the same as those noted in question 3 above.

7. All staff members liked the wheelchairs and believed they were convenient to use.

8. Some mentioned the possibility of being pinched when the seat ascended and descended. They also found that the back portion of the seat sticks up past the armrests in the upper position and thought that it should be rounded to reduce potential injury on transferring.

Notably, even the residents who said that the modified wheelchairs did not help them stand appeared to stand easier with the modified wheelchairs. Both the nurses and the researchers noticed this. The nurses commented that the residents do not readily adjust to change and prefer "old" procedures.

Many residents who required partial assistance to stand from standard wheelchairs could stand with no help from the nurses using the new chairs. When transferring total-assist residents, the nurses could simply start them into the seated posture and then steady them as the seat descended. They needed only to lift a little under the arms of these residents to help them stand.

All residents put their hands on the front portion of the armrest to steady them as they ascended and descended. If the seat were to tilt to a more extreme angle, it would interfere with their handhold.

It was standard procedure for the nurses to lock both wheels when transferring patients. This does not, however, eliminate the necessity for a latch that allows only the seat to rise when the wheels are locked. This design criterion is being investigated for the torsion spring design.

All staff members were very excited when the wheelchairs were used and wanted to know how long it would be until they could be purchased.

Conclusion

Electromyogram Test

It was found that the modified wheelchairs generally reduced the maximum and total muscle exertion required to ascend to a standing position, but the greatest reduction occurred when the user descended to a sitting position. This is of special interest to people with osteoporosis, for whom the impact of "dropping" into the seat is painful. Based on the EMG averages, the tension spring design performed the best overall.

User Test

Overall, the staff members and residents liked the amount of lift provided throughout the range of motion by the torsion spring and the ease of descent and smoothness of the tension spring.

The hydraulic seat-locking mechanism was preferred by all residents and nurses because it could be locked at any position and they knew whether the seat was locked or not. With the latch mechanism, it was not always obvious if the seat was locked or unlocked.

The modified wheelchairs were helpful to the residents and gave some residents the ability to ascend to a standing and descend to a sitting position without assistance. The chairs also greatly reduced the lifting force generated by a staff member to transfer residents. This reduced the nurses' back stresses and potential back injury. These improvements became more evident as both the residents and nurses gained confidence in the operation of the lift-seat wheelchair.

Recommendations

The following areas are recommended for further research and development:

1. Provide more variability in the lifting force.
2. Incorporate a hydraulic seat-lock mechanism on all lift-seat wheelchairs.

3. Install guards or other devices that would reduce the probability of injury from pinch points as the seat pivots.
4. Make sure all corners and edges are rounded or padded to reduce injury potential.
5. Make sure the sitting area is not too narrow, as was the case in the torsion spring design.
6. Incorporate a system to prevent actuation of the torsion spring lift seat without the wheels in a "brake-on" mode.

This study has shown that wheelchairs with a lift seat can be very beneficial to wheelchair users and attending personnel. They allow individuals with limited leg strength to rise from and move to a seated position without assistance and reduce the assistance required to transfer residents. It is proposed that this will reduce the frequency of back injury to nurses and assistants.

Acknowledgments

The authors thank Susan Wright and the staff at St. Joseph Villa for their assistance in the field evaluation of these wheelchairs. The authors also thank Roanna Keough for her assistance in the preparation of this manuscript.

References

Alexander, N.B., Schultz, A.B., & Warwick, D.N. (1991). Rising from a chair: Effects of age and functional ability on performance biomechanics. *Journal of Gerontology, 46,* 91–98.

Bak, D.J. (1989). Articulated wheelchair lifts body and spirit. *Design News, 45,* 116–117.

Joyce, M.E. (1989). Wheelchair enables disabled child to sit, stand, or play with ease. *Design News, 45,* 29.

Kamentz, H.L. (1969). *The wheelchair book: Mobility for the disabled.* Springfield, IL: Thomas.

Kelly, P.L., & Kroemer, K.H.E. (1990). Anthropometry of the elderly: Status and recommendations. *Human Factors, 32,* 571–595.

Nash, R.S.W., Davy, M.S., & Orpwood, R. (1990). Development of a wheelchair-mounted folding standing frame. *Journal of Biomedical Engineering, 12,* 189–192.

Tom Houston is a real stand-up guy, thanks to the versatile vertical wheelchair he devised. (1989, August 28). *People Weekly,* pp. 91–92.

Wheeler, J., Woodward, C., & Ucovich, R.L. (1985). Rising from a chair. *Physical Therapy, 65,* 22–26.

Chapter 15

Development of a Functional Test Battery for Carpal Tunnel Syndrome

One-Jang Jeng and Robert G. Radwin

Learning Objectives

On completion of the chapter, the reader should be able to

- Understand how the quantitative measurement of functional deficits associated with carpal tunnel syndrome (CTS) can be used to monitor for CTS signs through statistical analyses.
- Understand issues regarding subject selection bias in estimating sensitivity and specificity of the test battery for CTS.

Key Words

Carpal tunnel syndrome
Functional deficits
Psychomotor task
Sensory threshold

Abstract

Two new tests developed for monitoring employees for functional deficits in CTS were designed, tested, and evaluated. These two computer-controlled tests, called the *Wisconsin test battery*, include the gap detection sensory threshold test and the rapid pinch and release psychomotor test. The tests involve tasks resembling functional aspects of common manual work activities and were designed to quantify sensory and motor function in the median nerve–innervated area of the hand. Like the routine tests for detecting hearing loss from exposure to excessive noise, it was hypothesized, the Wisconsin test battery could be used for monitoring workers exposed to risk factors associated with CTS. The results showed the functional tests were reliable and able to differentiate well-defined CTS cases from control subjects. An industrial population was studied to evaluate the functional test battery. Results indicate these tests correlate with electrophysiologic and clinical findings, but more study is needed, involving a larger, unbiased sample in a longitudinal study, to determine whether performance changes in the functional test battery are reliable and valid for monitoring industrial workers for CTS.

Assessment of the Problem

CTS is one of the most prevailing peripheral entrapment neuropathies (Phalen, 1972) and is a major cause of reported occupational illness (Franklin et al., 1991; Centers for Disease Control, 1989). It results from a combination of ischemia and compression of the median nerve in the carpal canal (Lundborg et al., 1982). CTS symptoms include pain, loss of motor function, and sensory deficits in the index finger, long finger, and thumb (Phalen, 1972).

The diagnosis of CTS is usually based on clinical and electrophysiologic signs (Dawson, Hallett, & Millender, 1983; Kimura, 1989; Phalen, 1966). Electrodiagnostic methods, such as nerve conduction studies (NCS), are currently considered the most accurate diagnostic tests for CTS (AAEM Quality Assurance Committee, 1993). Electrodiagnostic studies often indicate a prolongation of the distal motor latency of the median nerve, slowing of median sensory nerve conduction velocity across the wrist, and denervation of the abductor pollicis brevis muscle (Kimura, 1989; Stevens, 1987). Conduction velocity is most abnormal when the myelin sheath is disrupted (Moody, Arezzo, & Otto, 1986). Increasing electrophysiologic deficits have been linked to increasing CTS severity (Mackinnon & Dellon, 1988). The obvious advantage of electrodiagnostic methods such as NCS and electromyography (EMG) is the absence of subjective reporting bias or any interference from more complex systems.

Aside from the expense, electrodiagnostic methods may not be suitable for routine in-plant monitoring. A recent investigation reported that only four out of 30 study subjects who had proven CTS were willing to undergo repeat NCS due to the mildly aversive nature of the stimulation (Gerr, 1994). It is clear there is a need for a measure of nerve function for monitoring CTS that has high sensitivity and specificity without some of the limitations associated with NCS. Such a test should be easily administered, noninvasive, have high retest reliability, and involve no discomfort.

Clinical history and physical examination using provocative tests such as Phalen's or Tinel's sign are easy to administer, but they are of limited value in routine monitoring for CTS. The Phalen's and Tinel's signs have sensitivities varying from 25% to 75% and specificities from 47% to 90% (Katz et al., 1990). *Sensitivity* is the conditional probability of a positive test, given that the person has CTS. *Specificity* is the conditional probability of a negative test, given that the person does not have CTS. Symptom surveys are commonly used in surveillance for CTS, but surveys have been shown to have high sensitivity but low specificity (Katz et al., 1991).

Two-point discrimination tests have long been used for assessing tactile sensory impairment (Dellon, Mackinnon, & Crosby, 1987; Moberg, 1990). These tests are reliable for measuring functional nerve regeneration but are not sensitive to the gradual decrease in nerve function created by external compression (Lundborg et al., 1982). Alternative sensory test techniques, such as Semmes-Weinstein

monofilaments testing, lack control of important variables (Levin, Pearsall, & Ruderman, 1978) and results may be dependent on examiner experience and training (Bell-Krotoski, Weinstein, & Weinstein, 1993). Many tactility tests are administered under manual control of the examiner, so the rate of impact and the extent of skin deformation can vary from one trial to the next (Bell-Krotoski & Buford, 1988; Bell-Krotoski, Weinstein, & Weinstein, 1993; Dellon, Mackinnon, & Crosby, 1987; Moberg, 1990).

Abnormal vibration sensation in the digits is believed to be related to a decrease in the number of large myelinated fibers in the median nerve (Bleecker & Agnew, 1987). Vibrotactile testing has been proposed for monitoring CTS, but the method suffers from numerous problems. Although the idea of vibrometry seems attractive, these tests were shown to lack sensitivity and specificity (Gerr, 1994; White et al., 1994; Winn & Putz-Anderson, 1990). Studies showed large variations of intra-individual vibration sensitivity thresholds, from –71% to 159% (Aaserud, Juntunen, & Matikainen, 1990) and from –59% to 58% (Fagius & Wahren, 1981). Daily variations in vibrometry have been shown to reduce specificity and sensitivity of the test (White et al., 1994). The effects of contact pressure, fatigue, and appropriate vibration stimulus waveforms for this test have not yet been clinically validated (Harada & Griffin, 1991). Furthermore, no relationship between vibrometry and NCS parameters has been observed (Merchut, Kelly, & Toleikis, 1990).

Just as subtle, noise-induced hearing loss can be identified early by using threshold shifts from routine audiometric tests administered in the workplace, it was hypothesized that a similar approach could be used for periodically monitoring workers exposed to risk factors associated with CTS. The gap detection sensory threshold test and the rapid pinch and release psychomotor test were therefore developed.

Design of the Test Battery

Gap-Detection Sensory Threshold Test

Radwin, Jeng, and Gisske developed an automated esthesiometer for measuring gap-detection sensory threshold in a tactile inspection task (1993). The test involves detecting the presence of a tiny gap in a highly polished surface. What distinguishes this test

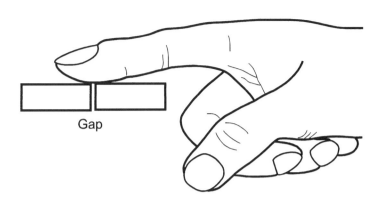

Figure 15-1. Schematic drawing for the gap-detection sensory threshold test.

Gap

from conventional tactility tests is that it measures performance in a functional tactility task that resembles tasks performed during manual work activities, such as sensing surface feature defects (e.g., scratches). Although test conditions are highly controlled, this test still permits natural finger probing. The gap esthesiometer permitted free finger probing while control of contact force was maintained through the use of a precision, constant-torque, balance beam system. Gap size was controlled using a micropositioner and digital encoder. The gap could be made as small as 0.001 mm, and finger contact was controlled within $1g$ for forces between $25g$ and $75g$.

The gap-detection test can estimate both dynamic and static stimulus sensory thresholds (Jeng & Radwin, 1995; Radwin, Jeng, & Gisske, 1993). The dynamic test involves probing the surface with the fingertip (Figure 15-1). The static test fixes the finger in a support that exposes the distal phalangeal pad while preventing the finger from exerting any force perpendicular to the stimulus platform or from moving the finger across the stimulus surface. The stimulus was automatically raised to contact the finger.

The gap was randomly set at zero or 1.6 mm for a static test, or at 0.16 mm for a dynamic test. A converging staircase method of limits was used for determining gap-detection sensory thresholds. This method concentrates responses around the threshold, which improves efficiency beyond the traditional method of limits. Gap-detection thresholds were estimated by convergence while titrating around the threshold using smaller and smaller discrete steps in gap size. Five gap step–size decrements were used. Each gap size was half the magnitude of the previous. A change in gap step size and direction occurred every time a response was different from the previous one. Subjects responded verbally if they could or could not detect a gap. The examiner entered the subject's response using the computer keyboard. A threshold determination took less than 5 minutes using the converging staircase method.

Rapid Pinch and Release Psychomotor Test

The rapid pinch and release psychomotor test requires use of the thumb and index finger to pinch two aluminum bars instrumented with strain gauges. The dynamometer was specially designed to measure force independent of the location of the fingers (Radwin, Masters, & Lupton, 1992). It eliminates possible errors due to different finger positions among trials. Figure 15-2 shows a schematic drawing of the task. The pinch force was calculated as the average force measured by the two dynamometer arms. Pulp pinch strength was measured to determine the maximal voluntary contraction (MVC) by taking the greater of two exertions of maximal effort.

Subjects were instructed to pinch and release as fast as possible while exceeding a predetermined upper force level (F_{UPPER}) and releasing under a lower force level (F_{LOWER}). All force measurements were normalized by expressing force in terms of percent MVC. Discrete visual and auditory feedback was provided after successful pinch or release trials. The task was performed using alternate hands for four conditions of F_{UPPER} (5%, 20%, 35%, and 50% MVC) for each hand. The lower force level was fixed

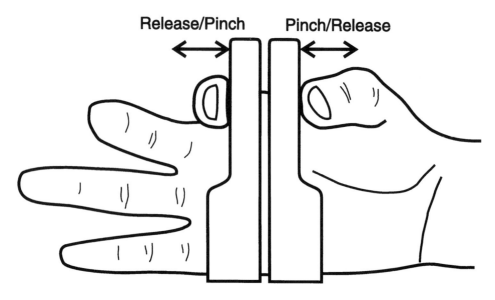

Figure 15-2. Schematic drawing for the rapid pinch and release psychomotor test.

at 2% MVC for all trials. The order of the experimental conditions was counterbalanced between subjects. Performance measures for the rapid pinch and release psychomotor test are listed in Table 15-1.

Test and Evaluation of the Battery

A series of studies were conducted for testing the apparatus and paradigm (Jeng, Radwin, & Rodriquez, 1994; Jeng & Radwin, 1995; Radwin, Jeng, & Gisske, 1993; Radwin et al., 1991; Rodriquez, Radwin, & Jeng, 1993). Comparisons were made between test performance of subjects with CTS and normals. These studies revealed functional deficits in

gap detection and rapid pinch and release performance associated with CTS. The objective was to evaluate whether the tests were reliable and valid for detecting CTS using a multivariate approach and whether the tests were suitable for use as a worker monitoring tool for CTS.

Test and Retest Reliability Studies

Sixteen normal subjects between 21 and 66 years of age were tested for important factors affecting gap detection thresholds (Jeng & Radwin, 1995). Factors investigated were finger contact force, static versus dynamic stimulus, hand dominance, learning

Table 15-1. Performance Variables for the Rapid Pinch and Release Psychomotor Test

Variable	Notation	Units
Pinch rate	R_P	Pinches/sec
Slope of pinch rate with respect to F_{UPPER}	$\Delta R_P/\Delta F_{UPPER}$	Pinches/sec/%MVC
Overshoot force	F_{OVER}	%MVC
Time above F_{UPPER}	T_{UPPER}	Msec
Time below F_{LOWER}	T_{LOWER}	Msec
Slope of the straight line between the time when F_{UPPER} and F_{LOWER} was exceeded during pinching	M_{INC}	%MVC/sec
Slope of the straight line between the time when exertion level fell below F_{UPPER} and F_{LOWER} during release	M_{DEC}	%MVC/sec

and fatigue effects, and test and retest reliability. Using the index finger for active probing revealed a threshold almost an order of magnitude more sensitive (mean, 0.19 mm; standard deviation [SD], 0.11 mm) than passive touch (mean, 1.63 mm; SD, 0.62 mm), which was similar to the two-point discrimination. Average thresholds decreased 24% as contact force increased from $25g$ to $75g$. As evidenced by no significant differences between six replicates after a practice trial, performance in the gap-detection sensory threshold test quickly stabilized and showed little learning effects over the period of the test. The results were highly repeatable, as evidenced by the high correlation ($r = 0.94$) between test and retest sessions. No significant threshold differences were observed between dominant and nondominant hands.

Jeng, Radwin, and Rodriquez studied the effects of force, hand dominance, test and retest reliability, learning, and intersubject variability for the rapid pinch and release psychomotor test using 13 subjects free from any hand disabilities or symptoms (1994). Dominant hands performed 4–8% better than the nondominant hands by having a greater pinch rate, a smaller overshoot force, and less time above the upper force level and below the lower force level. The test also showed a high test-retest reliability ($0.56 < r < 0.95$). Performance stabilized quickly and required little or no practice.

Case-Control Study

A case-control study was conducted to investigate the optimal use of the gap-detection sensory threshold test and the rapid pinch and release psychomotor test for differentiating between individuals with well-defined CTS and control cases.

Carpal Tunnel Syndrome Diagnoses

All CTS and control subjects were examined and received nerve conduction tests. Nerve conduction tests and CTS diagnosis were performed by two qualified physicians using the same test protocol. These included median nerve motor latency and amplitude (8 cm), median nerve antidromic sensory latency and amplitude (13 cm), median nerve transcarpal latency and amplitude (8 cm), and ulnar nerve motor latency (8 cm). Motor latencies were

measured to the negative peak using a sensitivity of 1 μV per division, and sensory latencies were measured to the negative peak using a sensitivity of 20 μV per division. Limb temperature was maintained above 32°C.

Criteria for accepting CTS subjects into the study included symptoms based on a history and physical examination and electrodiagnostic parameters compatible with a lesion of the median nerve in the carpal tunnel. The diagnosis of CTS was made on a case-by-case basis rather than judged by a simple cutoff from any of the electrodiagnostic parameters. In all cases, no history or physical evidence was suggestive of a confounding neurologic disorder, such as peripheral neuropathy, cervical radiculopathy, or other nerve entrapments.

Results

Ten referred outpatients diagnosed with CTS volunteered for the study. Eight patients had bilateral CTS, providing a total of 18 CTS hands. Although it was not intended to exclude male or left-handed subjects, the CTS subjects were all female and right-handed, ranging from 27 to 76 years of age. Eight asymptomatic control subjects were recruited from the university community by posting advertisements. The control group consisted of five women and three men, ranging from 30 to 52 years of age. Six of the eight control subjects described themselves as right-handed and two as left-handed.

Average differences in performance between the CTS and control groups for the gap-detection sensory threshold test are contained in Table 15-2. Analysis of variance (ANOVA) using age as a covariate demonstrated that all main effects of group, contact force, and stimulus were statistically significant ($p < 0.01$). There was also a significant interaction between group and stimulus ($F(1,32) = 9.78, p < 0.01$). CTS subjects had 104% greater average thresholds than the normal subjects for the dynamic stimulus ($F(1,31) = 13.64, p < 0.001$). CTS subjects also had 51% greater average static sensory thresholds than the normal subjects ($F(1,31) = 13.41, p < 0.001$). The average dynamic sensory threshold decreased 24% and static sensory threshold decreased 16% as contact force increased from $25g$ to $50g$ for all hands ($F(1,32) = 15.22, p < 0.001$).

Age was a significant covariate ($F(1,31) = 9.20, p < 0.01$) for the gap-detection threshold, which con-

Table 15-2. Gap-Detection Thresholds for Control and Carpal Tunnel Syndrome Subjects*

| Contact Force | Group | Gap-Detection Thresholds (mm) | | | |
| | | Dynamic Sensory Function | | Static Sensory Function | |
		Mean	SD	Mean	SD
25g	Carpal tunnel syndrome	0.45	0.18	2.88	1.15
	Control	0.24	0.13	1.79	0.62
50g	Carpal tunnel syndrome	0.36	0.20	2.29	0.65
	Control	0.16	0.10	1.63	0.50

*All main effects of group, contact force, and stimulus were statistically significant ($p < 0.01$).

Table 15-3. Statistical Summary of Psychomotor Performance Variables for $F_{UPPER} = 20\%$ MVC

Variable (units)	Group	Number	Mean	SD	F test
MVC (N)	Carpal tunnel syndrome	18	31.1	9.1	$F(1,31) = 8.10, p < 0.01$*
	Control	16	43.3	16.4	
R_P (pinches/sec)	Carpal tunnel syndrome	18	3.6	0.7	$F(1,31) = 8.98, p < 0.01$*
	Control	16	4.7	1.0	
$\Delta R_P/F_{UPPER}$ (pinches/sec/%MVC)	Carpal tunnel syndrome	18	−0.024	0.019	$F(1,31) = 18.93, p < 0.001$
	Control	16	-0.051	0.018	
F_{OVER} (%MVC)	Carpal tunnel syndrome	18	22.7	10.7	$F(1,31) = 10.64, p < 0.01$*
	Control	16	13.5	5.5	
T_{UPPER} (msec)	Carpal tunnel syndrome	18	121	26	$F(1,31) = 20.72, p < 0.001$*
	Control	16	84	23	
T_{LOWER} (msec)	Carpal tunnel syndrome	18	73	21	$F(1,31) = 15.80, p < 0.001$
	Control	16	45	22	

*Age was a significant covariate to the correspondent analysis of variance model.
MVC = maximal voluntary contraction.

tributed 11% of the total variance to the model. The Pearson product correlation indicated that age was significantly correlated with static sensory thresholds ($r = 0.47$, $p < 0.01$) but was not correlated with dynamic sensory thresholds ($r = 0.19$, $p > 0.1$). Older subjects tended to have slightly greater static sensory thresholds than younger subjects when other factors, such as subject group and contact force, were controlled.

Significant differences were observed between CTS patients and control subjects for several performance variables in the rapid pinch and release psychomotor test (Table 15-3). The change in pinch rate with respect to force as F_{UPPER} increased from 5% MVC to 50% MVC, $\Delta R_P/\Delta F_{UPPER}$ (pinches per second per %MVC), was estimated from a linear regression slope using F_{UPPER} as the independent variable and R_P (pinch rate) as the dependent variable. The correlation coefficients for these regression models ranged between 0.5 and 0.9.

Table 15-4 gives the Pearson correlation coefficients between gap-detection thresholds, rapid pinch and release test variables, and electrophysiologic parameters. Both gap-detection thresholds and rapid pinch and release test variables were significantly correlated with median nerve motor, sensory, and transcarpal latencies. For example, scatter plots used the dynamic sensory threshold against median sensory latency and the pinch rate against median motor latency (Figure 15-3). Fitted linear regression lines were included in the plots to describe the relationship between the functional test variables and the electrophysiologic parameters. Furthermore, they had poor correlation with ulnar nerve motor

Table 15-4. Correlation Between Electrophysiologic Parameters and Functional Test Variables

| | Median Nerve Latencies | | | Ulnar Nerve Latencies | |
	Motor	Sensory	Transcarpal	Motor	Age
Gap-detection test					
Dynamic threshold	0.783[a]	0.805[a]	0.659[a]	0.039	0.191
Static threshold	0.716[a]	0.706[a]	0.532[a]	0.049	0.470[b]
Psychomotor pinch test					
R_P	−0.619[a]	−0.759[a]	-0.572[a]	−0.107	−0.282
$\Delta R_P/\Delta F_{UPPER}$	0.599[a]	0.729[a]	0.619[a]	0.175	0.093
F_{OVER}	0.387[c]	0.357[c]	0.372[c]	−0.133	0.392[c]
T_{UPPER}	0.572[a]	0.595[a]	0.630[a]	−0.096	0.484[b]
T_{LOWER}	0.622[a]	0.701[a]	0.506[b]	−0.147	0.250
Pinch strength test					
Strength	−0.313	−0.214	−0.293	0.076	−0.300

[a]$p < 0.001$.
[b]$p < 0.01$.
[c]$p < 0.05$.

latency ($p > 0.1$). Pinch strength did not have a significant correlation with any electrophysiologic parameters (see Table 15-4).

Stepwise discriminant analysis was performed to determine the combination of functional test variables that would best classify the CTS subjects from the control subjects. Of all the functional test variables, only time below F_{LOWER} and $\Delta R_P/\Delta F_{UPPER}$ were selected into the final discriminant function.

For 18 diagnosed CTS cases, 13 cases were correctly assigned to their corresponding category. Therefore the sensitivity of the discriminant function for detecting CTS was 0.72. Fifteen of the 16 control cases were correctly assigned to their corresponding category. So the specificity of the discriminant function was 0.94. The resulting discriminant function canonical variable was

$$CTS = -1.07 + 32.23 \times \Delta R_P/\Delta F_{UPPER}$$
(pinches × second^{-1} × %MVC^{-1}) +
$0.04 \times T_{LOWER}$ (msec)

$$(F(2,31) = 15.29, p < 0.001)$$

Test results with a canonical variable value greater than 0 would be interpreted as having CTS. The mean canonical variable value for control subjects was −1.02, and +0.91 for the CTS subjects. A histogram based on the discriminant function for all subjects is plotted in Figure 15-4.

An alternative approach was adopted to further investigate the use of the Wisconsin test battery for CTS. Cutoff for normal values was obtained from the mean and standard deviation of the control group for each test performance variable. Each performance variable was treated as an individual score. A 95% confidence interval was defined as the upper boundary for normal test values. Therefore the criterion for a CTS case for each variable was the normal mean plus 1.96 × SD. For individual scores, the dynamic sensory threshold at $25g$ had the best sensitivity and specificity of any individual variables, resulting in a sensitivity of 0.44 and a specificity of 0.94. Combinations of all the variables were tried to obtain the scoring system. A positive case was defined as at least one positive test score for any of the variables. Results of this analysis are contained in Table 15-5.

Discussion

Strong correlations were observed between median nerve conduction latencies, the gap-detection thresholds, and most of the rapid pinch and release psychomotor test performance variables. Although the gap-detection sensory threshold test simply tested sensory function, the rapid pinch and release psychomotor task integrated motor and sensory function. A strong correlation was expected between the

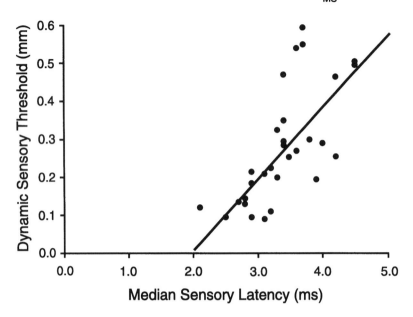

A

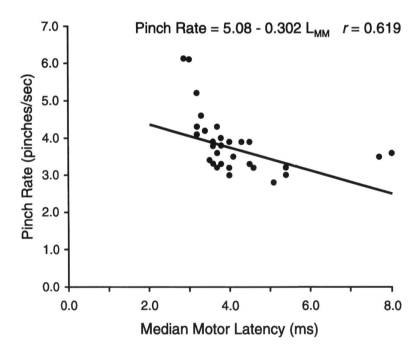

B

Figure 15-3. Scatter plots and fitted linear regression lines for **(A)** dynamic sensory threshold (from the gap-detection sensory threshold test) against median nerve sensory latency (L_{MS}) and **(B)** pinch rate (from the rapid pinch and release psychomotor test) against median motor latency (L_{MM}).

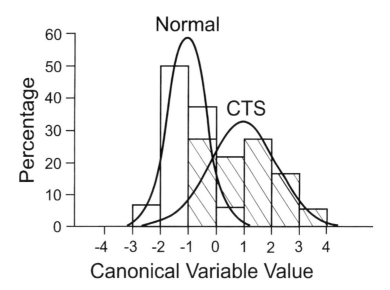

Figure 15-4. Histogram of canonical variables for CTS and control subject samples. Canonical variable is $-1.07 + 32.23 \times \Delta R_P / \Delta F_{UPPER} + 0.04 \times T_{LOWER}$. The normal distribution curves were constructed to best fit the frequency distributions of the two subject samples.

sensory thresholds and sensory latencies. Because the correlation between median nerve sensory latencies and motor latencies was 0.72 ($p < 0.001$), the high correlation between sensory thresholds and motor latencies might have occurred because the hands with high sensory latencies also tended to have high motor latencies. There was also a strong correlation between psychomotor performance parameters and motor and sensory latencies. This may have occurred because the rapid pinch and release psychomotor test involves not only fine-motor control but also sensory feedback.

The linear discriminant function provides a direct estimate of the canonical variable to predict whether a case belongs to the CTS or the normal category. Two psychomotor parameters, $\Delta R_P / \Delta F_{UPPER}$ and T_{LOWER}, were selected from the stepwise discriminant analysis. Although the dynamic sensory threshold was by itself the second best diagnostic indicator, it was not selected into the discriminant function. This occurred because the dynamic sensory threshold was highly correlated with the rapid pinch and release psychomotor test variables. Consequently, after $\Delta R_P / \Delta F_{UPPER}$ was entered into the discriminant function, the dynamic sensory threshold was deleted.

Analyses using different test combinations suggested that none of the individual variables alone was sensitive enough to detect CTS. The test paradigm involved both the gap-detection sensory threshold test

and the rapid pinch and release psychomotor test, for an upper normal boundary of $1.96 \times SD$ above the control group mean, resulting in a sensitivity of 0.78 and a specificity of 0.81 (see Table 15-5). Shifting the criteria obtains different sensitivities and specificities and reduces the test variables to only the rapid pinch and release psychomotor test, depending on the economics of misses and false positives in a CTS monitoring program.

Although this research has demonstrated that the Wisconsin battery may be suitable as a monitoring test for CTS, the research has several limitations. Due to practical considerations, subjects recruited in the patient and control groups might have been confounded with unequal distribution of gender, age, and other factors. Because two CTS subjects had unilateral CTS, each hand had to be treated as an individual subject. Eliminating two unilateral CTS cases to construct a complete block design would have reduced the CTS data by 12% due to the relatively small sample size. The magnitude of the difference between the CTS and control subjects for the functional tests suggests that the results are robust despite the potential subject correlation bias. A limited number of CTS subjects and control subjects were tested; therefore, a misclassification by the functional tests could change the sensitivity and specificity for detecting CTS. CTS subjects were recruited from patients referred to the study after electrophysiologic

Table 15-5. Sensitivity and Specificity for Different Test Combinations and Cutoff Criteria

Cutoff Criteria		Test Combination				
		Dynamic Sense	Static Sense	Dynamic and Static Tests	Psychomotor Test	All Tests
Mean	Sensitivity	1.00	0.94	1.00	1.00	1.00
	Specificity	0.50	0.50	0.31	0.13	0.13
Mean + 1.96 × SD	Sensitivity	0.44	0.44	0.61	0.67	0.78
	Specificity	0.94	0.88	0.88	0.94	0.81
Mean + 2.58 × SD	Sensitivity	0.44	0.33	0.50	0.44	0.56
	Specificity	0.94	1.00	0.94	1.00	0.94

confirmation. The sensitivity of the functional tests for detecting CTS may have been elevated because the disorders were well developed (Sox et al., 1988). Control subjects were confirmed by the absence of CTS symptoms, negative NCS results, and absence of other disorders that might have elevated the test specificity. Although commonly used, this case-control subject selection approach has what is referred to as a *spectrum bias* (Ransohoff & Feinstein, 1978). A test that is highly sensitive to well-developed diseases or disorders may not necessarily be able to detect them in the early stages. Additional study was necessary to determine whether the Wisconsin test is reliably capable of detecting CTS early with sensitivity and specificity.

Industrial Population Study

The purpose of the industrial population study was to evaluate the Wisconsin functional test battery using a general worker population with high prevalence of CTS. Subjects were tested for functional deficits, medical evaluation, and nerve conduction parameters in sequence. Performance in the Wisconsin test battery was compared against the medical findings.

The experiment was conducted in a Midwestern U.S. food processing plant. Volunteers were recruited by nurses in the employee health department and were queried for CTS symptoms. Potential subjects were identified and categorized into three groups: (1) those without any self-reported CTS-related symptoms, (2) those having symptoms compatible with CTS but no records of clinical confirmation, and (3) those having CTS symptoms and clinically diagnosed as having CTS but not having undergone carpal tunnel release surgery. This categorization was used to ensure that the subject selection procedure would have a wide distribution and enough positive cases for data analysis. Volunteers who had peripheral neuropathies, fractures, severe burns, arthritis, diabetes, and carpal tunnel surgery were not included. There were a total of 14 women and 13 men in this study. Their ages were between 23 and 57 years old (mean, 40.2 years).

Medical Evaluation

Every participant completed a questionnaire with the assistance of a physician. The questionnaire included information related to demographics, prior injuries of the upper extremity, past medical history (e.g., diabetes, arthritis, thyroid disease, Raynaud's disease, and renal disease), and the temporal pattern and circumstances associated with possible symptoms for each hand. Symptoms such as tingling, numbness, pain, perceived weakness, and clumsiness were evaluated. A self-reported hand diagram was completed by the subject with the examiner in attendance. Semmes-Weinstein monofilament (five-filament kit) testing was performed using the volar aspect of the distal thumb, index, and little finger (Bell-Krotoski, 1990). Callus present on examination was noted. Thenar atrophy, defined as concavity of the thenar muscle group along the plane parallel to the palm, was scored as absent or present.

Electrodiagnostic Evaluation

NCS were completed bilaterally for all subjects. Testing consisted of median and ulnar transcarpal

Table 15-6. Subject and Hand Distribution in the Symptom and Nerve Conduction Studies (NCS) Categories

		Median Nerve NCS	
		−	+
CTS Symptoms	−	16 subjects	5 subjects
		23 hands	6 hands
	+	11 subjects	9 subjects
		14 hands	11 hands

CTS = carpal tunnel syndrome.

studies using palmar stimulation and a 3-cm bar pickup electrode at 8 or 10 cm at the wrist; orthodromic median and ulnar motor studies with the G1 disc electrodes over the thenar and hypothenar eminences at 8 cm and the G2 disc electrodes over the thumb and little finger, respectively; and antidromic median digital sensory studies of the index finger with ring electrodes at 13 cm. Sensory nerve action potentials were recorded with filter settings of 20 Hz and 2 kHz, a sweep speed of 2 msec per division, and a sensitivity of 20 mV per division. Latency was measured to the negative peak, and amplitude was measured from baseline to peak. Compound muscle action potentials were recorded with filter settings of 2 Hz and 10 kHz, a sweep speed of 5 msec per division, and a sensitivity of 5 μV per division for amplitude and 500 μV per division for latency. Latency was measured to the onset of the negative peak, and amplitude was measured from baseline to peak. All studies were performed by two experienced electromyographers on a Teca TD-5 electromyograph (Teca Corporation, Pleasantville, NY).

Category Assignment

All the experimenters were blinded to individual subject medical records and results from the other two evaluations. Results of the medical and electrodiagnostic evaluation were independently reviewed, and the final determination of the presence or absence of CTS symptoms, as well as the existence of positive NCS results for each hand, was made. NCS− was defined as no electrodiagnostic evidence of median mononeuropathy. NCS+ was defined as electrodiagnostic evidence of median mononeu-

ropathy. The criteria for NCS− were median motor latency less than or equal to 4.5 msec at 8 cm, median sensory latency less than or equal to 3.7 msec at 13 cm, and a difference between median and ulnar transcarpal latencies less than 0.5 msec. Judgment of the NCS outcome did not depend on satisfying all these criteria. Symptom− was applied to hands with no CTS-related symptoms based on examination. Symptom+ was applied to hands with symptoms compatible with CTS. Table 15-6 lists the distribution of the hand categorization for all subjects. Hands were treated as individual members in all statistical analyses to account for unilateral and bilateral CTS cases.

Results

Two-way ANOVA with age as a covariate was used for evaluating functional performance according to symptom and median nerve electrodiagnostic evaluation. Age was not a significant covariate for any of the functional test variables ($p > 0.1$). Gap-detection sensory thresholds differed significantly from NCS− to NCS+ categories (Table 15-7). The average gap-detection sensory threshold (mean, 0.25 mm; SD, 0.07) was 32% greater for the NCS+ category than the NCS− category (mean, 0.19 mm; SD, 0.06). The average gap-detection sensory threshold was not significantly different between symptom+ and symptom− hands ($p > 0.1$). There were significant differences between NCS+ and NCS− categories and between symptom+ and symptom− categories for $\Delta R_P / \Delta F_{UPPER}$ and T_{LOWER}. Hands lacking CTS symptoms had a significantly greater R_P but less F_{OVER} than hands with CTS symptoms ($p < 0.05$).

Pearson product correlations were obtained between the electrodiagnostic parameters and the functional test variables (Table 15-8). Because the majority of median and ulnar transcarpal latencies were measured at 8 cm, data for the transcarpal latencies measured at 10 cm (12 of 54 hands) were not included in the correlation analysis. In general, there were significant ($p < 0.01$) correlations between median nerve latencies and functional performance variables ($0.3 < r < 0.6$).

Stepwise discriminant analysis was performed to determine the combination of functional test variables that would best classify the four categories, including symptom−/NCS−, symptom−/NCS+, symptom+/NCS−, and symptom+/NCS+. Different categorical combina-

Table 15-7. Means for the Functional Performance Variables in Four Subject Categories

	Symptom⁻ NCS⁻	Symptom⁺ NCS⁻	Symptom⁻ NCS⁺	Symptom⁺ NCS⁺	F Value[a]
Number of subjects	16	11	5	9	
Number of hands	23	14	6	11	
Gap-detection threshold (mm)	0.18	0.20	0.23	0.27	4.85[b]
Pinch rate (pinches/sec)	4.8	4.3	4.7	3.5	7.58[c]
Pinch rate change with respect to change in force (pinches/sec/%MVC)	−0.050	−0.035	−0.032	−0.023	10.36[c]
Overshoot force (%MVC)	14.9	20.8	19.5	24.7	3.69[d]
Time above the upper force level (msec)	83.4	95.3	103.9	101.2	2.44
Time below the lower force level (msec)	54.3	61.2	61.0	74.2	5.65[a]

[a]F statistics were calculated using one-way analysis of variance, treating subject categories as the independent variable.
[b]$p < 0.01$.
[c]$p < 0.001$.
[d]$p < 0.05$.
NCS = nerve conduction study; MVC = maximal voluntary contraction.

tions were applied to dichotomize subjects for investigating the use of the functional tests for best differentiating positive cases from negative cases according to different case definitions (Table 15-9). The gap-detection sensory threshold and the psychomotor test variables were initially included in the analysis. Several case definitions were explored to find the canonical variables that best differentiated the positive cases from the negatives. When the definition included symptom⁻/NCS⁺, symptom⁺/NCS⁻, and symptom⁺/NCS⁺ groups as positive cases, the stepwise discriminant analysis selected $\Delta R_P/\Delta F_{UPPER}$ into the discriminant function, which had a sensitivity of 0.74 and specificity of 0.83 (see Table 15-9). Canonical variables established in the case-control study as applied to the industrial population study data are also included in Table 15-9.

Discussion

High correlations were observed between the median nerve distal sensory, distal motor, and transcarpal latencies and the functional performance variables when all hands were pooled together. The results were consistent with previous findings (Rodriquez, Radwin, & Jeng, 1993; Jeng et al., 1994) and the case-control study described earlier in this chapter. The correlation coefficients between the NCS median nerve latencies and the functional perfor-

mance variables were less in the current study ($0.3 < r < 0.6$) than in the previous studies ($0.5 < r < 0.8$). This may have been because previous studies selected only well-defined CTS cases and control subjects. In the current study, the distribution of cases were less dichotomous but more realistic.

Stepwise discriminant analysis was used as an objective procedure to select functional performance variables for best differentiating positive cases from negative cases in the case-control study and the industrial population study. The case-control study selected $\Delta R_P/\Delta F_{UPPER}$ and T_{LOWER} for the optimal discriminant function, which are both from the rapid pinch and release psychomotor test. The usefulness of the gap-detection sensory threshold test in the case-control study was unclear. Stepwise discriminant analysis in the current study selected $\Delta R_P/\Delta F_{UPPER}$ and the gap-detection threshold for the canonical variable to differentiate symptom⁻/NCS⁻ hands from symptom⁺/NCS⁺ hands. The difference in the canonical variables very likely reflects the difference of subject selection criteria in these two studies.

The subject selection procedure in the industrial study is believed to better represent the target work population. The subject selection procedure for the case-control study ensured that the CTS patients were recruited only if they did not have any other upper-extremity peripheral nerve entrapment or disorders that might confound the functional perfor-

Table 15-8. Correlation Coefficients and Statistical Significance Levels for the Electrophysiologic Parameters and Functional Performance Variables

	Median Nerve Latencies			Ulnar Nerve Latencies	
	Sensory	**Motor**	**Transcarpal**	**Motor**	**Transcarpal**
Gap-detection threshold	0.583[a]	0.552[a]	0.507[a]	0.356[b]	0.201
Pinch rate	−0.452[a]	−0.357[b]	−0.446[b]	−0.135	−0.307[c]
Change in pinch rate	−0.571[a]	−0.410[b]	−0.507[a]	0.104	0.316[c]
Overshoot force	0.379[b]	0.278[b]	0.270	0.175	0.233
Time above F_{UPPER}	0.327[c]	0.345[c]	0.310[c]	0.099	0.047
Time below F_{LOWER}	0.580[a]	0.486[a]	0.455[b]	0.300[c]	0.373[c]

[a]$p < 0.001$.
[b]$p < 0.01$.
[c]$p < 0.05$.

Table 15-9. Sensitivity and Specificity of Functional Performance Variables Used (1) in the Canonical Variables from the New Stepwise Discriminant Analysis and (2) to Be Fitted into the Discriminant Function Derived from a Previous Case-Control Study

Symptoms, NCS

(−/−)	(−/+)	(+/−)	(+/+)	**Canonical Variable***	**Sensitivity**	**Specificity**
\multicolumn{7}{l}{**(1) Canonical variables from stepwise discriminant analysis**}						
−	+	+	+	$2.77 + 71.81 \times \Delta R_p/\Delta F_{UPPER}$	0.74	0.83
−	−	+	+	$2.59 + 67.22 \times \Delta R_p/\Delta F_{UPPER}$	0.72	0.76
−	+	−	+	$2.61 + 67.56 \times \Delta R_p/\Delta F_{UPPER}$	0.71	0.68
−	−	−	+	$5.92 - 1.35 \times \Delta R_p$	0.82	0.81
−	—	—	+	$0.93 + 8.29 \times$ threshold $+65.00 \times \Delta R_p/\Delta F_{UPPER}$	0.91	0.87
\multicolumn{7}{l}{**(2) Current data applied to the canonical variables established from the previous study**}						
−	+	+	+	$-1.07 + 32.23 \times \Delta R_p/\Delta F_{UPPER}$ $+0.04 \times T_{LOWER}$	0.71	0.74
−	−	+	+	Same as above	0.72	0.66
−	+	−	+	Same as above	0.82	0.62
−	−	−	+	Same as above	0.91	0.58
−	—	—	+	Same as above	0.91	0.74

*Case positive when canonical variable >0, case negative when canonical variable ≤0.
NCS = nerve conduction studies.

mance associated with CTS. The CTS cases in the previous study were diagnosed by clinical evaluations, NCS, and needle EMG. The subject selection procedure for the industrial study did not exclude workers who might have hand problems other than CTS. Future work will investigate potential confounding effects of other musculoskeletal disorders and the utility of using both the gap-detection sensory threshold and the rapid pinch and release psychomotor test for differentiating CTS from other work-related cumulative trauma disorders. It is anticipated that the gap-detection sensory threshold test will serve to differentiate between CTS and non-CTS cumulative trauma disorder cases.

The major limitation of the current study is the relatively small sample size ($n = 54$ hands). Any misclassification by the functional tests would significantly change the sensitivity and specificity for detecting positive and negative cases. Therefore, further studies require larger samples, and longitudinal studies are needed to verify the sensitivity and specificity of the test used in the general working population. The psychological impact on the individual workers and the potential cost to both the employers and the employees of having either false-positive or false-negative cases should not be overlooked.

Conclusion

This chapter reviewed the development and evaluations of the Wisconsin functional test battery for CTS through a series of studies. The normative studies showed that the gap-detection sensory threshold test and the rapid pinch and release psychomotor test were easily administered, required little learning, and had high test and retest reliability. The case-control study showed that the functional test battery was able to detect average differences between CTS and control subject groups, and performance was correlated with conduction parameters of the median nerve. The major limitation of this study was subject selection bias. The sensitivity and specificity for detecting CTS may have been elevated because only two extremes of the distribution of CTS severity were sampled.

The industrial population study categorized subjects according to positive or negative CTS symptoms and positive or negative NCS results from a relatively small worker sample. The selection procedure ensured that the subject sample had enough positive and negative cases for evaluating the efficacy of the functional test battery, but the distribution was biased. The results showed that the functional test battery had reasonable sensitivities and specificities for CTS using a sample of the general worker population. Further studies should be done to incorporate a larger random sample to justify the utility of the functional test battery for detecting CTS in a work setting. A prospective study could minimize the inter-subject variance by establishing the baseline for all participating subjects in high–CTS-risk jobs. The relationship between changes of performance in the functional test battery and the development of CTS could then be investigated.

The diagnosis of CTS requires both medical examination and thorough electrophysiologic evaluation, but the test battery is noninvasive, convenient, and inexpensive to administer. Once the utility of this test is established, workers who show

significant deficits in the functional test battery should be referred to qualified health care providers for medical evaluation.

References

Aaserud, O., Juntunen, J., & Matikainen, E. (1990). Vibration sensitivity thresholds: Methodological considerations. *Acta Neurologica Scandinavia, 82,* 277–283.

American Association of Electrodiagnostic Medicine Quality Assurance Committee, Jablecki, C.K., Andary, M.T., So, Y.T., et al. (1993). Literature review of the usefulness of nerve conduction studies and electromyography for the evaluation of patients with carpal tunnel syndrome. *Muscle and Nerve, 16,* 1392–1414.

Bell-Krotoski, J. (1990). Light touch–deep pressure testing using Semmes-Weinstein monofilaments. In J.M. Hunter, L.H. Schneider, E.J. Mackin, & A.D. Callahan (Eds.), *Rehabilitation of the hand* (3rd ed.). St. Louis: Mosby.

Bell-Krotoski, J., & Buford, W. (1988). The force/time relationship of clinically used sensory testing instruments. *Journal of Hand Therapy, 1,* 76–85.

Bell-Krotoski, J., Weinstein, S., & Weinstein, C. (1993). Testing sensibility, including touch-pressure, two-point discrimination, point localization, and vibration. *Journal of Hand Therapy, 6,* 114–123.

Bleecker, M.L., & Agnew, J. (1987). New techniques for the diagnosis of carpal tunnel syndrome. *Scandinavian Journal of Work Environment and Health, 13,* 385–388.

Centers for Disease Control. (1989). Occupational disease surveillance: Carpal tunnel syndrome. *Morbidity and Mortality Weekly Report, 38,* 485–489.

Dawson, D.M., Hallett, M., & Millender, L.H. (1983). *Entrapment neuropathies.* Boston: Little, Brown.

Dellon, A.L., Mackinnon, S.E., & Crosby, P.M. (1987). Reliability of two-point discrimination measurements. *Journal of Hand Surgery [Am], 12,* 693–696.

Fagius, J., & Wahren, L.K. (1981). Variability of sensory threshold determination in clinical use. *Journal of Neurological Science, 51,* 11–27.

Franklin, G. M., Haug, J., Heyer, N., et al. (1991). Occupational carpal tunnel syndrome in Washington State, 1984–1988. *American Journal of Public Health, 81,* 741–746.

Gerr, F.E. (1994). *Quantitative assessment of carpal tunnel syndrome. Final performance report 5K01OH00098-03.* Cincinnati, OH: National Institute for Occupational Safety and Health.

Harada, N., & Griffin, M.J. (1991). Factors influencing vibration sense thresholds used to assess occupational exposures to hand transmitted vibration. *British Journal of Industrial Medicine, 4,* 185–192.

Jeng, O.-J., & Radwin, R.G. (1995). A gap detection tactility test for measuring sensory deficits associated with carpal tunnel syndrome. *Ergonomics, 38,* 2588–2701.

Jeng, O.-J., Radwin, R.G., & Rodriquez, A.A. (1994). Functional psychomotor deficits associated with carpal tunnel syndrome. *Ergonomics, 37,* 1055–1070.

Jeng, O.-J., Radwin, R.G., Harmon, R.L., & Lotz, B.P. (1994). Carpal tunnel syndrome psychomotor and sensory functional tests. *Proceedings of the 12th Triennial Congress of the International Ergonomics Association, 3,* 240–243.

Katz, J.N., Larson, M., Fossel, A.H., & Liang, M.H. (1991). Validation of a surveillance case definition of carpal tunnel syndrome. *American Journal of Public Health, 81,* 189–193.

Katz, J.N., Larson, M.G., Sabra A., et al. (1990). Carpal tunnel syndrome: Diagnostic utility of the history and physical examination findings. *Annals of Internal Medicine, 112,* 321–327.

Kimura, J. (1989). *Electrodiagnosis in diseases of nerve and muscle: Principles and practice* (2nd ed.). Philadelphia: F.A. Davis.

Levin, S., Pearsall, C., & Ruderman, R. (1978). Von Frey's method of measuring pressure sensibility in the hand: An engineering analysis of the Weinstein-Semmes pressure anesthesiometer. *Journal of Hand Surgery, 3,* 211–216.

Lundborg, G., Gelberman, R. H., Minteer-Convery, M., Lee, Y. F., & Hargens, A.R. (1982). Median nerve compression in the carpal tunnel: Functional response to experimentally induced controlled pressure. *Journal of Hand Surgery [Am], 7,* 252–259.

Mackinnon, S.E., & Dellon, A.L. (1988). *Surgery of the peripheral nerve.* New York: Thieme.

Merchut, M.P., Kelly, M.A., & Toleikis, S.C. (1990). Quantitative sensory threshold testing in carpal tunnel syndrome. *Electromyography and Clinical Neurophysiology, 30,* 119–124.

Moberg, E. (1990). Two-point discrimination test. *Scandinavian Journal of Rehabilitation Medicine, 22,* 127–134.

Moody, L., Arezzo, J., & Otto, D. (1986). Evaluation of workers for early peripheral neuropathy. *Seminars in Occupational Medicine, 1,* 153–162.

Phalen, G.S. (1966). The carpal-tunnel syndrome. *Journal of Bone and Joint Surgery [Am], 48,* 211–228.

Phalen, G.S. (1972). The carpal-tunnel syndrome. Clinical evaluation of 598 hands. *Clinical Orthopaedics and Related Research, 83,* 29–40.

Radwin, R.G., Jeng, O.-J., & Gisske, E.T. (1993). A new automated tactility test instrument for evaluating hand function. *IEEE Transactions on Rehabilitation Engineering, 1,* 220–225.

Radwin, R.G., Masters, G. P., & Lupton, F.W. (1992). A linear force summing hand dynamometer independent of point of application. *Applied Ergonomics, 22,* 339–345.

Radwin, R.G., Wertsch, J.J., Jeng, O.-J., & Casanova, J. (1991). Ridge detection tactility deficits associated with carpal tunnel syndrome. *Journal of Occupational Medicine, 33,* 730–735.

Ransohoff, D.F., & Feinstein, A.R. (1978). Problem of spectrum and bias in evaluating the efficacy of diagnostic tests. *New England Journal of Medicine, 299,* 926–930.

Rodriquez, A.A., Radwin, R.G., & Jeng, O.-J. (1993). Median nerve electrophysiologic parameters and psychomotor performance in carpal tunnel syndrome. *Electromyography and Clinical Neurophysiology, 33,* 311–319.

Sox, H.C. Jr., Blatt, M.A., Higgins, M.C., & Marton, K.I. (1988). *Medical decision making* (pp. 103–145). Boston: Butterworth.

Stevens, J.C. (1987). AAEE minimonograph no. 26: The electrodiagnosis of carpal tunnel syndrome. *Muscle and Nerve, 10,* 99–113.

White, K.M., Congleton, J.J., Huchingson, R.D., et al. (1994). Vibrometry testing for carpal tunnel syndrome: A longitudinal study of daily variations. *Archives of Physical Medicine and Rehabilitation, 75,* 25–28.

Winn, F.J., & Putz-Anderson, V. (1990). Vibration thresholds as a function of age and diagnosis of carpal tunnel syndrome: A preliminary report. *Experimental Aging Research, 16,* 221–224.

Chapter 16

Consumer Product Case Study: Development of Child Safety Seats for Children with Hip Dysplasia

Janet Stout Everly, Marilyn J. Bull, and Karen Bruner Stroup

Learning Objectives

On completion of this chapter, the reader should be able to

- Cite an example of product development for injury prevention.
- Illustrate the steps involved in the development, including evaluation and usability testing.

Key Words

Dynamic crash testing
Product development
Safe transportation
Special needs

Abstract

We illustrate the process of responding to the need for a commercially available product to provide safe and proper motor vehicle transportation for children with hip dysplasia. Through a multidisciplinary team, resources and requirements for product design were assessed, adapted, and readied for dynamic crash testing. The dynamic crash test process was undertaken to evaluate the performance of modifications to an existing commercial product. The modified car safety seat was then made available for loan to children with hip dysplasia in a hospital setting and is available commercially nationwide to serve the needs of children unable to fit into conventional car safety seats.

Introduction

Proper protection for people during motor vehicle travel usually is defined, discussed, and understood by considering the needs of able-bodied children and adults. How vehicles are designed, which occupant protection products are developed, and how safety standards are revised are set by a research and education agenda that concentrates on individuals free from disability. To continue this focus conveys a message that buckling up is only for able-bodied children and adults who can use conventional occupant protection systems.

Dedicated work to help ensure proper occupant protection of children with special needs is critical as health care reform transforms and redefines the limits of medical care. Prevention of secondary injury to children with disabilities can be accomplished through concerted effort to ensure that proper restraint equipment is used and installed correctly and through appropriate research, development, and testing, when needed, to ensure that proper and safe transportation can be provided. Medical care costs can be better contained through this preventative orientation.

Rehabilitation specialists, pediatricians, therapists, transportation providers, nurses, and other professionals have roles in encouraging and creating new resources for occupant protection for children with special needs. Encouraging and creating new resources will help to broaden the field of resources and standards of practice for properly protecting children with special needs during travel.

Team Development

At Riley Hospital for Children, Indiana University Medical Center, a multidisciplinary team of medical and health professionals was developed through experience that grew out of staff joining together on weekly orthopedic rounds to assess needs of pediatric patients before hospital discharge. Included on these rounds were representatives from many discipline areas, including occupational therapy, respiratory therapy, orthopedics, and child passenger safety through the hospital's Automotive Safety for Children Program. Providing for the safe transportation of children with casts consistently surfaced as an issue with medical staff and child passenger safety specialists and was voiced as a concern by parents, who were visited by the orthopedics team on an individual basis. Many parents told the team some of the steps they had considered, including laying children on the floor of vans or on the seats of cars or lapholding the child, because fit into a car seat or safety belt often was not possible. From these multidisciplinary rounds a key relationship formed between occupational therapy staff and staff from the hospital's Automotive Safety for Children Program as the orthopedics team wrestled with questions about providing safe transportation home for children in casts. Occupational therapists and technicians provided critical expertise for evaluating the positioning needs of children and for developing resources and action steps that could be taken to meet those needs. Staff from the Automotive Safety for Children Program provided expertise for car safety seat selection and a broad knowledge of available occupant protection products on the market.

Assessment

Defining the Problem

The initial work to develop a resource for safe transportation of children with hip dysplasia was tempered by the time period, the mid-1980s. Use of car safety seats had only recently been mandated in Indiana, so the simple idea of using car safety seats was relatively new for most parents. Convincing people to use car safety seats consistently and correctly was a major focus of most education efforts throughout the country. The multidisciplinary team of medical and health professionals participating in weekly orthopedic rounds recognized the unsuitability of available safety seats for special populations of children.

Establishing Design Objectives

Our design objectives for a safety seat that would accommodate children in hip spica casts considered these broad criteria: (1) to limit product design costs by exploring use of a commercially available car seat rather than pursuing development of a new product and (2) to develop a car safety seat that would fit both infants and toddlers.

Assessment of Existing Products

Initial investigations focused on evaluating commercially available car safety seats that had already been crash tested and found to meet the requirements of Federal Motor Vehicle Safety Standard 213 (Code of Federal Regulations, 1994, 571.213. Standard No. 213; Child restraint systems, Office of the Federal Register, National Archives and Records Administration, U.S. Government Printing Office, Washington, DC). Through input from parents and members of the multidisciplinary team, the following positioning and safety concerns were identified. Children with hip dysplasia do not fit into standard car safety seats because the cast that is used to help correct this condition does not allow proper fit into the car seat plastic shell, which typically has raised sides to help contain the child's body inside the car seat. The casted child's legs are abducted so widely that the child's back, head, and neck are positioned too far forward to rest against the padding of the car safety seat. The danger is that harness straps may not be able to be positioned properly on the child's shoulders and hips. The harness straps may not hold the child securely into the car safety seat, and therefore, head and knee excursion levels may exceed what is considered safe. These assessments were made through clinical experience, which provided opportunities to fit children into car safety seats and communication with families about problems with achieving proper fit of children with hip spica casts into conventional convertible-style car safety seats. A wide variety of inserts, such as pillows or foam, are sometimes used in a misguided attempt to compensate for the lack of fit in standard safety seats. The use of these inserts, although well intentioned, compromises the child's secure fit into the car safety seat. Many parents of infants added pillows inside infant car seats, which often made it difficult to use the harness strap system or to secure the infant at all. The awkward fit of the infant in a hip spica cast into a car safety seat also makes it difficult to position a car safety seat facing rearward, as recommended and tested by the manufacturer. A potentially disastrous consequence of not being able to position children with hip spica casts into standard car safety seats is the choice of many users to simply lay the child on the vehicle seat or floor unrestrained.

Design

Development of Performance Criteria

Requirements for the design and crash performance of car safety seats in the United States are set forth in Federal Motor Vehicle Safety Standard 213. Crash performance is carried out under laboratory conditions that simulate speeds at 30 mph and $20g$ in frontal collisions. The multidisciplinary team accepted this standard, therefore applying the same criteria for product performance for children with special needs that is used for child safety seats for able-bodied children.

Test and Evaluation

Dynamic crash testing was carried out by the Child Passenger Protection Research Program at the University of Michigan, Ann Arbor. The concepts for crash testing were outlined, car safety seats for testing were secured, and testing procedures were carried out by staff with background and experience in biomechanical engineering. Staff from the multidisciplinary team were not present during the crash testing. Reports of the crash tests were provided to the team in written, videotape, photograph, and slide formats.

The initial crash test was intended to evaluate the workability of simply adding a stiff foam block into the base of a popular child safety seat, the Cosco Safe-T-Seat (Cosco, Inc, Columbus, IN). A test dummy was seated on the block and secured with harness straps. This design failed the performance criteria. The test dummy's head exceeded acceptable limits for head and neck excursion on impact, suggesting the potential for head or neck injury in a crash situation.

Second Design

Team and Assessment

Input from the team members, which now included the University of Michigan Child Passenger Protection Research Program, redefined the design objectives. A new design objective became the development of a car safety seat with reduced side panels and seat base that would allow for the fit of a child into the back padding of the car seat for support of the head, neck, and back. No commercially available car safety seat would accomplish this fit; therefore, modification of existing products was undertaken.

The primary requirements for modification were guided by these considerations: (1) The restraint system could not be an infant-only car safety seat because the small size of these restraints would limit its usability; (2) the restraint system should be a five-point harness, which would allow greater control in the adjusting and fit of the harness system to the child's body, compared to the T-shield or convertible car seat fitted with an arm rest; (3) the metal frame of the convertible car safety seat would remain uncompromised in any alteration of the shell; (4) the five-point harness system would not be compromised in any shell alteration; and (5) the outer plastic shell of the car safety seat could be cut away to a point that would accommodate the abducted hips.

Design Process

Two car safety seats met the five requirements listed above: the Century 100 (Macedonia, OH) (Figure 16-1) and the Strolee 612 (no longer available).

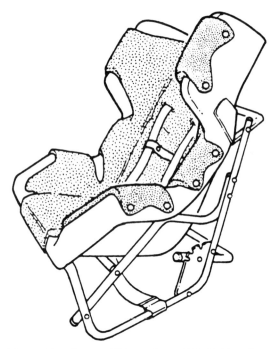

Figure 16-1. Century child restraint model 100 (Macedonia, OH). (Reprinted with permission from M.J. Bull, K. Weber, & K. Stroup. [1986]. Safety seat use for children with hip dislocation. *Pediatrics, 77,* 873–875. Reproduced by permission of *Pediatrics.*)

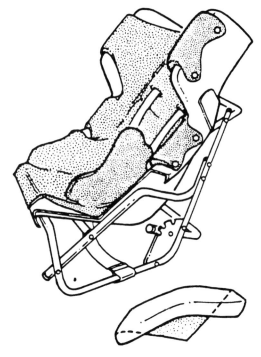

Figure 16-2. Padding detached and lower side of plastic shell removed. (Reprinted with permission from M.J. Bull, K. Weber, & K. Stroup. [1986]. Safety seat use for children with hip dislocation. *Pediatrics, 77,* 873–875. Reproduced by permission of *Pediatrics.*)

These two seats were modified by cutting away the lower sides of the plastic shell (Figure 16-2) (Stroup, Weber, & Bull, 1989). The plastic cut was filed smooth and covered by the original padding of the car safety seat. The padding was secured by duct tape to the car seat shell on its underside (Figure 16-3).

Test and Evaluation

Several pediatric patients with hip spica casts were fitted into these modified systems to field test comfort and fit. Dynamic crash testing was required, however, to assess the safety of the modification before these devices could be made available for actual use by children. Testing was completed again at the University of Michigan in collaboration with the Child Passenger Protection Research Program. Results of the dynamic tests showed that the modification of both shells did not alter the satisfactory performance of each car safety seat. The modified

car safety seats were found to be suitable for transporting children with hip spica casts.

One of the tested car safety seats, the Strolee 612, soon became unavailable as an option when the manufacturer went out of business. Although many Strolee 612 models were still available, it was not an acceptable course of action to pursue this model as a choice for alteration because it would not be possible to secure parts or support from the manufacturer, should questions arise.

Consequently, the other tested seat, the Century 100, was put into operation in a pilot loan program through the Automotive Safety for Children Program at Riley Hospital. Local professional organizations provided the means to purchase a quantity of Century 100 car safety seats that could be modified and made available for loan to pediatric patients. After a trial period of evaluation at Riley Hospital, instructions for modification were made available through pamphlets, telephone consulting, presentations, and publications.

Meanwhile, efforts continued unsuccessfully to secure a distributor for the modified Century 100 car safety seat to make this product more accessible to children throughout the country. As use of car safety seats increased in all states in late 1984, all manufacturers began to change existing products to better meet consumer needs. By 1986, the Century 100 model had been discontinued, which necessitated further product design and testing.

Third Design

Team and Assessment

At this point, a child safety seat manufacturer joined the team. Engineers from a major car seat manufacturer, acting as independent consultants, agreed to pursue steps to make the product commercially available. The objective for product design at this point was to create a product that did not require modification and was commercially available.

Design Process

The design of the Spelcast (formerly called the Evenflo 410), with its low-cut sides, made this seat an ideal replacement for the modified Century 100. The modification process for reducing the sides of the shell and the seat base of the Spelcast replicated that of the previous design.

Test and Evaluation

Crash testing again was conducted at the University of Michigan Child Passenger Protection Research Program. Crash tests were carried out with a 20-lb test dummy fitted with a plaster cast and secured into the Spelcast facing rearward and with a test dummy the size of a 3 year old, weighing 33 lb (15 kg) and measuring 38.4 in. (975 mm) tall, casted and secured facing forward in the Spelcast. Results of the crash tests demonstrated that the Spelcast provided satisfactory protection for infants and toddlers in hip spica casts.

Conclusion

The design engineer, having the knowledge of technology, standards, and the market, became the inde-

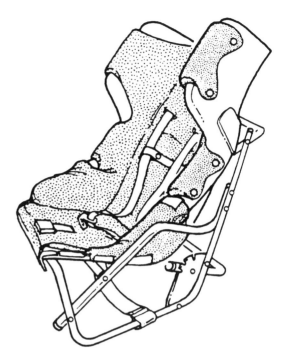

Figure 16-3. Padding replaced and taped securely to outer side of seat. (Reprinted with permission from M.J. Bull, K. Weber, & K. Stroup. [1986]. Safety seat use for children with hip dislocation. *Pediatrics, 77,* 873–875. Reproduced by permission of *Pediatrics.*)

pendent distributor for the Spelcast. The Spelcast improved on the consistency and aesthetics of the modification and served a population greater than that served by Riley Hospital.

The process of developing the Spelcast as a product has been a long term effort with continued challenges and changes in the availability of distributors and resources. When the Evenflo 410 shell became unavailable commercially, the Spelcast moved to a new manufacturer, Snug Seat (Matthews, NC). Snug Seat's design of the Spelcast has maintained the original concept of low-cut sides for optimal positioning of the child with leg abduction.

A major effort in getting this product to the users (i.e., hospitals, rehabilitation centers, and parents) was an affiliation with the National Easter Seal Society through the Kids Are Riding Safe, Special Kids Are Riding Safe project, supported by the National Highway Traffic Safety Administration. This project seeded the development of hospital-based car seat loan programs that serve the protection needs of all children. Products such as the Spelcast were part of their inventory. Another tool for informing parents and health care providers about safe transportation of children with orthopedic problems was an original video, *Safely Home* (1988), which demonstrated the correct use and installation of the Spelcast and other devices. Subsequent grant awards from General Motors through the National Highway Traffic Safety Administration to the National Easter Seal Society have significantly increased the availability and distribution of the Spelcast through hospitals, rehabilitation centers, and other developmental agencies nationwide.

The field remains wide open for continued investigation and product development. Future research and development of occupant protection systems for people with special needs should address these medical issues: (1) halo cervical spine immobilizers; (2) ambulance transportation, especially protection of infants in isolettes; (3) lap tray design for use in wheelchairs during transportation; (4) development of crashworthy wheelchairs and insert hardware; 5) development of crashworthy hardware for securing medical equipment during transportation; and (6) safe devices for providing neck support during transportation for persons with low muscle tone or poor head control.

This case study in usability testing exemplifies the creative process of analysis, design, test, and evaluation. Analysis involves identifying problems and learning about existing occupant protection resources. Product design involves having the courage of conviction in the usability of the product for a large audience beyond immediate patient contacts. Test and evaluation are critical and essential steps in the design process, which may include field testing with clients, gaining user input, and safety testing. Important in this ongoing developmental process were problem investigation, knowledge of existing products, and communication with researchers, grantors, manufacturers, health care providers, and families. Persistence and commitment have been critical to achieving the goal of maintaining the availability of the Spelcast. With

the Spelcast, dynamic crash testing documented the validity of the modification and helped to avoid questions pertaining to liability of the designers for the modification. Most important, dynamic crash testing ensured that children in hip spica casts could be assured of a safe ride in motor vehicles. Final evaluation involved loaning car safety seats to casted children and learning of successful transportation from their families.

Research alone is inadequate if others are not informed of successes and failures. Dissemination of information through publications, presentations, and conferences is critical to allow the most benefit to others.

Acknowledgments

Dynamic crash tests were supported by a grant award from the James Whitcomb Riley Memorial Association. Support from the Indiana Governor's Council on Impaired and Dangerous Driving, Office of Traffic Safety and the National Highway Traffic Safety Administration is gratefully acknowledged.

References

Bull, M.J., Weber, K., & Stroup, K. (1986). Safety seat use for children with hip dislocation. *Pediatrics, 77,* 873–875.

Bull, M.J., Stroup, K.B., Stout, J., & Zickler, C. (1989). Special children, special car seats. *Contemporary Pediatrics, November,* 122–136.

Safely Home. (1988). Indianapolis, IN: Automotive Safety for Children Program, Riley Hospital for Children.

Stout, J.D., Bull, M.J., & Stroup, K. (1989). Safe transportation for infants and preschoolers with special needs. *Infants and Young Children, October,* 67–73.

Stout, J.D., Bull, M.J., & Stroup, K. (1989). Safe transportation for children with disabilities. *American Journal of Occupational Therapy, 43,* 31–36.

Stout, J.D., Bandy, P., Feller, N., et al. (1992). Transportation resources for pediatric orthopaedic clients. *Orthopaedic Nursing, 11,* 26–30.

Stroup, K.B., Weber, K., & Bull, M.J. (1989). Safe transportation solutions for children with special needs. 31st Annual Proceedings, American Association for Automotive Medicine, New Orleans, LA.

Section VI

Americans with Disabilities Act

Chapter 17

Clinical Ergonomics and the Americans with Disabilities Act: An Introduction

Barbara L. Kornblau

Learning Objective

On completion of this chapter, the reader should be able to

- Understand the rules and functions of ergonomic consulting in light of the Americans with Disabilities Act (ADA).

Key Words

Consultation
Americans with Disabilities Act

Abstract

This chapter explains the roles and functions of the ergonomic consultant in the arena of the ADA— specifically, how ergonomic consultants can tailor their skills to promote compliance with the ADA. The author assumes readers have a rudimentary understanding of basic ADA concepts.

Introduction

Williams Widgets, a major employer in its community, never expected to see an applicant like Mrs. Brown apply for the electronic assembly position it advertised in the local paper. Mrs. Brown arrived on time for her appointment. She had a solid work history, showing more than 10 years of experience as an electronics assembler, the most recent of which was working with similar assembly items. She received excellent references from her prior employer and appeared to be the most qualified candidate.

What caused Williams Widgets to wonder about such a highly qualified candidate as Mrs. Brown? Mrs. Brown was the first candidate ever to apply for this position from a wheelchair.

Mrs. Brown's condition raised numerous questions for her future employer. How could she perform all her job duties from a wheelchair? Could she reach the assembly line from her wheelchair? What if she could not fit her wheelchair under the conveyor belt? Would she be able to reach the conveyor belt's emergency shutoff button?

Ben, a skilled biomedical repair technician who worked for a hospital for 12 years, found himself released to work by his physician after recovering from a back injury. His doctor gave him some restrictions, limiting his standing to no more than 20 minutes and his lifting to 25 lb, with no repetitive bending or stooping permitted. A dedicated employee, Ben wants to return to his previous job at the hospital but worries that he will be unable to manage at his work station within his physical restrictions.

How will Ben do his job if he can no longer perform repetitive bending? Will his standing and lifting restrictions prevent his return to work? Can the job be adapted to allow for his restrictions?

Sally always dreamed of a garden wedding overlooking the ocean. She finally found the perfect spot, at a beautiful ocean-side resort, where waves flirt with the rocks behind the garden of her dreams. There is one drawback: The steps leading down to the garden might as well be a mountain to Sally. She can make a grand entrance in her flowing, white bridal gown, but after the ceremony, she worries, her arthritis may prevent her ascending the steps to leave.

Can Sally have access to the resort hotel's garden? The resort hotel wonders whether the area can be adapted to enable Sally's exit.

Although the answers to these questions may seem obvious to a skilled ergonomic consultant, most employers, employees, and owners of public accommodations do not find the answers so obvious. Faced with these situations, few human resource professionals know what to do or whom to turn to for assistance. Owners and managers of hotels, restaurants, movie theaters, hospitals, office complexes, retail establishments, and other public accommodations find themselves without solutions to these increasingly common dilemmas. Yet because of the enactment of the ADA, the answers to these questions hold increasingly greater significance for employers and operators of public accommodations (ADA, 1990). Because ergonomic consultants can answer these questions for employers and operators of public accommodations, the ADA can facilitate a marriage between the ergonomic consultant and businesses and industry to create a new source of revenue for the ergonomic consultant from ADA consultation services.

Congress passed the ADA to provide the Mrs. Browns, Bens, and Sallys of the United States with an opportunity to enter the stream of independent living. To individuals with disabilities, the ADA extends the same civil rights protection guaranteed under the law to all individuals regardless of race, creed, sex, national origin, and religion. The ADA prevents discrimination against individuals with disabilities in the areas of employment, public accommodations, transportation, state and local government services, and telecommunications.

The ADA mandates that employers make reasonable accommodations to enable qualified workers with disabilities to perform work functions. It requires that businesses and places of public accommodation provide reasonable accommodations to make programs and facilities usable by individuals with disabilities. (Chapter 18 includes a resource list for readers who want more specific knowledge about the ADA.) This chapter explains the roles and functions of the ergonomic consultant in the ADA arena; specifically, how ergonomic consultants can use their skills to promote compliance with the ADA. In meeting this challenge, the author assumes that the reader has a rudimentary understanding of the ADA's basic requirements.

Introducing the ADA to a Business

The ADA presents employers with new, rather confusing terminology. They need assistance in understanding the basics of the ADA. Although those in top management generally have acquainted themselves with the rudiments of the ADA, this information has not necessarily filtered down to other employees. Employee education is the first line of defense against ADA litigation. An introduction to the ADA for all employees can prevent unwanted, unintentional acts of disability discrimination in the workplace.

Employers need to educate their front-line supervisors in the basic ADA requirements as a way of promoting a proactive approach to ADA compliance and furthering a better awareness of and a change in attitude toward individuals with disabilities. In this circumstance, the role of educator suits the ergonomic consultant. One need not possess the training of an attorney to review the ADA's basic terminology and basic requirements at a level that is meaningful to front-line personnel. Yet this basic understanding can mean the difference between a flexible supervisor open to a subordinate with a disability and a "we've-always-done-it-this-way" supervisor, whose actions may push the parties into litigation.

As an educator, the ergonomic consultant can teach company employees to identify essential job functions. Teaching company representatives to identify and write drafts of the essential functions of the company's positions benefits employers in reasonably accommodating existing employees and in hiring new employees (EEOC, 1992).

Ergonomic consultants can also be helpful in educating employees so companies can develop their own internal teams of job analysts. Internal job analysts can identify essential functions and develop functional job descriptions useful in hiring and accommodations.

Employers who provide goods and services to the public may also fall within the scope of public accommodations, which makes them subject to the ADA's Title III requirements for access. Ergonomic consultants can introduce places of public accommodation to their Title III obligations, to ensure access to the goods, services, facilities, privileges and services they provide (ADA Title III, 1991).

The Selection Process

The ADA changes the way employers can conduct themselves during the selection process. Because the ADA prevents employers from asking medical questions before making an offer of employment and from using pre-employment physical examinations, employers now need other methods of selecting the employee who can perform the job (EEOC, 1994).

The ergonomic consultant can assist employers in developing agility tests, which employers may legally administer before making a job offer, and preplacement screenings, which employers may give after making an offer of employment. Ergonomists with specialties in physical or occupational therapy or other health-related fields should exercise caution when it comes to developing agility tests. If health care professionals develop these tests, or if health care professionals train the test administrators, the company may find the agility test, which is given before extending an offer of employment, labeled an impermissible medical test (EEOC, 1994).

In developing preplacement screenings, ergonomic consultants must familiarize themselves with the standards set forth in the ADA and make sure their test meets the standard. Because any test that may tend to screen out individuals with disabilities must fall within the standard of being "job related and consistent with business necessity," ergonomic consultants may want to perform a job analysis and base the items tested on the results of the job analysis (EEOC, 1992). Testing protocols must allow for reasonable accommodation during the actual screening process (ADA Title I, 1991). For example, test administrators should be prepared to provide written instructions for individuals with hearing impairment, oral instructions for individuals with dyslexia, and possible alternative methods for completion of tasks for the individual with physical impairments.

Another avenue of assistance in the employee selection process includes job interview techniques. The ADA makes it illegal for employers to ask any questions of an applicant that seek medical information or information about the individual's disability (EEOC, 1994). An ergonomic consultant can teach interviewers to ask questions designed to match the applicant's abilities to the job's requirements based on the job analysis. The ergonomic consultant can also teach the interviewer how best to approach the issue of reasonable accommodation during the interview. Furthermore, disability awareness sessions may also smooth the interview process for the interviewer who faces a wheelchair user or someone with a prosthetic arm for the first time in his or her life.

Sensitivity Training

Ergonomic consultation benefits employers by ensuring that employers make individuals with disabilities feel comfortable in the workplace. For the ergonomic consultant, sensitizing coworkers and supervisors to individuals with disabilities and promoting ideas for accommodation are important consultation roles. Dispelling myths about the abilities and needs of individuals with disabilities and encouraging positive working relationships promote successful placement of qualified candidates. The ergonomic consultant may accomplish this through formal presentation or informal work groups established to solve specific accommodation problems. In both situations, involvement of an individual with a disability in the training process provides optimal benefits to all involved. A major focus of any training should include the assurance that qualified candidates with disabilities meet the same standards for performance and production as nondisabled workers (ADA Title I, 1991).

Reasonable Accommodation

The ADA gives the term *reasonable accommodation* a broad definition, to include, for example, raising the height of a desk so that a worker's wheelchair can fit underneath, acquiring special equipment (such as a speaker phone) for someone with limited upper-extremity mobility, and allowing the worker with a disability to work a modified work schedule so that he or she may go to therapy.

Ergonomic consultants have long made changes to the way workers perform their jobs. Designing or redesigning tools and equipment or work stations is certainly not new to most skilled ergonomic consultants. What is new is the "packaging" of this product: Some of the same ergonomic changes to the workplace can be called *reasonable accommodations* when they are made to match the workplace to the worker with a disability.

With the ADA firmly in place and with ergonomic consultants now producers of reasonable accommodations, ergonomic consultants have a new and broader market for their services. The need for reasonable accommodation under the ADA brings the ergonomist a wealth of opportunity for individual or case consultation. Consultation occurs when a company needs accommodation for a specific individual, as opposed to an industry- or company-wide design change. It may also occur on referral from private sector rehabilitation providers, as in a workers' compensation case, or from an insurance carrier for an individual who receives disability insurance benefits. In these situations, the ergonomic consultant finds that returning to work is the motivation behind the reasonable accommodation referral.

A consultation performed pursuant to a request for reasonable accommodation under the ADA requires making specific reasonable accommodation for a particular individual with a disability. The ergonomic consultant must remember that an individual with a disability will probably not function physically in the same manner as the "average" person from the anthropometric tables. In these individual case consultation situations, ergonomic consultants must base their solutions and specific changes not on anthropometric measurements but rather on consideration of the individual worker's needs. As the ADA states, reasonable accommodation decisions must be made on a case-by-case basis (ADA Title I, 1991). The specific limitations of the person in question dictates those needs. Thus, ergonomic consultants who pursue reasonable accommodation consultation need to know how people with disabilities function.

As part of the process of identifying reasonable accommodations, the Equal Employment Opportunity Commission (EEOC) reminds readers to get input from the individual with the disability. The EEOC views the individual with a disability as an expert on his or her disability and the reasonable accommodation he or she requires (EEOC, 1992). The ergonomic consultant must remember that the reasonable accommodations process should include an interactive dialogue among the individual with the disability, the employer, and any consultant involved in the process (EEOC, 1992).

The ergonomic consultant must keep in mind that the need for reasonable accommodation extends beyond employment (U.S. Dept. of Justice, 1992). As previously mentioned, privately owned places of public accommodation must also make reasonable accommodations to facilitate and enable access to its goods and services. Although some people assume that all these accommodations are structural, requiring the services of an architect, in reality, ergonomic consultants can play a significant role. Ergonomic consultants can give valuable, cost-effective solutions to places of public accommodation seeking to provide access for their customers. As in the employment context, many reasonable accommodations involve finding other ways to accomplish a task or alternatives to structural building changes to enable access.

Although a portion of Title III of the ADA (the title that addresses places of public accommodation) looks like a building code, most of these provisions apply to alterations or new construction only (ADA Title I, 1991). Existing places of public accommodation must make only readily achievable changes to their premises. The ergonomic consultant can develop readily achievable changes and other reasonable accommodations, which need not necessarily include structural changes (U.S. Dept. of Justice, 1992).

If a customer finds himself or herself unable to see the overnight depository at the bank from wheelchair level, for example, rather than lower the entire overnight depository opening, an ergonomic consultant might recommend installing a mirror. If a customer were unable to reach an item from the grocery store shelf, an ergonomic consultant could recommend that the store provide the customer with a reacher or install a push-button flashing-light system in the aisles to which a stock clerk would respond. Neither suggestion constitutes a structural change, but both provide viable alternatives that allow access to goods and services.

Under Title II of the ADA, state and local governments must also provide reasonable accommodations to enable access to their programs and services

(ADA Title II, 1991). This may include access to employment as well as programs. Ergonomic consultants find that their knowledge and skills are useful to assist state and local governments in making programs and services accessible to individuals with disabilities. For example, suppose an individual with a disability were called for jury duty. The ergonomic consultant could suggest the redesign of the jury box to allow access for a juror who uses a wheelchair for mobility. When state and local governments fail to make their programs and services accessible, as required by Title II, ergonomic consultants may fill the role of expert witness in litigation to enforce the law's access and reasonable accommodation requirements.

Determining Essential Job Functions

Some ergonomic consultants consult in an educational framework for employer and employee training to determine essential function in-house, whereas others may find employers asking them to make the determination for the employer. The ergonomic consultant may play a key role in assisting employers in determining a job's essential functions. Under the ADA, an employer must make reasonable accommodation for qualified individuals with disabilities, meaning individuals who can perform the essential functions of a position with or without a reasonable accommodation (ADA Title I, 1991). Thus, determination of essential functions can determine whether or not the employer must make an accommodation at all. If the individual with a disability cannot perform the essential functions of a job with or without an accommodation, he or she is not entitled to the ADA's protection (ADA Title I, 1991).

The ADA defines a job's essential functions as those that the individual holding the position must be able to perform unaided or with the assistance of a reasonable accommodation. As with the determination of essential functions under the ADA, whether a job task falls under the essential function umbrella remains a factual determination made on a case-by-case basis. To make this determination, one must inquire as to whether the person actually performs the function, if the position exists to perform the function, how many other employees perform the function, and whether a high degree of expertise or skill is required to perform the job task (EEOC, 1992).

If a person takes a job as a proofreader, for example, he or she must be able to proofread. On the other hand, a person who takes a job as a receptionist in an office with 10 other secretaries need not worry that his or her disability prevents him or her from driving a car. Driving a car is probably not an essential job function because the other 10 secretaries could meet any driving needs that may arise occasionally, or a courier could perform delivery duties.

Should a dispute arise as to whether an employer appropriately designates a task as an essential job function, the EEOC (the government agency that investigates ADA employment-related complaints) looks at evidence to determine whether a particular function is essential. According to the regulations and technical assistance manual, the evidentiary indicators include the written job description that was prepared before advertising or interviewing for the position (ADA Title I, 1991; EEOC, 1992).

Although the ADA does not require employers to write job descriptions, a carefully prepared job description may rescue employers who face claims of employment discrimination. Besides the potential risk management function, the written job description serves other purposes. A job description written in specific, functional terms leaves prospective employees with enough information to determine whether they can perform the job's essential functions, thereby allowing them to self-select out of jobs they know they cannot perform.

Job Analysis Consultation

Before the ADA, it was not common practice in the personnel field to write detailed, functional job descriptions. The trend until now has been to write task-oriented job descriptions filled with phrases such as "must be able to load trucks" rather than "must lift 50-lb bags of fertilizer and carry them a distance of 10 feet up an inclined ramp." The first phrase fails to give the reader much information about the job, whereas the second gives the reader detailed information that allows the applicant with a disability to compare his or her own abilities with the job's requirements. Just how does the employer begin the task of rewriting job descriptions?

Some companies may want the ergonomic consultant to instruct its own employees to perform job analysis, but in many situations it makes more sense for ergonomic consultants to perform the actual job analysis themselves. Many people find job analysis a perplexing process or a tedious task. Employees who are trained to perform the job analysis may find a particular job too complicated to analyze. Some in-house job analysts are biased toward the attitude that "everything we do is essential" and are unable to distinguish essential from marginal functions.

The ergonomic consultant can come to the employer's rescue by analyzing jobs at the workplace to determine the job's essential functions. From this job analysis, the ergonomic consultant can develop a job description written in specific, functional terms, describing the essential functions of the job. Employers find this detailed job analysis useful for meeting many needs, such as giving specific information about the job to physicians, pension or retirement boards, health care professionals, workers' compensation boards, judges, attorneys, and insurance company representatives. Ergonomic consultants can use the information gleaned from the job analysis to develop postoffer preplacement screenings and agility tests. Restricted duty or light duty jobs may be developed from the job analysis information by combining tasks from various positions. Job analysis information can also assist employers in developing injury prevention programs by identifying work-related tasks that may contribute to musculoskeletal injuries, thus allowing the employer to further investigate those tasks.

The job analysis gives applicants, employers, human resource professionals, and other professionals information useful in developing reasonable accommodations to enable individuals with disabilities to perform the essential and marginal tasks of their jobs. The information gleaned from the job analysis also helps the individual with a disability to identify jobs that he or she can perform and the reasonable accommodations that he or she may require to perform them.

Direct Threat Consultation

The ergonomic consultant brings to the employer another benefit from the job analysis: the identification of hazards that may pose a direct threat to an employee. The ADA allows employers to not hire employees who present a direct threat to themselves or others (ADA Title I, 1991). Under the law, how-

ever, employers may not base the direct threat on myths, misperceptions, and fears but must instead rely on real evidence of the threat (EEOC, 1992). Thus, if an employer suspects a direct threat in the workplace, it would be wise to engage ergonomic consultation services. Through job analysis and other aspects of the ergonomic consultation process, the consultant may discover aspects of the individual's disability that pose a direct threat to the individual with the disability or to others.

According to ADA regulations, should the employer find that a direct threat exists, before eliminating the individual with a disability from its employ, the employer first must try to reduce the risk by means of reasonable accommodation (ADA Title I, 1991; EEOC, 1992). Once again, the ergonomic consultant can provide the employer with valuable assistance to meet this challenge. In instances where the ergonomic consultant finds a hazard in the workplace or where an individual poses a direct threat because of his or her disability, the ergonomic consultant can provide consultation services to eliminate the hazard or threat.

The ergonomic consultant might, for example, suggest performing a task in a different manner, which would reduce the individual's risk. Alternatively, he or she might suggest that an employer redesign a work area to eliminate or reduce a risk to an individual or other workers. The consultant might suggest changing fluorescent lighting to another light source to prevent seizures triggered by fluorescent lighting. Another adaptation might be changing an auditory fire warning device to a visual signal for an individual with a hearing impairment.

Restricted Duty Programs and Creating Access to Jobs

Although the ADA does not require employers to develop light duty or restricted duty programs, employers may find it an alternative for avoiding litigation. Often, alternative programs save the company workers' compensation and short- and long-term disability dollars and provide other benefits to the employer. The ergonomic consultant can assist employers in developing restricted duty programs by using information obtained from the job analysis to find jobs the employer can easily adapt. The consultant may discover, for example, that parts of several jobs can be combined to form a single restricted duty job, or the consultant may recommend accommodations to a cashier position so that cashiers sit in swivel chairs at barstool height rather than stand, which could cause or aggravate lower-extremity ailments.

The ergonomic consultant can facilitate job placement and return to work by using job analysis information to create lists that categorize jobs into those that do not require excessive lifting, do not require standing, or do not require reaching overhead. This gives employers information, so they can match employees and potential employees who have restrictions and limitations with jobs they can perform.

Consultation with Architects

Ergonomic consultants can review plans with architects and interior designers to determine whether the plans allow individuals with disabilities to use the goods, services, and facilities offered at the site. Should the plans not provide access, the consultant can suggest cost-effective accommodations, which may not involve costly structural changes, such as rearranging furniture.

As an example of a nonstructural accommodation, a hospital began construction on a building designed to house, among other nonpatient functions, the human resources department. When construction was well under way, someone realized that, although wheelchair users could fit through the doorways of the interview rooms, once inside the rooms, they could not close the door or maneuver around. After much panic and discussion about tearing out walls, the architects called in an ergonomic consultant to brainstorm a nonstructural solution. The consultant suggested simply placing the desks in the interview rooms flush with the wall to allow an open area in the middle of the room, which would provide enough space for a wheelchair user. The relieved architect, interior decorator, and project manager approved the consultant's suggested accommodations, which kept the walls intact and the project within budget.

Ergonomic consultation with architects can extend outside the employment arena to cover Title III public accommodation matters in existing buildings. As places of public accommodation move to comply with the ADA or seek to remodel existing construction, they need the services of an architect. The ergonomic consultant can work hand in hand with the architect to develop cost-effective, workable solutions to access issues in existing or remodeled places of public accommodation (see Chapter 20).

Consultation with Attorneys: The Expert Witness

Attorneys for employers and employees find ergonomic consultants valuable members of the litigation team in ADA litigation. Under the rules of evidence, only someone who is qualified as an expert witness may render an opinion in court; a fact witness may testify only about facts of which he or she has firsthand knowledge (Fed. R. Evid. 702). The ergonomic consultant serving as an expert witness may provide the court with information to help in making its decision. Attorneys for an employer may hire the ergonomic consultant to testify that a particular accommodation offered by the employer accommodates the employee or, conversely, that the requested accommodation would present safety risks or fail to enable the employee's performance of job duties.

The ergonomic consultant's role as expert witness extends to both sides of the fence. Just as the employer's attorney finds the ergonomic consultant a valuable team member, so does the employee's attorney. For example, the consultant may testify on behalf of an employee as plaintiff that a particular accommodation meets both the employee's needs and the employer's budget and space requirements.

The ergonomic consultant can play a valuable role in promoting settlement of cases when he or she identifies accommodations to which both the employer and employee agree. With job analysis information in hand, ergonomic consultants can help employers save the cost of unnecessary litigation by providing detailed information about the job, which may be used during the mediation process to develop reasonable accommodation. In fact, ergonomic consultants may find themselves consulting with mediators during the actual mediation session to identify ergonomic solutions and suggest reasonable accommodation that may end the dispute.

In situations in which ADA disputes are subject to mandatory arbitration (under securities laws, for example, all ADA matters dealing with stock brokerage firms must be resolved through arbitration), ergonomic consultants may find themselves giving arbitrators the reasonable accommodation ideas that become part of the arbitrator's decision. An arbitrator's decision is final and binding on the parties.

In addition to ADA cases involving employment, ergonomic consultants can play a valuable role as expert witnesses in matters involving the Title III public accommodation provisions. Through testimony, ergonomic consultants can provide proof to the court that reasonable accommodation can or cannot be made to the place in question. They can also testify as to the costs of the accommodation and the relative degree of ease with which accommodations can be made. Further, as in the employment cases, ergonomic consultants can add valuable information about accommodations in public places to the mediation process to facilitate settlements of Title III ADA disputes.

Conclusion

This chapter has outlined potential consultative roles for egonomists who wish to enlarge their practice into the arena of the ADA. Health care ergonomists have unique skills with which to provide educational services in basic concepts, hiring prac-

tices, and sensitivity training regarding the ADA. Other areas of practice require interventions such as reasonable accommodations, job and task analysis, restricted duty assignments, and consultation or structural changes. For all of these roles, as well as that of the expert witness, the health care ergonomist must adequately prepare himself or herself by carefully studying documents and cases related to the ADA. This is a challenging and rewarding arena for the innovative health care ergonomist.

References

Americans with Disabilities Act. (July 26, 1990). Pub. L. No. 101-336.

ADA Title I Regulations. (1991). 29 CFR §1630.01 et seq. and Appendix.

ADA Title II Regulations. (1991). 28 CFR §39.101 et seq.

ADA Title III Regulations. (1991). 28 CFR §36.101 et seq.

Equal Employment Opportunity Commission. (1992). *A technical assistance manual on the employment provisions (Title I) of the Americans with Disabilities Act.* Washington, DC: EEOC.

Equal Employment Opportunity Commission. (1994). *Enforcement guidance on pre-employment medical inquiries under the ADA.* Washington, DC: EEOC.

Fed. R. Evid. 702.

U.S. Department of Justice. (1992). *The Americans with Disabilities Act Title III technical assistance manual.* Washington, DC: U.S. Department of Justice.

Chapter 18

The Americans with Disabilities Act: Legal Ramifications of ADA Consultation

Barbara L. Kornblau

Learning Objective

On completion of this chapter, the reader should be able to

- Understand the various legal issues affecting ergonomic consultation and the Americans with Disabilities Act (ADA).

Key Words

Malpractice
Consultation

Abstract

This chapter familiarizes the ergonomic consultant with some of the legal issues affecting ergonomic consultation in the ADA context. The author provides guidance for the ergonomic consultant's handling of these and other concerns. The chapter is not intended as a substitute for competent legal counsel. The reader is encouraged to seek the advice of an attorney with any questions that arise based on the issues presented.

Introduction

Mani's Manufacturing makes high-technology surgical implements. An innovative leader in the field, Mani's Manufacturing runs five plants, employing more than 750 people.

William Worker, a 10-year veteran employee, was injured on the job 3 months ago. As a result of his injury, he lost the use of his left, nondominant hand. Having reached maximum medical improvement, William notifies the company of his desire to return to his former position as a senior designer in the main assembly plant.

After extensive discussions with William, the company decides William cannot do his job as it presently exists. William suggests that the company hire an ergonomic consultant to look into changing the way the job is performed or redesigning the work station. The company is not sure it wants to set a precedent for other employees by complying with this request.

Conversations with the company attorney convince Mani's Manufacturing of the benefits of hiring an ergonomic consultant. The company's attorney explains that under the ADA (Public Law 101-336, 1990), Mani's Manufacturing must try to make reasonable accommodations to enable William to return to his job. According to the company's attorney, using the services of an ergonomic consultant is one way to demonstrate a good faith effort to provide reasonable accommodations for William. The company heeds its attorney's advice and calls an ergonomic consultant.

This hypothetical situation raises several questions for the ergonomic consultant who receives such a phone call. What is the consultant's role with employers? What happens if the ergonomic consultant makes a recommendation that does not work? What if the ergonomic changes make William's medical condition worse? What if Mani's Manufacturing fails to follow the ergonomic consultant's recommendations? Can the ergonomic consultant incur liability by virtue of his or her recommendations? How does the manufacturer protect itself from liability? How does it avoid problem situations?

Liability and Malpractice

Ergonomic consultants sell their advice as their trade. Like any other consultant, they provide advice to clients based on their knowledge, experience, and expertise. Because the clients purchase the advice from the consultants, clients may decide how they wish to use the advice. They may follow the consultants' advice, follow a portion of the advice, or reject the advice and do something else altogether.

Under the ADA, for example, an ergonomic consultant advising a company about ADA compliance strategies might recommend that a company develop functional job descriptions for all its positions. The ADA does not require the company to do this. The client company or consultee pays the ergonomic consultant for a report outlining his or her recommendations on implementation of an ADA compliance program, but the company remains free to decide whether it will follow the advice.

As advice givers, ergonomic consultants present themselves to their clients as experts in the field. The company seeking the ergonomic advice relies on the consultant for accurate, up-to-date, complete, and appropriate information. Failure to provide the client with the proper information in the proper manner may render the ergonomic consultant liable for malpractice. Given that the consultant makes recommendations about ergonomic solutions but does not implement them, the consultant can open himself or herself up to malpractice by exercising poor judgment in the giving of advice, especially if it is something about which the consultant lacks adequate knowledge.

Although it is often mentioned, few people know exactly how to define *malpractice*. Malpractice is a negligent tort (i.e., a wrong committed against another person that causes damages) perpetrated by a professional—in this case an ergonomic consultant—that causes damages (*Black's Law Dictionary*, 1979). In the case of an ergonomic consultant, the damage could be done to a specific individual when the consultant advises a company to do something that causes damages to an individ-

ual (e.g., William Worker). The damage could also affect the company, for example, if the consultant's incorrect advice causes the company to incur the wrath of the U.S. Department of Justice for failure to comply with Title III accessibility requirements (28 CFR §36.101 et seq., 1991).

Malpractice may occur in several other contexts. If a company follows the ergonomic consultant's advice and, in the process of doing so, harms someone, the consultant may be liable for malpractice. Ergonomic consultants may find themselves liable for malpractice if they fail to stay current with the latest changes in ADA laws and regulations and provide a consultee with incorrect information, thus causing harm.

In other situations, liability for malpractice may arise because the ergonomic consultant omitted some significant or relevant information. Suppose an ergonomic consultant is hired to assist a restaurant in making physical changes to its facilities to comply with the accessibility requirements of Title III of the ADA. The consultant fails to inform the facility about certain requirements for accessibility. As a result, the facility fails to comply with the ADA, and a disgruntled customer decides to sue the restaurant.

The ergonomic consultant may face malpractice litigation for harm that resulted to the company being advised because he or she failed to ask the company the right questions. In a related scenario, the ergonomic consultant may take on the company's liability to a third party, where harm results to a third party due to the consultant's failure to ask the right questions. If the consultant failed to ask appropriate questions about the specific operations of a particular piece of equipment, for example, he or she could take on the liability if an employee were injured while operating the machine with an adaptation the consultant suggested.

Simply put, malpractice is negligent performance by a professional. A malpractice action may be brought against any professional, including health care professionals, engineers, ergonomists, lawyers, and accountants.

To sustain a case of liability for malpractice, the plaintiff must prove all four of the following elements (Prosser, 1971):

1. A duty to act in a particular way
2. Conduct below the standard of care
3. Damages
4. Actual cause

First, the parties must have a relationship between them that created a duty to act in a particular way (Christoffel, 1982). Second, the plaintiff must prove that the ergonomic consultant's conduct fell below the professionally reasonable standard of care, thereby breaching the duty to act in a particular way. Third, the plaintiff must prove that he or she suffered real damages. Finally, the plaintiff must prove that the ergonomic consultant's breach of duty actually caused the damages suffered (Burghardt et al., 1996; American College of Legal Medicine, 1995; Scott, 1990; Stromberg et al., 1988; Calloway, 1985; Christoffel, 1982; Prosser, 1971).

A Duty to Act in a Particular Way

The ergonomic consultant owes a duty to those with whom he or she establishes a professional relationship. Thus, the consultant owes a duty of care to the client company with whom he or she consults, and probably to any reasonably foreseeable "patient" or client worker affected when the company follows the consultant's advice (Prosser, 1971). This duty of care also extends to the individual worker about whom the consultant provides case consultation.

The duty of care owed applies to acts of omission and acts of commission. This means that the ergonomic consultant can be liable for damages caused by things he or she does as well as things he or she fails to do (American College of Legal Medicine, 1995; Scott, 1990; Calloway, 1985). For example, if an ergonomic consultant failed to advise the client company to install grab bars and raised toilet seats in the bathrooms, as required under Title III, this could give rise to malpractice through an act of omission. If the ergonomic consultant improperly redesigns a work station as a reasonable accommodation under Title I's employment provisions, causing the worker further injury, the ergonomic consultant could face a malpractice action based on an act of commission.

The ergonomic consultant's duty compels him or her to exercise the reasonable care and skills expected of an ergonomic consultant. To define "reasonable care and skills expected of an ergonomic consultant," the courts will inquire as to whether a reasonably prudent ergonomic con-

sultant would have acted in a similar manner, given the same set of circumstances (Burghardt et al., 1996; American College of Legal Medicine, 1995; Hopkins and Anderson, 1990).

Most companies hire an ergonomic consultant because they need some ergonomic advice and they have limited knowledge or expertise in this area. These clients rely on the ergonomic consultant's expertise when they hire him or her. They consider the ergonomic consultant an expert who is competent to give advice in the area of ergonomics.

Because the ergonomic consultant holds himself or herself out as an expert, the consultant must understand the limits of his or her expertise, knowing when to refer the client to someone with greater knowledge and skills. The consultant should be aware of his or her credentials and the limitations that these credentials may impose (Hopkins and Anderson, 1990). A particular consultation situation may demand someone with more specialized or different credentials.

Suppose, for example, that a company seeks an ergonomic consultant to assist with making reasonable accommodations under Title I's employment provisions. If the company seeks advice on the proper seating at the worksite for an individual with a complicated disability, such as severe cerebral palsy, the consultant should be well versed in seating and be able to perform an assessment of the biomechanical problems affecting this individual. An understanding of seating includes a knowledge of the range of variables available in the wheelchair market and the features and functions of accessories currently in distribution. The consultant should also know how cerebral palsy affects a person's ability to function while seated. An ergonomic consultant coming from a background in engineering may find himself or herself referring the company to an ergonomic consultant with a background in occupational therapy if the situation requires technical, medical, or functional capacity information outside his or her realm of knowledge.

Suppose a company contracts with an ergonomic consultant to develop work-site modifications for a particular division in the plant that is plagued with cases of cumulative trauma. Shortly thereafter, one of its employees requests to return to work after an injury for which he or she has received workers' compensation. The returning employee requests specific reasonable accommodations to enable her to perform her job. The company asks the ergonomic consultant whether the worksite modifications just made would be adequate reasonable accommodations under the ADA for the returning worker.

This is a tricky question because it may call for a legal conclusion from the ergonomic consultant, who is not an attorney. Further, the consultant may not be familiar with the inner workings of the ADA and might give incorrect advice. The ADA law, its regulations and technical assistance manuals, and case law present an ever-changing wealth of information, which influences the consultant's course of action in ADA matters. In this case, it would be prudent for the consultant to refer the company either to an attorney who specializes in labor and employment law to learn more about the legal ramifications of the ADA or to a consultant more knowledgeable about reasonable accommodations and the ADA.

Failure to refer a consultee who requires more expertise than the consultant possesses could constitute malpractice. The consultant should make sure that the professional to whom the consultee is referred is competent and has appropriate credentials. If, despite the consultant's efforts, the client sues him or her, the defense is strengthened by the fact that the consultant appropriately referred the client to another competent professional.

If an ergonomic consultant holds himself or herself out as an expert in a particular area, the consultant must meet the standards of an expert in that area. The courts will look at the standard of care or the level of proficiency against which the consultant's conduct should be measured. Because little legal precedent exists to define the standard of care the ergonomic consultant must follow, the courts probably will look to the standards of practice of similar professions, such as the American Occupational Therapy Association (AOTA) *Standards of Practice* and the AOTA *Code of Ethics*, if the ergonomic consultant comes from the occupational therapy field (AOTA Standards and Ethics Commission, 1994; Hopkins & Anderson, 1990; Calloway, 1985). If the ergonomic consultant comes from an engineering field, the courts would look to the engineering profession's standards of practice and code of ethics for guidance in determining standard of care.

Breach of Duty

The second element of malpractice, breach of duty, occurs when the ergonomic consultant's conduct falls below the applicable standard of care. Expert witness testimony helps form the basis of proof at trial to help the court or jury to determine the standard of care and whether the consultant's conduct fell below that standard, thereby breaching a duty of care owed. Thus, the court hears from an expert witness—another ergonomic consultant—who gives his or her opinion of the standard of care that the consultant on trial allegedly fell below.

Given that ergonomic consultation has been an interdisciplinary or transdisciplinary field, the ergonomic consultant may find himself or herself in court facing an ergonomic consultant from another field as the expert witness. This expert witness testifies as to his or her opinion of the standard of care and level of knowledge against which the consultant's conduct should be measured. Because he or she comes from a different field, the expert witness may have more knowledge of the area at issue and may present a different standard of care from that demanded by the practitioner's own field. Should this happen, the ergonomic consultant on trial will likely find himself or herself in the difficult position of trying to prove that his or her behavior fell within the standard of care of another profession of which he or she is not a member and not qualified to act.

This possibility points to the importance of ergonomic consultants knowing the limits of their breadth of knowledge. With interdisciplinary practice a reality, consultants must be prepared to defend their actions within the boundaries and scope of their knowledge.

Under the doctrine of *respondeat superior*, the ergonomic consultant may find himself or herself liable for activities that his or her subordinates, rather than the consultant, perform. This Latin term means "let the master answer" (*Black's Law Dictionary*, 1979; Burghardt et al., 1996). Because the employer consultant is in the best position to supervise and direct acts of his or her employee within the scope of employment, under *respondeat superior,* the law imputes liability to the employer if the employee performs in a negligent manner. The law also considers a manager to be in the position of authority to supervise and control his or her subordinate employees, imputing to the manager liability for the employee's negligent performance. Liability may even rest with the employer or manager under the doctrine of *respondeat superior* for acts of which the supervisor had no knowledge (Burghardt et al., 1996). Thus, an ergonomic consultant who hires another ergonomic consultant in an employer-employee relationship, or in a manager-supervisor-subordinate employee relationship, may find him- or herself liable for the negligent activities of his or her subordinates. The doctrine of *respondeat superior* does not apply to independent contractors, however, because the doctrine is grounded on the right of control, and technically under the law, independent contractors work on their own, without control from a supervisor (Scott, 1990; Calloway, 1985).

The ergonomic consultant may be liable for the actions of subordinates under the theory of negligent supervision. Under this theory, the ergonomic consultant may find himself or herself liable for negligent supervision if he or she assigns others to perform ergonomic consultative services for which they lack the qualifications and then fails to properly supervise the consultants (Stromberg et al., 1988). For example, suppose a bank were to contract with an ergonomic consulting firm to develop reasonable accommodations under the ADA. The Chief of Ergonomic Consulting assigned this project to an ergonomic consultant with a specialty in workplace lighting and video display terminals (VDTs). Although the assigned consultant could make excellent recommendations about lighting and VDTs, suppose he or she failed to make appropriate suggestions on issues of access for customers with disabilities—the bank's main concern—because of a lack of knowledge about and experience with the ADA. In this situation, if a customer sues the bank for Title III access violations, the consulting firm and the Chief of Ergonomic Consulting may face a malpractice action. Thus, just as ergonomic consultants must understand the boundaries of their own knowledge and skills, they must also understand the boundaries of their subordinates' knowledge and skills.

Further, the interdisciplinary-transdisciplinary nature of ergonomic consulting uniquely complicates supervision issues: Supervisors must feel confident about the scope of skills of their subordinates before assigning tasks to an ergonomic consultant from a different profession, lest they set themselves up for accusations of negligent supervision. Although each discipline brings its own perspective and skills to ADA-related ergonomic consulting, the supervisor remains responsible for ensuring the adequacy of the individual consultant's breadth and depth of knowledge of relevant ADA-related information.

On the other hand, the interdisciplinary-transdisciplinary quality of ergonomic consulting may prove beneficial in ADA consulting. The ADA sets forth broad mandates for access as well as policy changes. The consulting demands and breadth of knowledge that the ADA requires can be addressed in a comprehensive manner by individuals from various backgrounds, including but not limited to engineering, design, industrial psychology, vocational rehabilitation, occupational health and rehabilitation nursing, and clinical rehabilitation. The varied perspectives may present an advantage to the consumer of ergonomic services, provided the ergonomic consultant is knowledgeable about the ADA and familiar with his or her own limitations.

Damages

The third element required to sustain an action for malpractice is damages or actual harm (Burghardt et al., 1996; American College of Legal Medicine, 1995; Scott, 1990; Stromberg et al., 1988; Calloway, 1985; Christoffel, 1982; Prosser, 1971). The harm caused by the ergonomic consultant may include physical harm to a patient or client or financial harm to a consultee company. Even if the ergonomic consultant acts in a clearly incompetent manner, no basis for a malpractice or negligence action can be found unless actual harm can be proved (Burghardt et al., 1996; American College of Legal Medicine, 1995; Scott, 1990; Prosser, 1971).

On the other hand, if the ergonomic consultant acts in a reasonable manner and makes appropriate recommendations in a case consultation, but the individual worker's performance does not improve, this harm alone does not constitute malpractice.

Suppose, for example, that you as an ergonomic consultant are called in to advise a company about specific reasonable accommodations for a worker with multiple sclerosis (MS) desiring to return to work after the initial diagnosis. The worker is having difficulty with visual focusing and balance. After extensive discussions with the worker, you recommend several accommodations commonly used with individuals with MS, including large print materials and a cane. You also recommend grab bars for the bathroom, and handrails accompanied by brightly colored tape on the floor where the level of the walkway changes.

Unfortunately, the worker's condition declines and the accommodations are of no help to her. In spite of the accommodations, the worker finds herself no longer able to work. The fact that the universally acceptable accommodations did not meet their stated purpose does not constitute malpractice. The reasonable accommodations put in place did not cause the worker's condition to decline. Rather, you acted within the acceptable standard of care expected in a similar situation and did not cause any damages.

Compare that situation to one in which the ergonomic consultant's accommodations or failure to suggest accommodations does cause injury to the individual worker. Suppose the county government, under its Title II (1991) obligation, calls in an ergonomic consultant to make reasonable accommodations for an individual who, after an acute flair-up of rheumatoid arthritis, wants to return to work in his office setting.

After a review of the job description and a brief conversation with the worker's supervisor, who spoke to the risk manager, who spoke to personnel, who spoke to the worker, the consultant makes some changes. She redesigns the work station to decrease repetitive motions, places the wrist in a neutral position, gives the worker a foot rest, recommends an "ergonomic chair," and adjusts the lighting. In spite of these accommodations, the worker experiences continued physical decline, especially in his feet and hips, and ends up out of work, totally disabled, and requiring a total hip replacement. His physician attributes the disability to the repetitive rising from a chair and walking back and forth to the customer counter at work. The worker sues the county under the ADA for failing to make effective accommodations in spite of his request and causing the decline in his condition.

Apparently, this job involved repeated rising from sitting and walking back and forth to the customer counter, but the job description did not indicate this requirement. The worker's rheumatoid arthritis affected her hips, knees, and feet. Had the consultant first conducted a full-scale job analysis and held a conversation with the worker, she would have discovered these key facts.

An obvious, necessary accommodation would have been to move the worker's desk closer to the customer counter to decrease the amount of walking and rising from a chair. A sit-stand or barstool-height chair would also decrease walking and the need to rise from the chair simply by allowing the worker to sit at the counter. The consultant failed to make these recommendations, though, and as a result of the failure to recommend appropriate reasonable accommodations, the county faces a lawsuit. Any losses sustained because of this lawsuit are considered damages in terms of the ergonomic consultant's malpractice situation.

Causation

The fourth element required to sustain a cause of action for malpractice is causation (Burghardt et al., 1996; American College of Legal Medicine, 1995; Scott, 1990; Stromberg et al., 1988; Calloway, 1985; Christoffel, 1982; Prosser, 1971). The plaintiff must show that the ergonomic consultant's negligent conduct was responsible for the plaintiff's (the consultee or company) injury. The standard is the "but for" test. That is, but for the consultant's negligence, the plaintiff's injury would not have occurred.

The previous example illustrates this point: But for the ergonomic consultant's failure to recommend the proper reasonable accommodations, the worker would not have experienced further physical decline, which her doctor blamed on the repetitive rising from sitting and the walking back and forth to the counter. But for the consultant's failure to recommend proper reasonable accommodations, the company would not be the defendant in an ADA lawsuit.

Other situations may arise in which, although someone suffers damage, the ergonomic consultant has not caused the damage. In one such scenario, a consultee suffers some kind of damage because the employer (consultee) fails to take the consultant's advice.

Suppose, for example, that a resort hotel contacts an ergonomic consultant to design a plan to make its programs and facilities accessible, as required by

Title III of the ADA. The ergonomic consultant presents to the resort hotel a thorough, comprehensive plan that makes all the physical facilities accessible and proposes policies to ensure access. The resort hotel decides to undertake only a few, select modifications from the plan and ignores the remaining recommendations. When an ADA lawsuit claiming violation of Title III of the ADA reaches the resort manager, he or she wants to sue the ergonomic consultant for malpractice. Because the resort ignored the ergonomic consultant's recommendations, however, the manager lacks the requisite causation. Put simply, the ergonomic consultant presented an adequate product and thus did not give rise to the resort's lawsuit. Rather, the resort caused its own problems by failing to follow the ergonomic consultant's advice.

Preventing Malpractice

The ultimate goal for any ergonomic consultant is to prevent malpractice from occurring. As an ergonomic consultant, you can take several steps to limit your liability for malpractice, especially in the area of ADA consulting:

1. Always practice according to the standards of your profession.
2. Learn everything you can about the ADA, and stay current.
3. Know the limits of your knowledge.
4. Refer to other professionals when appropriate.
5. Maintain current knowledge of relevant regulations (OSHA, workers' compensation).
6. Maintain malpractice insurance.
7. Document ergonomic recommendations in writing.
8. Make formal written agreements detailing the parameters of the ergonomic consultation task.

First, the ergonomic consultant must always practice according to the standards outlined in the professional code of ethics, standards of practice, and state licensure laws and regulations. These documents can help to establish the standard of care to which the ergonomic consultant will be held, so the consultant must not fall below those baselines.

Before beginning to practice as an ADA ergonomic consultant, learn everything possible about the ADA and stay current with that information. Although you need not become an "ADA lawyer," you should understand ADA regulations as well as changes in regulations and emerging case law that may affect the advice you give in the ADA arena. If you plan to engage in ADA consulting, at the very least, your library should include copies of the regulations for Titles I, II, and III, as well as the technical assistance manuals for each title. Newsletters may also provide updated information on ADA changes, and several reporting services provide case law updates as well as complete texts of cases as the courts decide them. (A brief list of helpful ADA resources may be found in Appendix 18-1.)

As preventive maintenance, the ergonomic consultant should attend professional education courses to keep current on practice techniques in the field and regularly attend professional meetings. Read professional journals to stay abreast of the latest research and ADA cases to cover all bases. Monitor how colleagues within the field or profession view the changing role of the ergonomic consultant in the ADA context.

Although you may learn a great deal about the ADA from readings, professional literature, and continuing education courses, if you are not an attorney accustomed to reading legal jargon and interpreting the latest case law, your knowledge and understanding of the ADA will probably be limited. Further, depending on your discipline, as an ergonomic consultant working with the population of individuals with disabilities, you may have limited knowledge about specific disabilities, the course of certain disease processes, the impact the disability has on the individual's life, and the scope of functional limitations an individual may have as a result of a particular disability.

Be aware of the need to refer a client or consultee to another professional when a situation arises beyond the boundaries of your knowledge. Ergonomic consultants from varying backgrounds must understand the limitations of their credentials. In a case consultation with an individual with severe disabilities, you may need to refer the case to an ergonomic consultant wearing a therapeutic hat, who has more knowledge about the specifics of the disability. You may find that an architect is the appropriate ergonomic consultant for certain reasonable accommodations involving complicated building design issues under Title III. Other ergonomic consultants may not have the background to realize that a computer's excessively low refresh rate contributed to an increase in epileptic seizures and migraine headaches. Regardless of the situation, ergonomic consultants need to be aware of consulting situations in which they are not the expert the client needs or desires and learn to say yes or no appropriately. Ergonomic consultants should always refer to competent, knowledgeable professionals when they fall short of the level of expertise needed to complete an ADA-related consulting assignment.

If an ergonomic consultant hires other ergonomic consultants to work for him or her, the consultant must select competent personnel with due care and carefully define their responsibilities. Do not delegate consultation tasks to unqualified individuals. The hiring ergonomic consultant must not assume that another ergonomic consultant's knowledge matches his or her own level of knowledge and experience about the ADA. Many consultants claim to "know" the ADA.

If an ergonomic consultant delegates consultation tasks to another ergonomic consultant, he or she must provide the consultant with appropriate supervision, if necessary. At the very least, he or she should monitor the subordinate consultant's performance and be sure to provide the subordinate consultant with enough information and authority to perform the assigned tasks.

Ergonomic consultants must stay up to date on state and local laws and regulations that affect the advice they give so their advice is accurate and current. Other laws affect how the ADA applies to a particular situation. Occupational Safety and Health Act regulations may affect what type of reasonable accommodations are acceptable in a particular setting. Where applicable, one must also consider how state-controlled worker's compensation laws affect ADA requirements. Social Security regulations must also be considered under Title I's employment provisions. Under the ADA, for example, an individual filing a claim asserts that he or she is a qualified individual with a disability who can do the essential functions of a job with or without reasonable accommodation (ADA Title I, 1991). By filing a claim with Social Security at the same time, the individual also asserts that he or she is unable to perform substantial gainful employment in the labor market—two competing interests. Thus, the individual claims he or she can work with reasonable accommodations and, at the same time, claims he or she cannot work at all. This dichotomy may place the ergonomic consultant, who is trying to make the accommodations, in the middle of the dispute, or it may obviate any need to make the accommodations at all if the person is not a qualified individual with a disability.

A state worker's compensation claim added to the already filed ADA and Social Security claims can further complicate the situation for the ergonomic consultant. Depending on the state law, the ergonomic consultant may find the worker unable to do his or her job but willing and able to do another job for the same employer. The employer may need an ergonomic consultant to assist the employee in making the transition back to the workplace, should the employee need some accommodations.

Family Medical Leave Act (FMLA) regulations (1993) may also affect ergonomic consulting, and local ordinances and other laws and regulations change continually. For example, the FMLA combined with the ADA may require the ergonomic consultant to make reasonable accommodations for individuals who are returning from a leave under the FMLA.

To protect against lawsuit, the ergonomic consultant should carry malpractice insurance. The malpractice carrier will pay the consultant's legal fees to defend an action. The ergonomic consultant should also maintain appropriate business records.

Detail the specific task on which you have contracted to consult. The specifics should be spelled out in writing, either by contract or by letter, so that the parties are clear about the tasks to be performed. You may also want to specify which tasks you are not performing (the tasks specifically excluded from the contract).

Documentation

The ergonomic consultant should always have the key tool to prevent malpractice suits—good documentation. Maintain detailed files on each consultee company and each case consultation. Take notes at all meetings with consultees, and write memoranda to the file detailing the meeting's subject, questions asked, and the suggestions or recommendations offered. Send a memorandum to the consultee company summarizing the meeting so that both parties have the same understanding of the advice given by the consultant. This protects you in the event that the consultee chooses not to follow your advice and later claims that you failed to advise the company properly. A file copy of memoranda sent to the client shows that the client was properly advised but chose not to implement the advice.

You may also want to send a copy of memoranda to the individual worker to further document your efforts. If the company is the client, however, you should be sure to get its approval before releasing information to the worker. The company may consider this information confidential.

When involved in case consultation, make specific notes about the patient or client, including findings and recommendations. Send your findings and recommendations to the consultee, and keep records for the consultee's file in your office. This protects the consultant from liability, should injury occur to the patient or client if the consultee elects not to follow your advice for reasonable accommodations or other modifications. In some situations, when the union may be promoting the ergonomic changes, for example, the consultee may be the individual worker rather than the company. In these situations, send a copy of the findings and recommendations to the worker.

Clinicians can also protect themselves by obtaining a physician's referral for certain types of case consultations. For example, if a clinician, such as an occupational or physical therapist, wishes to perform a functional capacities assessment as part of a case consultation, he or she should first obtain a physician's referral. In theory, by making the referral, the physician is approving the assessment for the client and should inform the clinician of any precautions the client may need to take during the assessment.

In states where clinicians are licensed, licensure regulations may not require a physician referral before an evaluation or treatment is done. Referrals may be required only for the purpose of billing insurance companies. If payment depends on an insurance carrier, the carrier may require the physician's referral. In other cases, the company for which one performs the consultation may pay for services directly, thereby obviating the need for a physician's referral. If the physician's referral is not required, however, the clinician should still consider obtaining a physician's referral to try to limit liability should a worker become injured during a physician-referred assessment.

Telephone calls should be logged and notes recorded in the consultee file with a brief explanation of the subject matter, questions asked, and suggestions offered. If a problem arises, document the steps you take to solve it. If you perform research to solve a problem, detail the methods and sources used in a memorandum to the file. If you confer or consult with an ergonomic consultant from a different discipline, you also should record notes of this conversation in the client's file. Always leave a paper trail that can be retraced and revisited in the future, if needed to help prove that you acted within an acceptable standard of care for an ergonomic consultant.

In all situations, the ergonomic consultant should document termination of services and the outcome reached. At the time of termination, the consultant should summarize the reason for the termination, the recommendations made, and the person to whom they were made.

Conclusion

The ADA presents a plethora of opportunities for ergonomic consultants knowledgeable about the ADA. This area of ergonomic consulting depends on a certain level of knowledge and a commitment to stay current in the area as legal precedents develop. The ADA's Title I employment provisions, Title II state and local government services provisions, and Title III public access provisions cry out for ergonomic consultants to assist business and industry, local governments, and places of public accommodations to comply with their obligations under the law. As multidisciplinary-transdisciplinary ergonomic consulting expands its scope, ergonomic consultants may find themselves at risk for malpractice. Companies have a right to expect an ergonomic consultant to perform to a certain level of expertise. Ergonomic consultants must maintain a current knowledge base of the ADA, practice according to the standards of their profession, and know their limitations both to avoid malpractice and to practice competently and confidently.

Other information about the ADA may be obtained from the sources listed in Appendix 18-1.

References

American College of Legal Medicine. (1995). *Legal medicine.* St. Louis, MO: Mosby–Year Book.

American Occupational Therapy Association Standards and Ethics Commission. (1994). Occupational therapy code of ethics. In American Occupational Therapy Association, *Reference manual of the official documents of the American Occupational Therapy Association* (pp. 117–120). Bethesda, MD: AOTA.

American Occupational Therapy Association Commission on Practice. (1994). *Occupational therapy standards of practice.* Bethesda, MD: AOTA.

Americans with Disabilities Act. (July 26, 1990). Public Law No. 101-336.

Americans with Disabilities Act Title I Regulations. (1991). 29 CFR §1630.01 et seq. and Appendix.

Americans with Disabilities Act Title II Regulations. (1991). 28 CFR §39.101 et seq.

Americans with Disabilities Act Title III Regulations. (1991). 28 CFR §36.101 et seq.

Black's law dictionary (5th ed.). (1979). St. Paul, MN: West Publishing.

Burghardt, R., Long, S., & Stanley & Fisher P.C. (1996). *Rehabilitation and the law.* Bethesda, MD: American Occupational Therapy Association.

Calloway, S. (1985). *Nursing and the law.* Eau Claire, WI: Professional Education Systems.

Christoffel, T. (1982). *Health and the law.* New York: Free Press.

Family Medical Leave Act Regulations. (1993). 29 CFR 825 §100 et seq.

Hopkins, B.R., & Anderson, B.S. (1990). *The counselor and the law.* Alexandria, VA: American Association for Counseling and Development.

Prosser, W.L. (1971). *Law of torts.* St. Paul, MN: West Publishing.

Scott, R. (1990). *Health care malpractice.* Thorofare, NJ: Slack.

Stromberg, C.D., Haggarty, D.J., Leibenluft, R.F., et al. (1988). *The psychologist's legal handbook.* Washington, DC: Council for the National Register of Health Service Providers in Psychology.

Appendix 18-1
Sources for Information about the ADA

Title I (Employment)

Equal Employment Opportunity Commission
(202) 663-4900 (Voice)
(202) 663-4399 (TTD)
Numerous publications about the ADA employment provisions, including the Title I technical assistance manual

Titles II (State and Local Government Services) and III (Public Accommodations)

U.S. Department of Justice, Civil Rights Division, Coordination and Review Section
P.O. Box 66118
Washington, DC 20035-6118
(202) 514-0301 (Voice)
(202) 514-0381 (TTD)
Numerous materials about the state and local government services and public accommodations provisions of the ADA; "Title II Highlights" and "Title III Highlights"; Title II and Title III technical assistance manuals

Job Accommodations Network (JAN)
West Virginia University
809 Allen Hall
Morgantown, WV 26506
(800) 526-7234
(304) 293-7186

Ask about the Project Enable computer bulletin board, where you can download the ADA, its regulations, and a wealth of articles and information.

National Easter Seal Society
70 East Lake Street
Chicago, IL 60601
(800) 221-6827
Numerous films and other materials about various aspects of the ADA, all of which are wonderful teaching tools

President's Committee on Employment of People with Disabilities
1331 F Street, NW, 3rd Floor
Washington, DC 20004
(202) 376-6200
Numerous publications, pamphlets, and other materials about the ADA

U.S. Chamber of Commerce
1615 H Street NW
Washington, DC 20004
(800) 638-6582
What Every Business Must Know About the Americans with Disabilities Act, *an excellent teaching tool*

Chapter 19

Industrial Setting Case Study: Ergonomics and Title I of the Americans with Disabilities Act

Donald S. Bloswick, Dana C. Jefferies, Susan Brakefield, and Mark Dumas

Learning Objectives

On completion of this chapter, the reader should

- Understand ergonomic job analysis, physical stress reduction through job redesign, and the establishment of essential job functions in an industrial setting.
- Be familiar with the use of ergonomic job analysis in developing hiring and promotion programs that comply with the Americans with Disabilities Act (ADA).
- Be comfortable with the methodology used to translate essential job functions into clinical evaluation procedures.

Key Words

Americans with Disabilities Act
Ergonomics
Post-offer screening
In-hire program

Abstract

Ergonomic consultation was provided to a major forest products company in the Northwestern United States to develop a procedure for selecting new hires (in-hire program) that complies with the requirements of the ADA. The program was based on an existing return-to-work program and focused on the ergonomic analysis of jobs, minimization of job stresses, and establishment of essential job functions. The program, although still under way, appears to have improved working conditions, allowed a more diverse workforce to be hired, and improved employee morale while increasing productivity. The overall goal of the program was to screen people *into*, not *out of*, jobs in this organization.

Introduction

This chapter presents a case study of the application of ergonomics in the development of an in-hire program that complies with Title I (Employment) of the ADA and other Equal Employment Opportunity Commission (EEOC) requirements. The program was established at a forest products company (lumber, plywood, and medium-density fiberboard) in the Northwestern United States. The company's 1,800 workers are distributed through its Seattle headquarters; Columbia Falls, Montana, regional office; and 11 manufacturing plants in Washington and Montana. This self-insured company is one of the largest employers in Montana and is entirely nonunion. In 1994, revenues were $578 million, and more than $70 million was spent on capital improvements between 1989 and 1994.

In 1986, the company began fine-tuning its return-to-work program. It was decided to evaluate every position in each mill to identify and quantify the physical demands placed on all hourly employees. The finished product was called the *Listing of Job (Position) Physical Demands*. These analyses were performed by a rehabilitation consultant. This evaluation process (1) facilitated recommendations to modify certain job tasks, making them easier, safer, and more productive; (2) demonstrated to the medical community that the company was truly interested in its employees; and (3) gave health care professionals information on job requirements to help them determine whether an individual is capable of returning to work and to help develop appropriate work hardening in the return-to-work process.

Around 1988 (pre-ADA), the company began to scrutinize its hiring practices. Although many factors were considered in the screening process, back x-rays were heavily weighted. It was determined that a more comprehensive job evaluation was needed to better identify criteria for physicians to use in the pre-employment physical examination process. A physical therapist who had been involved with the company's back safety program and was knowledgeable about processes at several plants worked with the company safety director to identify the physical demands of each position.

The evaluation process began with the physical therapist's review of existing Job Safety Analyses and physical job demands and was broadened to include interviews with supervisors and employees who perform the tasks. It was also decided to videotape every job to provide a record of the job and to give treating physicians information on actual job activities as part of the return-to-work process.

In 1989, back x-rays were eliminated from the pre-employment physical examination. The company began looking for an alternate method to compare the capabilities of the worker to the requirements of the task. At about this time, the company safety director became aware of the ADA, which was to go into effect on July 26, 1992, for companies with 25 or more employees and on July 26, 1994, for those with 15–24 employees (EEOC, 1990, 1992, Section I, p. 6). This company was required to meet the 1992 date.

The ADA's employment provisions prohibit discrimination against disabled individuals who can, with or without reasonable accommodation, perform the essential functions of the job. An employer must make reasonable accommodation if it would not impose undue hardship on the operation of the employer's business. Reasonable accommodation includes but is not limited to (1) making facilities accessible and usable, (2) restructuring or modifying the job or work schedule, (3) acquiring or modifying equipment, examinations, and training material, and (4) providing readers or interpreters. Undue hardship is defined as significant difficulty or expense in light of the employer's size, resources, nature, and structure of the operation. The definition of an essential function is quite complex, but the *Technical Assistance Manual on the Employment Provisions of the ADA* (EEOC, 1992, Section II, pp. 13, 14) indicates that a function is considered essential if

> (1) the position exists to perform the function, (2) a limited number of other employees are available among which the function could be distributed, and (3) the function is highly specialized, and the employee is hired for his or her special ability or expertise to perform the function.

The ADA requires that the essential functions of a position be delineated in such a way that applicants may describe or demonstrate their ability to perform these essential functions before being hired. After a conditional offer of employment is made, the quantitative description of essential functions may also be used to assess the applicant's ability (actually, the employee's ability, because this is done post-offer) to perform the jobs or tasks associated with the position as part of a medical examination. If the applicant has the ability to perform the essential functions of the job, it must be determined if there is direct threat—defined as a significant risk of substantial harm to the health or safety of the individual or others which cannot be eliminated or reduced by reasonable accommodation (EEOC, 1992). Determination of direct threat must be based on "individualized assessment of objective and specific evidence about a particular individual's present ability to perform essential job functions" (EEOC, 1992, Section IV, p. 7).*

The identification and evaluation of these essential functions requires an understanding of ergonomics. The task requirements must be quantified in such a way that the applicant's ability to perform the

---

*For a full explanation of the hiring process, testing of applicants, pre- and post-employment inquiries, and medical examinations in compliance with the ADA, see the *Technical Assistance Manual on the Employment Provisions of the ADA* (EEOC, 1992).

essential functions can be evaluated and compared to established, objective criteria.

An initial review of the ADA and its comprehensive requirements was somewhat intimidating, but after a thorough review it became apparent that the company had already completed much of the groundwork for an ADA-compliant in-hire program. A team of experts was formed to assist in final program development. The team consisted of the company safety director, physical therapists working with the different facilities, physicians already involved in the medical evaluation process, and ergonomic consultants. The ergonomic consultants were retained primarily to (1) review the essential function analysis, (2) ensure agreement between the videotapes and the Job Task Analyses, (3) ensure agreement between the Job Task Analyses and the Job Summary, and (4) consult and advise on actual measurement and assessment techniques. The focus of the program changed from identifying criteria for physicians in the pre-employment physical process to ensuring compliance with the ADA.

Analysis

Position Analysis

Some initial clarification is in order. Applicants are considered for specific positions in a plant or facility. Each position may consist of one or more jobs, and each job consists of tasks. At one facility, the Laborer position consists of the following jobs: bander-helper, basement cleanup, breakdown hoist operator–secondary sorter, planer–dry chain, sticker placer, labeler, and horizontal helper. At this facility, the basement cleanup job alone consists of the following tasks: Blow down assigned areas with air wand, pick up debris and good boards, sweep floor and shovel and rake debris from around conveyors, clean lunch and rest rooms, feed logs from pond to sawmill, use chain saw to cut long boards, oil chains and grease bearings, pick up clubs and bunks, and fill in at employee break times on other jobs. At a different facility, the Green Chain Puller position, however, consists of only one job and three tasks. The Green Chain Puller position is used as an example throughout this discussion.

The physical therapist (1) videotaped all tasks, (2) performed task analyses for all jobs associated with each entry-level position in each facility (Job Task Analysis), and (3) worked with plant personnel to develop a Job Summary, including a list of the essential functions for jobs within that position. For each position, the ergonomic consultant reviewed the videotape, Job Task Analysis, and Job Summary.

Videotape

Videotaping included front, back, and side views with specific observation of requirements of the lower extremities, low back, neck, upper back, and upper extremities. Basic guidelines for the use of videotaping in task analysis are included as Appendix 19-1 of this chapter. Still photographs were also taken with a 35-mm camera to document the task.

Job Task Analysis

The Job Task Analysis addressed the issues listed below. A position may consist of only one job or several jobs, and each job may consist of one or more tasks.

1. Listing of position title, work schedule, date of analysis, analyst, and the position's education or training requirements
2. Position description in terms of the specific jobs
3. Work pace (self-paced, machine-paced, incentive, quota)
4. Lifting requirements (weight, object description, frequency, locations)
5. Carrying requirements (weight, object description, frequency, distance)
6. Push-pull requirements (weight, object description, frequency, distance)
7. Postures, such as sit, stand (maximum consecutive time, maximum daily time, ability to change positions)
8. Movements, such as bend, turn, twist at waist, kneel, squat, crawl, climb (frequency)
9. Balance or agility; the test should involve a task simulation
10. Upper-extremity functional requirements, such as reach, grasp, pinch, finger manipulation, and neck movement (frequency)

11. Use of equipment or tools
12. Environmental exposure, such as chemicals, confined spaces, high elevations, ionizing and nonionizing radiation, noise, slippery surfaces, vibration, wetness, dust, heat, cold, requirement for special clothing
13. Special conditions (need to work with others, work alone, work with minimal supervision)
14. Communication skills required (speaking, phone use, public contact, writing, reading) (A notation is made if the applicant has difficulty following directions during the assessment.)
15. Possible ergonomic considerations (potential ergonomic stressors were noted and potential abatements suggested even at this early stage of the analysis)

Basic equipment required to perform the Job Task Analysis includes the following:

1. Video camera, tape, tripod, batteries, lights (see Appendix 19-1)
2. Still camera, film, flash
3. Tape measure and stop watch (or digital wrist watch)
4. Force gauges (Chatillon Model DPPH 100KG, Greensboro, NC, and Wagner force dial push-pull force gauge, Model FDK 60, Wagner Instruments, Greenwich, CT) were used to measure lift, push, and pull forces.
5. Grip and pinch dynamometers (Jamar hand dynamometer, 200 lb force, Jamar, Clifton, NJ; 1-lb pinch gauge, Therapeutic Instruments, Clifton, NJ) were used to determine perceived grip and pinch requirements, which are difficult to measure directly. The pinch grip force required to pull an object can be estimated from pull force and coefficient of friction (CoF) with the equation

$$\text{Grip force} = (\text{Pull force}/2)/\text{CoF}$$

The Job Task Analysis for the Green Chain Puller position in one facility is included as Appendix 19-2. The person filling this position removes plywood veneer from a moving conveyor and grades and stacks the veneer on wheeled carts. For this position there is only one job (the position and the job are basically the same) consisting of several tasks. The frequency terms are assigned the following meanings: rare (1–10% of total time), occasional (11–33%), frequent (34–66%), continual (67–100%). These categories are used throughout the evaluation process.

Job Summary and Essential Job Function List

The Job Summary for the Job Task Analysis associated with a position consists of a listing of the jobs associated with a position, discussion of job task demands, and the essential job functions. (For a full definition of essential job functions see EEOC, 1992.) Note that every essential function may not show up in the listing of the essential job function list for a position. If an essential function noted on one Job Task Analysis is more stressful than an essential function on another Job Task Analysis, only the more stressful would be included for testing purposes. For example, if one essential function was a frequent lift of 40 lb from the floor to a 50-inch height and another was a frequent lift of 30 lb from 10 up to 30 in., only the first, more stressful, essential function would be included.

A Job Summary for the Green Chain Puller position is included as Appendix 19-3.

Employment Evaluation Process

The intent of the Employment Evaluation Process is to (1) comply with the ADA while attempting to match the worker and the job (by assessing whether an applicant can perform the essential job functions), (2) gather baseline medical data to be compared to injury statistics, (3) provide additional medical information to the physician, and (4) to identify areas of weakness or muscle tightness that may put a worker at risk of injury so that exercises can be recommended. The Employment Evaluation Process consists of three phases: (1) pre-offer process, (2) post-offer functional assessment and physical therapy evaluation, and (3) post-offer essential job function evaluation.

Pre-Offer Process

Applicants are first interviewed at Job Services, where they complete the job application and their references are checked. All applicants are shown the Job Summary and given the opportunity to describe or demonstrate how they would perform the essential job functions. Ideally, three to five applicants are sent to the facility, where they are interviewed by plant personnel. The job is shown to them, and they are again given the opportunity to describe or demonstrate how they would perform the essential job functions (with or without reasonable accommodations). The most qualified applicant is then made a conditional offer of employment, in writing, subject to his or her successful completion of the Employment Evaluation Process and Drug Screening. In this chapter, the term *applicant* is used to define individuals throughout the process, even after the conditional offer of employment has been made. The same physical therapist that prepared the Job Task Analysis performs the Functional Assessment.

Post-Offer Functional Assessment and Physical Therapy Evaluation

The functional assessment for each individual follows the same general protocol and consists of a measure of pulse rate, grip and pinch strength and endurance, lifting capabilities, balance, trunk flexibility, abdominal strength, hamstring and hip flexor flexibility, ability to squat repetitively, and full-body range of motion. Physically demanding activities are interspersed with less stressful ones. The instructions for each employment candidate are identical (Appendix 19-4). Note that, *although the Functional Assessment Worksheet used by the physical therapist is essentially the same for all positions (Appendix 19-5), only the information relevant to the position as noted on the Employment Entrance Examination Essential Job Functions list (Appendix 19-6) is recorded and compared to the task requirements.* Other information, such as pulse rate and endurance, is provided to the physician to assist in the medical evaluation and is used as a baseline for each applicant. Overall results, without identification of individual applicants, can be used to aid in future development of the Functional Assessment Process.*

Pulse rate is an indication of cardiovascular condition. Initial pulse rate is taken and documented after the introductory instructions. It is recognized that the employee may be nervous and pulse rate

may be somewhat higher than expected. Pulse rates are documented after each physically demanding activity, and a 1-minute recovery heart rate is also taken and documented on the form. A jump in pulse rate is expected after physically demanding activities, and a drop in pulse is expected at 1 minute. Recovery heart rates are helpful in determining general cardiovascular condition. A drop of 30–40 beats per minute is considered good, and a drop of 40–60 beats per minute or more is considered excellent (Bailey, 1978). A termination pulse rate is also taken and would generally be expected to be higher than the initial pulse rate (see Appendix 19-5).

Repetitive, forceful use of the upper extremities is common in the industry. In many instances, it has not been possible to eliminate this requirement through ergonomic redesign; therefore, grip and pinch strength are evaluated. Grip dynamometer and pinch dynamometer capabilities are measured at the beginning, middle, and end of the Functional Assessment and Physical Therapy Evaluation to give adequate time for the muscles to recover between tests. Grip and pinch strength are expected to stay the same or increase by the middle of the Functional Assessment and Physical Therapy Evaluation (due to warmup) and may drop minimally by the end. A drop of 20% from beginning to end might indicate a low level of endurance. In such a case, the applicant would be given instruction for exercises or techniques to increase his or her endurance. Samples of maximum grip and pinch capabilities are measured during a 3-minute test at 15 repetitions per minute for 3 minutes. The actual pinch-grip test frequency and duration are based on an observation of general task requirements (see Appendix 19-5). Therefore, the number of blanks used on the form would be appropriate to the job task in question.

Maximum lifting capabilities are determined using a weighted box beginning at 5 lb and adding approximately 5 lb per lift until the applicant determines that he or she has reached his or her safe maximum capability. Applicants are informed when there is a minimum lifting requirement. Body mechanics and changes in body mechanics are closely observed to determine frequent and occasional maximum lifting capabilities that can be performed without significant risk of substantial harm to the individual. Instructions in body mechanics may be provided if an applicant demonstrates body mechanics that are thought to be unsafe by the Assessment Specialist (e.g., twisting,

---

*It is important to note that clinical judgment is applied throughout the process and is crucial in determining critical variables, such as endurance descriptions and contributions of items such as pinch and grip strength to the medical evaluation for a specific job. Clinical judgments must be defensible and soundly based on the literature.

jerking, a combination of forward bending and twisting) or if the employee reports pain or discomfort. If body mechanics are observed to be unsafe, and the applicant is not able to adapt, the activity is terminated. Observations include endurance, indicated by the need for rest, strain, or signs of fatigue in the upper extremities, back, or lower extremities. Pulse rate and 1-minute recovery are taken after this activity (see Appendix 19-5). Observations are made regarding trunk flexibility in flexion and extension, hamstring and hip flexor flexibility, and abdominal and back extensor strength.

Doolittle et al. (1988) recommend that an individual lift no more than 20% of his or her maximum for repetitive efforts and not more than 75% for occasional efforts. Ayoub (1982) suggested that workers could safely lift 50–60% of their maximum for dynamic lifts (no mention of frequency) and later suggested that workers not exceed 75% of their maximum ability (Ayoub, Selan, & Jiang, 1984). This issue remains in debate because some researchers have found that excess strength did not serve to decrease medical incidents compared to those who just met the job requirements (Keyserling et al., 1980). To take the conservative route and to gather information on this issue ourselves, the authors measure the applicant's maximum lifting capability as well as her ability to perform the essential functions of the job. Observations of strain, need for rest, flexibility, and so on are made to identify areas that may be tight or weak, and applicants are instructed in exercises to stretch or strengthen specific areas.

The ability to squat fully or move to one knee and back, while maintaining a neutral back position and maintaining good endurance of the lower-extremity muscles, is evaluated during repetitive squatting (10 repetitions). The applicant is instructed in appropriate back position, and the activity is performed in front of a mirror to allow the applicant to observe his or her ability to complete the task as instructed. Signs of fatigue may include bringing the shoulders forward of the hips as the movement to resume standing is initiated. This observation also allows early intervention through exercise.

Full-body range of motion is observed, and any discrepancies from normal are documented. Some of the jobs require full-neck range of motion using a hard hat; therefore, the evaluation is conducted with the applicant wearing a hard hat. During cervical range of motion, if tightness is noted through the scalene mus-

cles during side bending or rotation, the employee is then given Adson's maneuver (Happenfeld, 1976, p. 127) to observe possible signs of neurovascular compression at the thoracic outlet. Shoulder range of motion includes full abduction, flexion, external and internal rotation with elbow flexion, extension, supination, and pronation; wrist flexion and extension; ulnar and radial deviation; and finger flexion and extension. Phalen's and Finkelstein's tests are also completed (Kasdan, 1991, p. 377, Fig. 23; p. 392). Trunk, hip, and knee range of motion is observed during the back screen, as well as repetitive squatting. Ankle range of motion, including ability to plantarflex and dorsiflex in standing, is also examined, and discrepancies from normal are documented. Full-body range of motion may or may not preclude safe performance of a job, depending on the specific essential job functions. This information serves as the individual's baseline. Stretching exercises may be provided based on the interest of the applicant. All information is shared with the physician, who provides the company with his or her advice regarding the individual's functional abilities and limitations and safety requirements.

The maximal grip, pinch, and lift capabilities are compared to the requirements included in the essential functions on the Job Summary. This maximal information and the information relating to pulse rate, fatigue, endurance, flexibility, and outcomes of Phalen's and Finkelstein's tests are intended to establish a baseline for each applicant, assist in developing exercise and conditioning programs, and aid in the future development of the Functional Assessment and Physical Therapy Evaluation Process.

Post-Offer Essential Job Function Evaluation

The Employment Entrance Examination Essential Job Functions form (see Appendix 19-6) is prepared from the Job Summary. On this form the physical therapist indicates whether the applicant meets or does not meet the requirements of the position as defined by the essential functions. This portion of the evaluation process compares the capabilities of the applicant with the requirements of the position. The assessment is based on additional testing, not on the therapist's opinion, given the results of the functional analysis.

Figure 19-1 illustrates the relationship between the Position Analysis (Job Task Analysis and Job Summary) and the Employment Evaluation Process

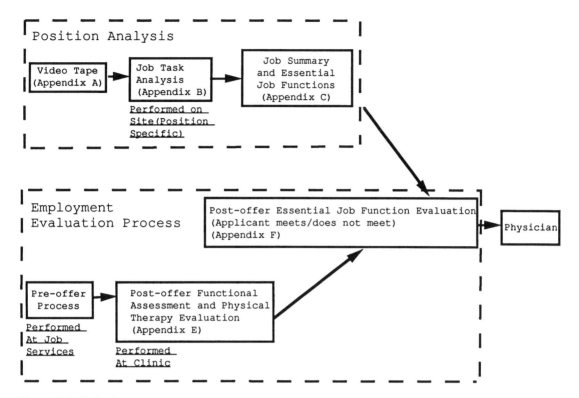

Figure 19-1. Evaluation process.

and how these are used to evaluate the applicant's ability to perform the essential job functions.

In summary, the company's hiring process follows these steps:

1. Specific position openings are listed with the local Job Service. The Job Summary and the essential job functions list can be used to help write the position advertisement.
2. The Job Service has a copy of the job summary, including the essential job functions for each entry-level position.
3. Applicants apply at the Job Service.
4. The application gives applicants an opportunity to self-identify as needing accommodation.
5. Selected applicants are sent to the specific plant with the open position.
6. Applicants are interviewed and their references reviewed. They are shown the job tasks associated with the position for which they are applying and asked to describe or demonstrate how they would perform the essential functions.
7. The most qualified applicant is then made a conditional offer of employment, in writing,

subject to his or her successful completion of the employment evaluation process, drug screening, and medical evaluation.

8. The applicant is scheduled for evaluation, which consists of a 90-minute functional assessment by the physical therapist. (As noted earlier, job-specific criteria have been established for each entry-level position in each plant.)
9. The applicant goes to a physician for completion of the medical evaluation portion. The examining physician receives the functional assessment results and the results of the essential function evaluation before his or her examination.
10. Based on the information provided by the physical therapist and the medical evaluation, the physician advises the company regarding the individual's ability to perform the job, with or without an accommodation, and whether the person can perform the job without posing a "direct threat" to the health or safety of himself or herself or others.
11. The company uses all information available in the hiring decision.

Test and Evaluation

It is important to evaluate whether a newly developed program has made an appreciable difference in the workplace. The primary goals of this in-hire program were to bring the company into compliance with the ADA, to initiate an ergonomics program, and to better match worker capabilities with job requirements and thereby reduce injuries. Secondary goals include identification of limited duty positions and increasing the diversity of the workplace. Although measurable outcomes that are statistically analyzed give the company more reliable information, preliminary information can include the number and types of changes that have been made, as well as anecdotal information gathered from workers, supervisors, and management.

Goal 1: Compliance with the Americans with Disabilities Act

In meeting the first goal (compliance with the ADA), the suggested administrative and performance-based measures to evaluate the program's impact could include identifying the number and percentage of positions for which essential functions have been identified, included on the Job Summary, and made part of the Functional Assessment. Other methods might be to have an independent ADA consultant review the process and offer his or her opinion as to whether the process meets the ADA requirements, as he or she sees them, or to use a checklist (developed internally or externally) on compliance with the ADA and determine the number and percentage of the items on the checklist that the company meets.

Goal 2: Integration of an Ergonomics Program

A number of ergonomic worksite improvements were made as a result of the ergonomic-based in-hire program; these address the second goal of the new program. One method of measurement would be to quantify the number and percentage of all company positions that have been modified to reduce musculoskeletal stress. Some of the engineering controls that have been implemented are as follows:

1. Scissor lifts, hoists, mobile cranes, and other material-handling equipment were installed to maintain optimum height for stacking lumber. Scissor hoists under the floor were used to locate workers in an optimum position.
2. Automation was used to reduce the physical stresses in plywood lay-up and to apply Universal Product Code labels to each board.
3. Single-wheeled wheelbarrows were replaced with totes or double-wheeled carts to reduce material handling stresses. Wheel types on plywood and lumber carts were changed from rubber to hard nylon to reduce the rolling friction.
4. Heaters, cooling fans, better lighting, and electrostatic precipitators were installed to improve the working climate.
5. Ergonomically designed operator control rooms and booths were installed for inspection and lumber classification operations.

Administrative controls to reduce musculoskeletal stress include the following:

1. Initial orientation procedures were modified to allow for work conditioning for physically demanding positions. Flexible scheduling was implemented during the return-to-work process for previously injured workers. Part of the work conditioning and flexible scheduling process included reduced work hours and job rotation.
2. On-the-job training was modified to include application of proper body mechanics, body awareness, stretching exercises, and home therapy.
3. A rotation program for Green Chain Pullers (a physically demanding job requiring workers to pull veneer from a conveyor line and stack it on carts) was implemented. This allowed the workers to rotate through five work locations in this position, which reduced the continuous stress on the arms and back and encouraged the use of different muscle groups. This process was carefully evaluated to avoid simply exposing more workers to risk factors.
4. Workers were instructed in proper lumber-pulling techniques to reduce grip strength requirements.

Other anecdotal evidence of the overall effort's impact indicates positive results:

1. In many cases, high physical demands were eliminated or reduced, working conditions improved, and, in some instances, job tasks were automated based on the ergonomic review during the Job Task Analyses for the different positions.
2. Existing employees, as well as new hires, benefit from worksite modifications. Documentation is not yet available, but it appears that employees appreciate what the company is doing to reduce the physical stress of job tasks.
3. Improved working conditions make employment at the company more suitable for the general population. Documentation is not yet available, but it appears that the company is able to hire a more diverse workforce.
4. The return-to-work process appears to be functioning well.
5. Documentation is not yet available, but the company anticipates that fewer musculoskeletal injuries will occur.
6. Productivity and product quality appear to be improved, although formal documentation is not available.

Another method of evaluating the impact the new program has made could include an evaluation of the incidence and severity of musculoskeletal disorders before and after program implementation using the Occupational Safety and Health Act 200 log of workers' compensation data. A survey of employees could be conducted, including job satisfaction, pain and discomfort, perceived ability to perform the job, and employee opinions about the relevance of the functional assessment process or the return-to-work program. An evaluation of the program might use any or all of the above measures before and after program implementation, probably through a retrospective record review.

Summary

This ergonomics program, supported by upper management, has improved working conditions for veteran employees as well as new employees. Without management support and employee involvement, compliance with the ADA would not have been possible. It must be emphasized that the ADA does not instruct employers on how to implement the ADA. The process described herein is an example of how one company interpreted and implemented the ADA guidelines. It also demonstrates how the results of job task analysis and essential job tasks can be combined to accomplish the multiple goals of complying with the ADA, matching worker capabilities with job demands, and reducing musculoskeletal injury risk factors.*

Acknowledgments

The authors would like to thank Roanna Keough for her invaluable assistance in the typing and assembly of this manuscript.

References

Ayoub, M.A. (1982). Control of manual lifting hazards: III. Preemployment screening. *Journal of Occupational Medicine, 24,* 751–761.

Ayoub, M.A., Selan, J., & Jiang, B. (1984). *Mini-guide for lifting.* Lubbock, TX: Texas Technical University.

Bailey, C. (1978). *Fit or fat* (p. 47). Boston: Houghton Mifflin.

Doolittle, T.L., Spurlin, O., Kaiyala, K., & Sovern, D. (1988). Physical demands of lineworkers. In *Proceedings of the Human Factors Society 32nd annual meeting* (pp. 632–636). Santa Monica, CA: Human Factors and Ergonomics Society.

Happenfeld, S. (1976). *Physical examination of the spine and extremities.* East Norwalk, CT: Appleton-Century-Crofts.

Kasdan, M.L. (Ed.). (1991). *Occupational hand and upper extremity injuries and diseases.* Philadelphia: Hanley & Belfus.

Keyserling, W.M., Herrin, G.D., Chaffin, D.B., et al. (1980). Establishing an industrial strength testing program. *American Industrial Hygiene Association Journal, 41,* 730–736.

U.S. Equal Employment Opportunity Commission. (1990). Americans with Disabilities Act of 1990. Public Law No. 101-336. Washington, DC: U.S. Government Printing Office.

U.S. Equal Employment Opportunity Commission. (1992). *A technical assistance manual on the employment provisions (Title I) of the Americans with Disabilities Act.* Washington, DC: U.S. Government Printing Office.

---

*It is important that the ergonomic consultant be fully aware of the requirements of the ADA, so that he or she does not confuse ergonomic intervention for the prevention of work-related musculoskeletal disorders with ADA requirements, although the two complement each other nicely.

Appendix 19-1
Videotaping Guidelines

Equipment Required

Video camera, blank tapes
Tripod
Batteries for camera (at least two)
Battery charger or AC adapter if taping projected to be longer than 1 hour
Clipboard and paper
Tape measure
Device to weigh objects
Writing utensils (pens, large markers for signs that must be visible on tape and other purposes)

Procedure

1. Record the following information at the beginning of the videotape and at the top of the written narrative diary of the tape:
   a. Name and location of facility
   b. Date and time of day
   c. Name of person using camera
2. It is important that the tape reviewer be able to easily follow the tape and the tape narrative diary. Key the narrative diary to the sequential numbers printed on the videotape. If you are using a camera without the capability to print the numbers on the tape, you may videotape a piece of paper with a number and the name of the task written on it immediately before the task is taped and refer to that name or number in the narrative diary and task description. If possible, also note the name of the task on the audio portion of the tape at the beginning of each task.

3. Taping procedure
   a. Tape the subject from the side and from the front for at least 5 minutes during normal "steady-state" performance of the task. Tape from the top and back if possible. Be sure that the camera frame includes the entire body and load (in the case of material handling) or workstation (in the case of tasks focusing on the upper extremity).
   b. Be sure the camera is still. Use a tripod. For material handling tasks, keep the camera approximately 36 in. above the floor. This should be about in the center of the movement pattern. Do not walk with the camera unless absolutely necessary to record the task. When you must change locations, move slowly and minimize recorded camera movement. Be sure the object has enough light on it to be clearly visible. If the camera has a high-speed shutter, turn it off: It requires too much light for most industrial tasks. If you are taping a worker with dark clothes on a light background, activate the "back-lit" capability on the camera.
   c. It is sometimes advantageous to tape several workers to determine the hazard level for workers with different anthropometries. If possible, try to tape one worst case (where the worker appears to be mismatched to the task), a best case (where the worker and job

are appropriately matched), and an average case (which seems to represent the "normal" situation). This is particularly important if you are analyzing the overall stress in the task. If you are more interested in the stress to a particular worker (e.g., determination of compensability in a workers' compensation case) you may want to focus on a worker of a particular height and weight.

d. It is frequently helpful to establish a reference length of known dimension on the videotape to help in later determination of forgotten dimensions. To minimize parallax and scale errors, this reference marker may be the ankle-knee or hip-knee distance because these points usually do not twist out of the camera view. Mark these points with pieces of reflective or white tape.

e. Try to tape the performance of sporadic task elements. These might include the loading of machines or parts bins, emptying parts bins, or moving pallets. (Although these may not be part of the initial analysis, they will assist in the overall determination of the task hazard.)

4. For each taped worker, determine the following parameters to the maximum extent possible:

a. Name, height, weight, and age of worker being taped

b. Length of time in the job being taped and other jobs performed

c. Length of time on previous jobs that may relate to any complaint of work-related musculoskeletal disorder

d. Existence of nonoccupational risk factors

Appendix 19-2

Job Task Analysis (Professional Therapy Associates, Inc., P.C.)

Position Title: <u>Green Chain Puller</u>   D.O.T. No: _____

Company: Plum Creek: _____

Contact Person/Title: _____

Date: <u>02-27-92</u>_____   Analyst: <u>Susan Brakefield, P.T.</u>

Schedule: <u>Shifts 4 people/shift; 3 shifts</u>_____   Days: <u>M-F</u>   Hrs/Day: <u>8</u>_____

    Hrs/Wk: <u>40</u>_____   Overtime Required: <u>Occasional Saturday</u>

Physical Demands: <u>Heavy</u>_____   Pay Schedule: <u>Tier II</u>_____

Education/Training Requirements: <u>6 weeks on-the-job training</u>

Position Description: <u>A rotation system has been established, with each employee working at four different locations, rotating every 2 hours.</u>_____

Tasks	% of Day per Shift
1. Sort and pull green veneer according to width, moisture, and usability, building square loads.	74%
2. Operate stacker, tally loads by width, trouble-shoot as bins become plugged.	25%
3. Clean around work area.	1%

Work Pace: _____ Self-paced _____ Incentive based _____ Quota system __x__ Machine paced: Chain runs 180 feet per minute.

Physical Demands

Lifting: In the position of first person on chain, stacking of veneer is done at least 75% of time. Sheets may be stacked 2–13 deep, with sheets 4–5 deep being most common. These stacks of veneer are then pulled off the conveyer onto a cart. About 65% of the time, the stack is picked up by one employee; turned around by step turn, pivot, or slight twist; and placed on the cart.

Lifting

| Weight | Frequency | | | | Objects | Lowest-Point Lift/Lower Height | Highest-Point Lift/Lower Height |
	Rare (1–10%)	Occasional (11–33%)	Frequent (34–66%)	Continual (67+%)	Sheets of Veneer	Cart (lowest part of cart)	Conveyor Height
1–10 lb				3–7 lb	1–2	6 in.	39 in.
11–20 lb				13–18 lb	4–5	6 in.	39 in.
21–35 lb			30 lb		4–8	6 in.	39 in.
36–50 lb		45 lb			Up to 10	6 in.	39 in.

Carrying

	Rare (1–10%)	Occasional (11–33%)	Frequent (34–66%)	Continual (67+%)	Objects	Max. Distance Carried
5–45 lb		Bilateral			Veneer carried up chain to place on cart	6 ft
Push/pull maximum force 20–35 lb				Pull	Veneer from chain conveyor to cart	6 ft

Description/Comments (objects, surfaces, etc.): Depending on the position on the chain and the number of pieces pulled, the need for stacking changes. The first persons on the chain work at a fast pace, with the back positions not as difficult.

Physical Demands

Postures/ Movements	Max. Consecutive Time	Total Daily Time	Position Change Optional?	Further Description
Sitting	20 mins	50 mins	Yes	Breaks, lunch
Standing (in place)	10–15 mins	2 hrs	No	Stacker moves feet constantly and
On feet	2 hrs	7 hrs	No	moves up and down chain as
Walking	20 ft	2 hrs	No	veneer is pulled from chain

	Never	**Rare**	**Occasional**	**Frequent**	**Continual**	
Bending				x		Placing veneer on low carts
Turning/ twisting				x		Turning with up to 45 lb veneer in hands to place on cart
Kneeling		x				Cleaning; fixing chain
Squatting		x				Cleaning; fixing chain
Crawling		x				Cleaning; fixing chain
Climbing		x				Stacker; 6-in. step up to chain
Balance/ agility					x	Quick turns/body mvmts required
Reaching (out)				x		Up to full arms' reach
Reaching (up)				x		Stacker gins; up to 63 in.
Reaching (down)					x	39 in.–6 ft; conveyor to cart
Wrist turning				x		
Grasping					x	
Pinching					x	22-lb lateral pinch side of veneer
Finger manipulation		x				
Foot controls	x					
Neck movements/ static posture		x				Normally within neutral position

Comments: Continuous firm grasp required during pulling, lifting, and carrying of veneer (Figure 19A-1)
Equipment/Tools: Wrenches, shovel, broom, "long knife" (7–17 lb)

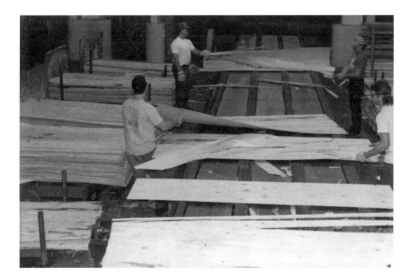

Figure 19A-1. Overhead view of Green Chain Puller.

Environmental Exposures

Inside: 100%   Temperature Range: 40–100°F
Outside: N/A   Comments:

	None	Slight	Moderate	Severe	Comments
Chemicals:					
Contact	x				
Consumption	x				
Inhalation		x			Dust
Confined spaces	x				
High elevations		x			
Ionizing radiation	x				
Moving objects			x		Conveyor belt; lift truck
Noise				x	Hearing protection required
Nonionizing radiation	x				
Safety equipment			x		Gloves; earplugs; apron optional
Slippery surface			x		Moist wood occasionally
Special clothing			x		Gloves; optional apron
Vibration		x			Stacker; chipper
Wetness		x			Moist wood

Special Conditions

_x_ Works with others   ___ Works alone   ___ Moderate Supervision
Communication Skills Required:
Speaking: __x__ In person _____ Phone _____ Public contact
Writing: <u>Not required</u>   Reading: <u>Instructions, warnings, and emergency signals</u>
General Comments: The most labor-intensive positions are the first people on either side of the chain, with high estimated metabolic demands in this area. Back position on the chain is still quite taxing, but not as demanding, because there is less stacking and pulling of heavy loads. The stacker operator position allows for standing, sitting, and resting from continuous upper-extremity use, becoming more difficult as bin becomes plugged.

Possible Ergonomic Considerations

1. Heaviest peel (wood strip peeled from log to be handled) should be run the second and third hour of work, allowing the first 2 hours as warmup.
2. Scissor lifts for carts to avoid forward-bend reach with up to 45 lb at 6-in. height. This could begin with the front four carts.
3. Bring work platform out between carts to decrease need to step down or reach out, allowing workers to place veneer on carts more evenly with less bending and throwing.
4. Use sit-stand stool by controls for stacker operator.
5. Rotate positions on the chain more frequently than every 2 hours; possibly every half hour.
6. Stretching program developed specifically for Green Chain workers to be done before beginning work and after breaks and stacker operation.

Appendix 19-3
Entry-Level Job Summary

Position: Green Chain Puller

This facility manufactures solid wood products in modernized manufacturing facilities. Teamwork, pride, and motivation are important personal attributes for applicants.

Although the plywood plant is considered state-of-the-art in this industry, the entry-level Green Chain Puller position is normally physically intensive. Entry-level employees are placed on an Extra Board status and assigned work on an on-call basis.

The successful applicant

- Must be available and willing to work different shifts, weekends, holidays, and overtime.
- Must be capable of receiving, interpreting, and applying oral or written instructions and directions.
- Must be capable of performing job tasks unaffected by temperature extremes (hot and cold) and often dusty and noisy environmental conditions.

At any given time, there are up to six employees in the plant or on call that can successfully perform this position.

Job Demands

This position exists for the sole purpose of maintaining the mill's production and to provide relief operators in various production capacities as needed so that safe and healthful working conditions are maintained.

During a normal 8-hour shift, employees stand up and move at least 90% of the time. Pushing and pulling, lifting, carrying, sweeping, and so on are common motions. Walking and working surfaces are normally even. Most tasks require repetitive use of bilateral upper extremities.

Essential Job Functions

Material Handling

1. Occasional lift up to 45 lb veneer from floor to 36 in.
2. Occasional carry of 45 lb veneer up to 10 ft.
3. Frequent lower up to 30 lb veneer from 39 in. to 6 ft in height.
4. Pull veneer from conveyor to cart 20–60 times per minute for 2 hours.
5. Place 43 lb of veneer to a 6-ft height six to eight times per hour.
6. Pull 20–60 times per minute.
7. Upper-extremity:
   a. Pinch with 17 lb of lateral pinch, 15 times per min for 3 min.
   b. Pull with either hand up to 35 lb of force on a continuous basis up to 15 times per minute for up to 3 minutes (Figure 19A-2).
8. Detecting audible or visual signals of evacuation for emergency.

As an equal opportunity employer, this facility does not discriminate on the basis of race, religion, color, sex, age, national origin, or disability.

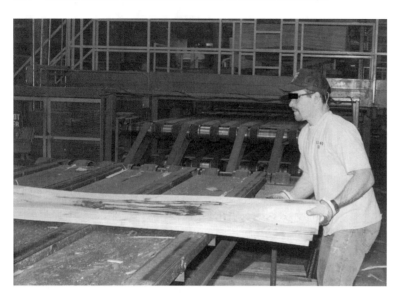

Figure 19A-2. Essential job function 7B "Pull with either hand up to 35 lb force up to 15 times per minute up to 3 minutes."

Appendix 19-4

Instructions to Candidates for Employment

The following information shall be clearly and concisely communicated to every employment candidate. The methods of communication may vary from case to case; use your own judgment to ensure that instructions are clearly understood.

Introduction

1. You are here as part of (Company) employment evaluation process. The process includes three parts:
   a. Functional Assessment (considered part of the medical evaluation)
   b. Medical Evaluation
   c. Drug Screening
   The Functional Assessment will be conducted here. You will visit the physicians at _____ for the remaining two parts.
2. My name is _____. I am a licensed _____ therapist. I am under contract with (Company) to evaluate entry-level positions in each of its mills to determine the essential job functions for each job task and to conduct a physical therapy functional evaluation.
3. You are applying for _____ position at (Company) _____ facility.
4. During the next 90 minutes, I will assess your physical status and your ability to perform the essential job functions identified for the job for which you are applying. There are more than 20 segments to the evaluation process. I will observe you the entire time.
5. Although you will lift weights during the evaluation, it is not a strength test. You will be evaluated on endurance, flexibility, cardiovascular conditioning, and the application of proper body mechanics.
6. I ask that you perform each task to establish your own "maximum safe capability." If you should experience pain, discomfort, or other signs of distress, please let me know immediately. I am asking for your personal best.
7. Please let me know if you have questions or concerns about the assessment process before we begin.
8. Are these instructions clear to you? If not, in what areas would you like further explanation?
9. Have you had the opportunity to observe the jobs for which you are applying?

Appendix 19-5
Employment Evaluation

Functional Assessment Worksheet

Employee Name: _____   Date: _____
SSN: _____   Phys. Name: _____

I. Pulse Rate

	Activity	Pulse Immediately After	Pulse 1 Minute After
Initial	_____	_____	_____
After	_____	_____	_____
After	_____	_____	_____
After	_____	_____	_____
After	_____	_____	_____
After	_____	_____	_____
Termination		_____	_____

II. Grip Dynamometer   Right _____ Left _____
Beginning of functional assessment

	Minute 1 R/L	Minute 2 R/L	Minute 3 R/L
1.	___/___	___/___	___/___
2.	___/___	___/___	___/___
3.	___/___	___/___	___/___
4.	___/___	___/___	___/___
5.	___/___	___/___	___/___
6.	___/___	___/___	___/___
7.	___/___	___/___	___/___
8.	___/___	___/___	___/___
9.	___/___	___/___	___/___
10.	___/___	___/___	___/___
11.	___/___	___/___	___/___
12.	___/___	___/___	___/___
13.	___/___	___/___	___/___
14.	___/___	___/___	___/___
15.	___/___	___/___	___/___

Middle of functional assessment; activity preceding: _____

	Minute 1 R/L	Minute 2 R/L	Minute 3 R/L
1.	___/___	___/___	___/___
2.	___/___	___/___	___/___
3.	___/___	___/___	___/___
4.	___/___	___/___	___/___
5.	___/___	___/___	___/___
6.	___/___	___/___	___/___
7.	___/___	___/___	___/___
8.	___/___	___/___	___/___
9.	___/___	___/___	___/___
10.	___/___	___/___	___/___
11.	___/___	___/___	___/___
12.	___/___	___/___	___/___
13.	___/___	___/___	___/___
14.	___/___	___/___	___/___
15.	___/___	___/___	___/___

End of functional assessment; activity preceding: _____

	Minute 1 R/L	Minute 2 R/L	Minute 3 R/L
1.	___/___	___/___	___/___
2.	___/___	___/___	___/___
3.	___/___	___/___	___/___
4.	___/___	___/___	___/___
5.	___/___	___/___	___/___
6.	___/___	___/___	___/___
7.	___/___	___/___	___/___
8.	___/___	___/___	___/___
9.	___/___	___/___	___/___
10.	___/___	___/___	___/___
11.	___/___	___/___	___/___
12.	___/___	___/___	___/___
13.	___/___	___/___	___/___
14.	___/___	___/___	___/___
15.	___/___	___/___	___/___

III. Pinch Dynamometer

Lateral pinch: Right _____ Left _____
Palmar pinch: Right _____ Left _____

Beginning of functional assessment

	Lateral Pinch			Palmar Pinch		
	Minute 1 R/L	Minute 2 R/L	Minute 3 R/L	Minute 1 R/L	Minute 2 R/L	Minute 3 R/L
1.	___/___	___/___	___/___	___/___	___/___	___/___
2.	___/___	___/___	___/___	___/___	___/___	___/___
3.	___/___	___/___	___/___	___/___	___/___	___/___
4.	___/___	___/___	___/___	___/___	___/___	___/___

5.	__/__	__/__	__/__	__/__	__/__	__/__
6.	__/__	__/__	__/__	__/__	__/__	__/__
7.	__/__	__/__	__/__	__/__	__/__	__/__
8.	__/__	__/__	__/__	__/__	__/__	__/__
9.	__/__	__/__	__/__	__/__	__/__	__/__
10.	__/__	__/__	__/__	__/__	__/__	__/__
11.	__/__	__/__	__/__	__/__	__/__	__/__
12.	__/__	__/__	__/__	__/__	__/__	__/__
13.	__/__	__/__	__/__	__/__	__/__	__/__
14.	__/__	__/__	__/__	__/__	__/__	__/__
15.	__/__	__/__	__/__	__/__	__/__	__/__

Middle of functional assessment; activity preceding: _____

| | *Lateral Pinch* | | | *Palmar Pinch* | | |
	Minute 1 R/L	Minute 2 R/L	Minute 3 R/L	Minute 1 R/L	Minute 2 R/L	Minute 3 R/L
1.	__/__	__/__	__/__	__/__	__/__	__/__
2.	__/__	__/__	__/__	__/__	__/__	__/__
3.	__/__	__/__	__/__	__/__	__/__	__/__
4.	__/__	__/__	__/__	__/__	__/__	__/__
5.	__/__	__/__	__/__	__/__	__/__	__/__
6.	__/__	__/__	__/__	__/__	__/__	__/__
7.	__/__	__/__	__/__	__/__	__/__	__/__
8.	__/__	__/__	__/__	__/__	__/__	__/__
9.	__/__	__/__	__/__	__/__	__/__	__/__
10.	__/__	__/__	__/__	__/__	__/__	__/__
11.	__/__	__/__	__/__	__/__	__/__	__/__
12.	__/__	__/__	__/__	__/__	__/__	__/__
13.	__/__	__/__	__/__	__/__	__/__	__/__
14.	__/__	__/__	__/__	__/__	__/__	__/__
15.	__/__	__/__	__/__	__/__	__/__	__/__

End of functional assessment; activity preceding: _____

| | *Lateral Pinch* | | | *Palmar Pinch* | | |
	Minute 1 R/L	Minute 2 R/L	Minute 3 R/L	Minute 1 R/L	Minute 2 R/L	Minute 3 R/L
1.	__/__	__/__	__/__	__/__	__/__	__/__
2.	__/__	__/__	__/__	__/__	__/__	__/__
3.	__/__	__/__	__/__	__/__	__/__	__/__
4.	__/__	__/__	__/__	__/__	__/__	__/__
5.	__/__	__/__	__/__	__/__	__/__	__/__
6.	__/__	__/__	__/__	__/__	__/__	__/__
7.	__/__	__/__	__/__	__/__	__/__	__/__
8.	__/__	__/__	__/__	__/__	__/__	__/__
9.	__/__	__/__	__/__	__/__	__/__	__/__
10.	__/__	__/__	__/__	__/__	__/__	__/__
11.	__/__	__/__	__/__	__/__	__/__	__/__
12.	__/__	__/__	__/__	__/__	__/__	__/__
13.	__/__	__/__	__/__	__/__	__/__	__/__
14.	__/__	__/__	__/__	__/__	__/__	__/__
15.	__/__	__/__	__/__	__/__	__/__	__/__

IV. General Lifting Capabilities

	Start Time	End Time

A.   Floor to 36-in. height   _____   _____
       Reports/Comments:
       Body Mechanics:
       Weights Achieved:

B.   Other lift _____   Pulse rate _____ 1 minute after _____

V. Balance Activities

A. Board Walk

  1. Forward/Backward Gait

    Arms: _____ at sides   _____ out from body

    Eyes: _____ looking at board   _____ to front

    Balance _____ number of wavers during forward

            _____ number of wavers during backward

    Step-Offs _____ number during forward

            _____ number during backward

    Attempts _____ to complete

  2. Heel-Toe Forward/Backward

    Arms: _____ at sides   _____ out from body

    Eyes: _____ looking at board   _____ to front

    Balance _____ number of wavers during forward

            _____ number of wavers during backward

    Step-Offs _____ number of during forward

            _____ number of during backward

    Attempts _____ to complete

  3. Crossover Ambulation

    Arms: _____ at sides   _____ out from body

    Eyes: _____ looking at board   _____ to front

    Balance _____ number of wavers during front crossover

            _____ number of wavers during back crossover

    Step-Offs _____ number during front crossover

            _____ number during back crossover

       Attempts _____ to complete

B. Golfer's Lift

    _____ 6 times right leg   _____ balance losses

    _____ 6 times left leg   _____ balance losses

    _____ able to maintain back position

    _____ able to follow directions

    Comments:

C. Stand-Kneel-Stand   _____ number completed

    Ability to follow directions

    Ease of movements

    Balance losses

    Hands on knees to resume stand

    Pulse _____ 1 minute after _____

    General Comments:

VI. Back Screen   Total Score _____
    Sitting toe touch (4)   _____
    Hamstring flexibility (right) (4) _____
    Hamstring flexibility (left) (4)   _____
    Sit-up 5 times (3)   _____
    Lower abdominals 1 minute (3) _____
    Back extension flexibility (4)   _____
    Back extension strength (3)   _____
    Hip flexion (right) (3)   _____
    Hip flexion (left) (3)   _____

VII. Repetitive Squat   _____ Repetitions Completed
    Speed: Slow _____ Moderate _____ Rapid _____
    Body Posturing: _____ able to maintain neutral back
    Use of UE:
    Signs of fatigue:
    Pulse _____   1 minute after _____

VIII. Full-Body Range of Motion

	Within Normal Limits	Discrepancy
Neck	_____	_____
Shoulders	_____	_____
Elbows	_____	_____
Wrist	_____	_____
Hand/Fingers	_____	_____
Trunk	_____	_____
Hips	_____	_____
Knees	_____	_____
Ankles	_____	_____

IX. Special Instructions Given:

Appendix 19-6
Employment and Medical Evaluation

Essential Job Functions

Employee Name: _____ Date: _____

SSN: _____

Assessment Specialist: _____

Green Chain Puller

Material Handling

	Meets	Does not meet	Not evaluated
1. Lift up to 45 lb from floor to 35 in. on occasional basis	_____	_____	_____
2. Carry 45 lb up to 10 ft on occasional basis	_____	_____	_____
3. Lower up to 30 lb from 39 in. to 6 ft on frequent basis	_____	_____	_____
4. Pull veneer from conveyor to cart 20–60 times per minute (Figure 19A-3)	_____	_____	_____
5. Place 45 lb of veneer to a 6-ft height (6–8 times per hour)	_____	_____	_____
6. Pull 20–60 times perminute maintaining neutral back position (no twisting, etc.)	_____	_____	_____
7. Upper-extremity:			
a. Pinch with 17 lb of lateral pinch, 15 times per min for 3 min.	_____	_____	_____
b. Pull with either hand up to 35 lb force on up to 15 times per min for up to 3 min.	_____	_____	_____
8. Detecting audible or visual signals of evacuation for emergency.	_____	_____	_____

General Observations

1. Pulse Rate:
2. Back Screen:
3. Grip and Pinch Strength/Endurance:
4. Upper Extremity Strength/Endurance:
5. Range of Motion:

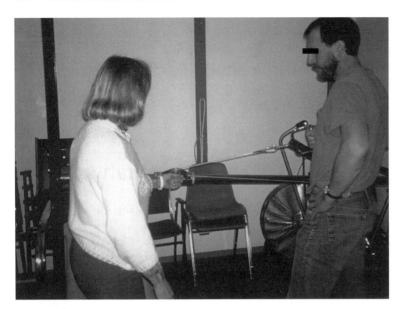

Figure 19A-3. Pull test in clinic.

6. General Lifting Capability   Occasional   Frequent
   a. Floor to 36 in.
   b. Other
7. Body Mechanics:
8. General Coordination:
9. General Conditioning: 1-minute recovery ranged from:
10. Blood pressure before and after assessment:

Chapter 20

Complying with the Americans with Disabilities Act: A Design Retrofit

Wm. L. Wilkoff, Paula C. Wilkoff, and Laura W. Abed

Learning Objectives

On completion of this chapter, the reader should

- Have increased awareness of the pervasiveness of barriers in interior and exterior environments.
- Understand how the technical guidelines provided in the Americans with Disabilities Act (ADA) can be used to target specific barriers and effect their elimination.

Key Words

Accessibility
Universal design
Barrier free
Accommodation

Abstract

Since the passage of the ADA, businesses have begun to hire design firms for the purpose of surveying their facilities to determine areas of noncompliance with the mandate. This case study details one such survey, analyzing points of noncompliance and the steps that must be taken to retrofit the facility. The chapter emphasizes the need for sensitivity in design as well as an understanding of the technical guidelines.

Introduction

The passage into law of the ADA in 1990 brought the promise of positive change for people with disabilities. It also signaled a turning point in commercial design, one that was long overdue. Although previous laws had been passed by federal, state, and local authorities that mandated accessible design, their effects were hindered by the limits of their jurisdiction; contradictions between local, state, and federal codes; and the lack of enforcement procedures. Some designers responded to these laws by incorporating barrier-free design into all their work, but others had little experience or practical knowledge of the concept. The ADA was the first mandate that truly required all commercial designers to practice their trade with the full breadth of anthropometric data in mind. Failure to comply would constitute an act of discrimination because the ADA is a civil rights law, a compelling reason for any designer to use more universal design strategies.

For the designer of public or work space, the task of retrofitting an existing space now has new ramifications. Any design needs to comply with the ADA while simultaneously addressing client needs. How is the designer to accomplish this task? In 1993, the Architectural and Transportation Barriers Compliance Board (ATBCB) issued a formal survey tool reflecting ADA standards for the purpose of evaluating compliance. Before its release, the *Uniform Federal Accessibility Standards* (UFAS) document was considered a "safe harbor" survey vehicle. UFAS, a product of the Rehabilitation Act of 1973, provided standards by which accessibility to government buildings and federally funded programs could be ensured. However, it did not address all aspects of accessibility covered in the ADA *Accessibility Guidelines* (ADAAG). Although a designer could technically satisfy the law with a UFAS survey before 1993, he or she would be overlooking certain items, such as visual alarms, that are specified in ADAAG but not in UFAS (Appendix 20-1 compares a sample survey form from each publication). This emphasizes an important point about the ingredients of a successful survey. Along with the survey tools, the designer must bring a certain sensitivity to the needs of the potential users of a space to effectively address the spirit as well as the letter of the law.

The present case study explores a project undertaken in March 1991 by a two-member survey team acting as ADA consultants to an architectural firm. The facility to be renovated was a financial institution occupying a 550,000-sq. ft. building in a campus setting. The area included interior and exterior parking facilities, office space, a bank, drive-through automated teller machine (ATM) units, a fitness center, a cafeteria, strolling paths, and picnic areas. The facility was primarily dedicated to employee use, making Title I (Employment) the primary concern of the ADA survey. The general public did, however, have access to certain exterior parking areas, the bank and ATM units, and the cafeteria; therefore, ensuring compliance with Title III (Public Accommodations) was also a goal of the survey.

Rather than being concerned with the specific ergonomic needs of one or more individuals, a survey of this type demands consideration of all possible users of a space. The designer must think in broad terms that encompass mobility, visual, auditory, dexterity, and cognitive disabilities. A perusal of ADAAG or a similar guide demonstrates how extensive the specifications have become over the years. The bulk of the specifications accommodate users of wheelchairs. This is true not because most people with disabilities are in wheelchairs, as many people believe, but because so many architectural barriers exist for them in the built environment. For that reason, many of the problems cited in a survey refer to reach range, height, width, maneuvering

space, or vertical level change. Other problems must not be overlooked, however, especially because the bulk of accommodations are universally beneficial. Lowered drinking fountains, elevator buttons, and paper towel dispensers can benefit children; people with strollers or temporary injuries use ramps and elevators as readily as people with wheelchairs; and visual and auditory alarms are a feature that can increase the opportunity for safe escape for everyone. The most important point is that a designer must look beyond the specifications, using personal sensitivity and sound judgment to make appropriate decisions that will afford comfort and convenience to the greatest number of people.

Analysis

To identify inaccessible building elements, the survey team studied both the interior and the exterior of the building, noting problems on a UFAS survey form modified to reflect ADA standards. (Table 20-1 shows a sample page from the modified form.) The team also made use of several other tools, including a copy of the ADAAG; a measuring tape or rule to identify critical clearances, heights, and widths; a small level to be placed on top of an adjustable triangle for measuring ramp angles, with markings on the triangle indicating the various mandated slopes (e.g., 1:12, 1:20, 1:50); and a fish scale, which is affixed to the inside doorknob so that when the door is opened from the outside, the scale registers the pounds of force (lbf) required to open the door. The fish scale has been recommended as an acceptable measuring device by the ATBCB. Since the completion of this survey, however, another tool, called Window Ease (A-Solution, Inc., Albuquerque, NM), has been made available for measuring pounds of force of a window or door. It consists of a calibrated rod with a plunger and a rubber ring. When the plunger is pushed in, the rubber ring moves along the calibrated rod to give an exact measure of pounds of force. This device is much more convenient to use than the fish scale.

As a result of the survey, a number of elements throughout the building and grounds were found to be inconsistent with existing standards. These are

Table 20-1. Modified UFAS Survey Form Reflecting ADAAG Requirements

Location	Noncompliance	UFAS Reference*	Priority Rating
Drinking fountains phase I and phase II	The drinking fountains in phase II comply, but the drinking fountains in phase I do not comply.	4.15	***
Public telephone in third-floor break room, phase I	Phone projects from the wall within an unacceptable height range; however, it is not mounted in a major path of travel for the room.	4.4.1	*** ***
	The highest operational part is 54 in. from the floor.	4.31.3; 4.2.5; 4.2.6	
Public telephone in cafeteria, phase I	Phone projects from the wall within an unacceptable height range; however, it is not mounted in a major path of travel for the room.	4.4.1	***
	Phone is missing volume control.	4.31.5	***

*Reference numbers are the same for both UFAS and ADAAG.

UFAS = *Uniform Federal Accessibility Standards*; ADAAG = Americans with Disabilities Act *Accessibility Guidelines*; *** = readily achievable, immediate action recommended.

described below and, when applicable, are supported by the text or reference number of the appropriate guideline from ADAAG. (To obtain information on how to use ADAAG, see Wilkoff and Abed, 1994).

Exterior Parking Facilities, Paths of Travel, and Entrances

Main Entry

The parking lot serving the main entrance to the building provided two designated handicapped parking spaces for visitors. These spaces were not wide enough to allow a wheelchair user or person with a prosthesis to easily enter or exit a vehicle. ADAAG recommends at least 96 in. of width for accessible parking spaces, with a 60-in.–wide adjacent access aisle (ADAAG, 1991, 4.6.3, A4.6.3). Further, the international symbol of accessibility was painted on the ground surface of each space, but vertical signs were not displayed. Designating spaces only with pavement symbols makes it difficult for drivers to locate accessible spaces, especially when other cars are parked adjacent to these spaces or drivers have limited trunk or back mobility. According to ADAAG, vertical signs are needed as well (ADAAG, 1991, 4.6.4).

The placement of the spaces also presented difficulties. Although they were near the main entrance, there was no accessible route. To reach the front door of the building one had to negotiate a curb to the sidewalk and several sets of stairs. There was in fact a gently sloped walkway that led to the main entry located 75 ft away, but no signage indicated the presence of or directions to this walkway. This accessible-route problem existed for the public transportation drop-off point as well.

The entrance to the main lobby of the building was through either a revolving door or double-leaf doors on either side. At the time of the survey, the acceptable opening force for exterior swinging doors was 8.5 lbf or less. These entry doors required 14–20 lbf to open.

Bank

The parking lot near the bank also provided two accessible spaces, but a built-up curb ramp extending into the area between the two spaces negated the function of a proper access aisle (Figure 20-1). This was clearly an attempt at sensitive design using limited knowledge. Although a ramp is necessary to negotiate the curb, a flat surface adjacent to a parking space is equally necessary to allow the user to enter or exit the car safely and without the risk of having a wheelchair roll away.

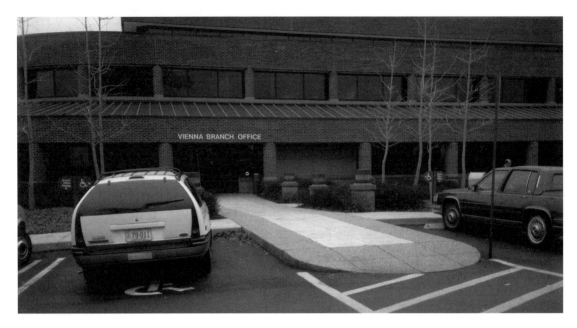

Figure 20-1. This built-up ramp extends into the access aisle, making it difficult for wheelchair users to safely exit or enter their cars.

Human Resources Center

The walkway leading to the Human Resources Center had a 1-in. rise where it met the sidewalk, which could prove to be an impediment for people with visual disabilities, canes, walkers, or wheelchairs (ADAAG, 1991, 4.5.2). The exterior entrance door required more force to open than the 8.5 lbf then considered acceptable, as did the interior doors of the vestibule, which required 9 lbf to open. The acceptable force for interior doors is 5 lbf (ADAAG, 1991, 4.13.11). Finally, the exterior door hardware was difficult to use. ADAAG states that operating mechanisms "shall not require tight grasping, pinching, or twisting of the wrist" and shall not require more than 5 lbf to operate (ADAAG, 1991, 4.27.4, p. 52). Although the survey team did not use devices for measuring torque or twisting force, they did use the "closed-fist" method. This is based on the first-hand experience of people with manual dexterity disabilities, who have suggested that team members use a closed fist to try operating hardware or controls. If they are unable to accomplish their task or can do so only with great difficulty, then they should consider the controls inaccessible. This is an example of a situation in which sensitivity is as helpful as objective measurement.

Interior Parking Facility and Path of Travel

The interior parking facility, which was for employee use only, provided three accessible parking spaces, each designated with the international symbol of access on the ground but no vertical stanchion displaying the symbol at the head of the space (Figure 20-2). The three spaces were scattered throughout the garage rather than being situated nearest to the elevator lobby entrance. None of the spaces had a dedicated adjacent access aisle or a delineated path of travel from the space to the elevator lobby entrance, thus creating a potentially dangerous situation as patrons travel between parked and moving cars. This is especially hazardous for those using wheelchairs because they are not tall enough to be seen easily in a rear view mirror. Although a curb ramp was provided to gain access to the elevator lobby platform, a nonaccessible parking space was located at the mouth of the ramp, effectively blocking access to it.

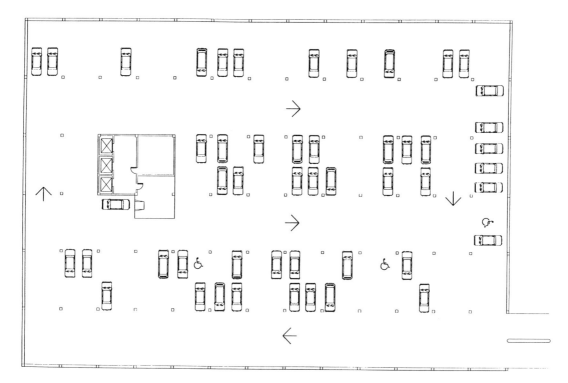

Figure 20-2. Interior parking facility before renovation. Note the scattered "accessible" parking spaces.

Dining Facilities

Executive Dining Room

The entrance to the executive dining room did not have the minimum 18-in. clearance space needed adjacent to the latch on the pull side of the door that would allow the door to swing toward an individual in a wheelchair without hitting the chair (ADAAG, 1991, 4.13.6).

Cafeteria Seating

The tables in the cafeteria had aprons (vertical supports located under the top surface and between the four legs) that extended too far down to allow a wheelchair user to pull close to the table without bumping his or her knees. ADAAG (1991, 4.32.3) requires a knee clearance of 27 in. above the finished floor (AFF). With the appropriate number of accessible tables, however, the existing table arrangement provided adequate aisles at least 36 in.

wide to afford access to a choice of seating in accordance with ADAAG (1991).

Food Counter and Vending Machines

The soft drink, snack, and ice dispensers were beyond the reach capabilities of wheelchair users and short people, as were portions of the salad bar area (ADAAG, 1991, 5.5). Most of the food vending machines also had operable parts out of reach range. A person's reach range is not determined solely by his or her maximum arm extension and trunk or back mobility. It also depends on environmental factors, such as how closely the wheelchair can be maneuvered to the operable parts and how high those parts are situated. In many cases, visibility is limited as well when dispensers, controls, and other equipment are beyond reach capabilities. ADAAG provides guidance concerning reach allowances, with a forward approach having a reach range of 15–48 in. AFF (ADAAG, 1991, 4.2.5), and with a side approach having a range of 9–54 in. AFF (ADAAG, 1991, 4.2.6).

Bank

Although the bank had adequate floor space with accessible aisles at least 60 in. wide that would allow passing and ease of movement for wheelchair users, the teller windows and customer service desks were all too high to reach from a wheelchair. At 44 in. AFF, they did not meet the mandate of having at least one teller window at a maximum height of 36 in. AFF (ADAAG, 1991, 7.2).

Human Resources Center

The Human Resources Center used a systems furniture arrangement that did not allow clear passage for prospective employees who might be wheelchair users. In many cases, the allotted aisle space was less than the 36-in. minimum width needed for a single wheelchair to pass down an aisle. Further, there was no provision for the 60-in. width required for two wheelchairs to pass each other. (For an in-depth discussion of space allowances for wheelchair users, see sections 4.2 and 4.3 of ADAAG, 1994.)

Restrooms and Locker Rooms

The restrooms throughout the building and in the fitness center locker rooms presented several barriers for people using wheelchairs. Although there were designated accessible stalls in the core men's and women's restrooms, they were not configured to allow for a side approach to the toilet and they lacked rear grab bars, as required by ADAAG (1991, 4.17). The toilet stalls in the locker rooms were too narrow (36 in.) to allow wheelchair access. The men's restrooms also did not have one urinal lowered to a maximum rim height of 17 in. AFF, a necessity for wheelchair users (ADAAG, 1991, 4.18.2). Knee clearance under the lavatory aprons was less than the required minimum of 29 in. (ADAAG, 1991, 4.19.2), and hot water pipes were not insulated to protect people in wheelchairs from burns (ADAAG, 1991, 4.19.4). Paper towel dispensers were higher than the allowed 48-in. maximum height (ADAAG, 1991, 4.27.3). Likewise, the bottom edges of the mirrors were higher than 40 in. AFF (ADAAG, 1991, 4.19.6). Neither the men's nor the women's locker room had a roll-in shower or transfer seat to allow

people in wheelchairs to shower (ADAAG, 1991, 4.21). Finally, accessible restroom facilities were not provided in or near the cafeteria.

Miscellaneous Elements

Elevators

There were no audible signals to indicate the direction of elevator travel, nor were there raised symbols or Braille on the hoistways (doorway recesses) to designate each floor (ADAAG, 1991, 4.10). Although the control panels inside the elevator cab did have raised symbols, they did not have the Grade II Braille required by ADAAG (1991, 4.30.4) to be used in signage. Unlike Grade I Braille, which uses raised dot patterns to represent different letters and numbers, Grade II uses a group of contractions designed to shorten Braille messages and is therefore suitable for signage. The cord on the emergency telephone handset was shorter than the recommended 29 in. (ADAAG, 1991, 4.10.14). Finally, the horizontal gap between the car platform and the landing edge was greater than 1.25 in., a possible hazard for someone using a cane, walker, or wheelchair that might become wedged in the gap.

Drinking Fountains

Only a portion of the building had accessible drinking fountains as described in ADAAG (1991, 4.15). Even if the existing number had met the required criterion of 50% accessible fountains per floor, they should have been dispersed throughout each floor so that no individual would have to travel too far to use one.

Telephones

With the coin slot at 64 in. AFF, the public telephone in the third-floor lounge was mounted too high to comply with the ADAAG standards (1991, 4.31). Likewise, the public telephone in the cafeteria was mounted at the same height and was missing a volume control. Both telephones also projected more than 4 in. from the wall at a height that was potentially dangerous for people with visual disabilities, who might bump into them. ADAAG specifies that "objects projecting from walls . . . with their leading edges between 27 in.

and 80 in. . . . above the finished floor shall protrude no more than 4 in. . . . into walks, halls, corridors, passageways, or aisles" (ADAAG, 1991, 4.4.1, p. 21). The telephones in question, however, were not considered protruding objects because they were in niches with passage space beside them rather than in the path of travel.

Alarms

Visual alarms were not present to alert people with hearing disabilities to possible emergency situations, as recommended (ADAAG, 1991, 4.28.3).

Interior Signage

Signage identifying permanent rooms (including core stairs) was placed on doors higher than the recommended 60 in. AFF (ADAAG, 1991, 4.30.6) and did not have tactile lettering and Grade II Braille. This was especially significant at the entrance to the computer room, where warning signage indicated protection by a halon fire suppression system.

Coat Rods

All coat rods were mounted at 62 in. AFF, out of reach range for individuals in wheelchairs and people of short stature.

Doors

Doors had doorknobs rather than levers or U-shaped handles, which are easier for people with manual dexterity difficulties.

Design

Using ADA guidelines as a reference, the survey team recommended design solutions to the problems outlined in the survey, prioritized in terms of safety, benefit to the greatest number of people, and cost-effectiveness. In prioritizing solutions, two references are especially useful. The first is the ADAAG itself, which suggests that solutions for public accommodations be implemented in the following order: (1) exterior accessibility for entrances, sidewalks, parking, and public transportation; (2) accessibility to goods and services, including such

retrofits as widening doors, rearranging furniture to create accessible paths of travel, providing accessible signage, and installing interior ramps; (3) restroom accessibility; and (4) any other retrofits necessary to attain accessibility. A reference such as *The New ADA: Compliance and Costs* (Kearney, 1992) is also helpful in identifying the cost of each compliant retrofit, prioritizing in terms of cost benefit, and establishing a budget.

In an institution of this size, it is commonly understood that implementation of accessible solutions will occur over time due to the scope of such a project. According to the ADA, the facility must make whatever accommodations it can without causing undue burden, and alternate methods of providing services may be used until such time as funds become available to complete accessible changes.

Exterior Parking Facilities, Paths of Travel, and Entrances

Main Entry

The accessible designated visitor parking spaces located near the stairway to the main entry were relocated to position them directly in front of the ramp entrance. Although this located the accessible spaces 75 ft from the main entry, it provided an accessible exterior path of travel through gently ramped walkways that bypass the entry stairs. A 5-ft–wide access aisle was placed between the two 96-in.–wide parking spaces, along with a curb ramp where the access aisle meets the curb. In addition, a portion of the roadway in front of the access aisle was delineated by diagonal painted stripes on the ground surface for use as a dedicated drop-off point for public transportation and private vehicles. In this way, individuals alighting from public or private vehicles can take advantage of the curb ramp and accessible route. Vertical parking signs displaying the international symbol of accessibility were located at the head of each accessible parking space at a height visible above a parked vehicle. No specific height is mandated by ADAAG, which states that vertical signs "can be seen from a driver's seat if the signs are mounted high enough above the ground and located at the front of a parking space" (ADAAG, 1991, A4.6.4, p. A7). The international

Figure 20-3. This curb ramp with flared sides provides easy and safe access to accessible parking spaces.

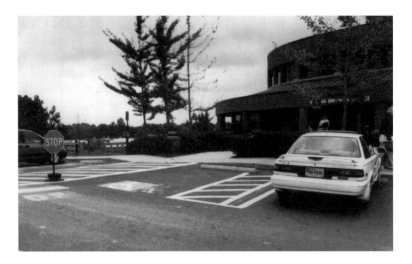

symbol also was painted on the ground at each accessible space.

Signs were strategically placed to designate the shortest accessible route to accessible entrances. To alleviate the heavy-door problem, an automatic door opener was installed on one set of double-leaf doors, permitting people to enter and exit the building without seeking assistance. Since the time of the survey, ADAAG (1994) has put the pounds of force requirement for opening exterior hinged doors on reserve until a means of compensating for a variety of internal building air pressures can be found. If the facility had been unable to afford an automatic device, technically they would no longer be out of compliance on this issue.

Bank

The built-up curb ramp between the two parking spaces was removed. In its place, a delineated, flat access aisle and a curb ramp with flared sides were provided to allow proper and safe access to the side-walk leading to the bank entrance (Figure 20-3).

Human Resources Center

The 1-in. level change between the concrete walk-way and the sidewalk was probably caused by set-tling of the sidewalk and was easily repaired by breaking up the first section of concrete and repour-ing a new surface with a gentle acceptable slope

(1:20 or less, according to ADAAG, 1991). An automatic door opener was installed to compensate for the heavy doors, an accommodation that went above and beyond the mandate. The interior doors of the entrance vestibule were adjusted to 5 lbf. In addition, the exterior doors were fitted with U-shaped handles to accommodate users with manual dexterity difficulties.

Interior Parking Facilities and Path of Travel

The primary concern with the indoor parking was the potential danger that an employee with a dis-ability might face in attempting to travel from the accessible parking space to the raised deck of the elevator lobby. The three accessible spaces, there-fore, were positioned as close as possible to the ele-vator entrance, and the curb ramp was relocated (Figure 20-4). A 60-in.–wide adjacent access aisle was included to allow sufficient space to enter or exit a vehicle. A dedicated path of travel, identified by crosshatching painted on the ground surface, was created from the parking spaces to the curb ramp. This not only protected the users of the spaces but also precluded other drivers from parking in front of the curb ramp entrance, as they had done before. The parking spaces were identified by a vertical sign showing the international symbol of access at the head of the space, suspended from the ceiling at a height visible above the parked vehicles.

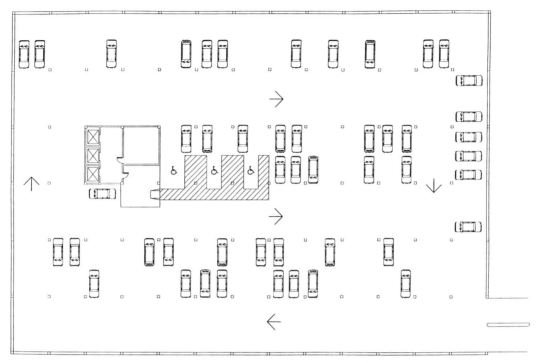

Figure 20-4. Interior parking facility after renovation. People with disabilities have a safe path of travel to and from the elevators.

Dining Facilities

Executive Dining Room

Because there is no feasible architectural means to create an 18-in. clear space on the latch side of the door, an automatic door opener should be installed to provide wheelchair users ready access. This has not been implemented yet and is a good illustration of a low-priority item because few people will benefit from it. The executive dining area serves only the top executives in the building, none of whom has a disability. In the event that an executive should entertain a guest with a disability, the guest would be escorted to the dining area and would therefore have assistance.

Cafeteria Seating

As the circulation path of travel worked well through and around the seating area, the major problem was the tables themselves. A minimum 27-in. vertical knee clearance is needed for people in wheelchairs to pull up to a table (ADAAG, 1991, 4.32.3). In compliance with ADAAG (1991, 5.1), 5% of the existing tables, dispersed throughout the seating area, were replaced with tables having an accessible configuration. This could have been achieved either by purchasing tables with a pedestal base or by reducing the apron on existing tables. The latter choice was made to maintain aesthetic conformity throughout the seating area (Figure 20-5). A symbol of accessibility was placed in a corner on the top surface of the modified tables.

Food Counter and Vending Machines

As the vending machines are replaced with newer models, machines will be chosen that address ADAAG (1991) standards by incorporating operating controls no higher than 48 in. AFF. This height accommodates people with a variety of reach capabilities and will soon become the industry standard.

The food counter dilemma, however, was not as easily solved. Standard cafeteria lines and salad bars present a difficult reach range problem that

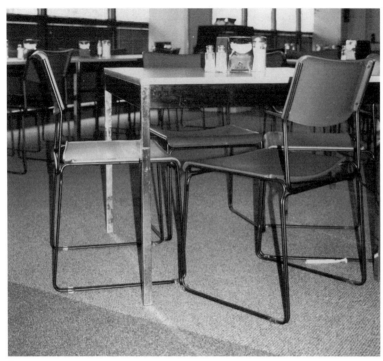

Figure 20-5. Note the difference in the size of the aprons on these tables. **(A)** This apron does not allow the necessary knee clearance for wheelchair users to eat at a comfortable distance from the table. **(B)** The apron has been cut away and the legs are supported with angled brackets.

A

would be addressed most effectively by replacing old equipment with a new configuration that more adequately considers human factors (Figure 20-6). Unfortunately, no manufacturer to date has created a line of equipment that successfully resolves the problem, leaving an issue that begs to be studied by ergonomists. An alternative accommodation was, therefore, implemented in the form of individualized service provided by the cafeteria staff. Dispensers for trays, napkins, and silverware were lowered to 48 in. AFF as well.

Bank

Ideally, one teller window and one portion of the service desk should be lowered to 36 in. AFF to accommodate wheelchair users (ADAAG, 1991, 7.2). However, ample maneuvering space throughout the facility allows people in wheelchairs to approach the service desk unimpeded to execute their banking needs. The ADA mandate states that an alternative accommodation is permissible when it is cost effective, and in a facility with so many retrofit needs, this solution allowed limited

funds to be allocated for more urgent problems. Although this solution achieves compliance with the mandate, using it and other alternative accommodations presents the risk of offending people with disabilities who are determined to maintain their independence by being totally self-sufficient. Unfortunately, the financial realities sometimes postpone the better alternative or render it impossible.

Human Resources Center

To be in compliance with Title I of the ADA, it is vital that prospective employees with disabilities have a clear interior path of travel from the building entry to and through the reception area and into the interview cubicles. The survey team recommended a major reconfiguration of the systems furniture to bring about this compliance. Space constraints in the existing location, however, rendered impossible a reconfiguration that would effect the required interior path of travel. Therefore, the whole department was moved to a more spacious location that allowed for adequate traffic

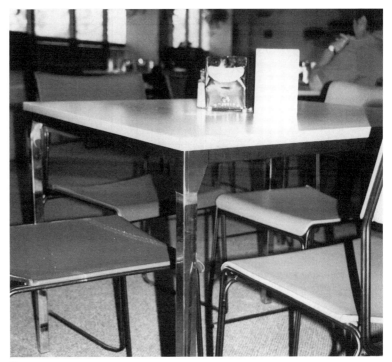

B

flow and space allowances that conformed to ADAAG standards. The original space has been reconfigured in an accessible manner for use by another department.

Restrooms and Locker Rooms

Ideally, all restrooms in the building would be retrofitted for accessibility. Unfortunately, various constraints often prohibit the ideal situation, and this building was no exception. Not only were the funds insufficient for such a step, but architectural infeasibility and local codes combined to make it impossible. Local building codes determine how many stalls are necessary per restroom, and using the combined space of two stalls to make one enlarged accessible stall sometimes means that local codes are not met. Because of these circumstances, the survey team recommended an alternate accommodation in the form of several properly dispersed accessible unisex restrooms. Again, it would be ideal to have one per floor, but as many as budget allows should be dispersed throughout the building. The first unisex restroom

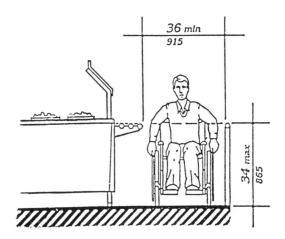

Figure 20-6. This figure, adapted from ADAAG, demonstrates the difficulty in reaching past a tray slide to the second row of items at a salad bar.

was installed near the cafeteria. Signage using grade II Braille and raised characters at existing restrooms is essential for directing users to accessible restrooms. An accessible unisex restroom includes entrance doors with either levers or U-

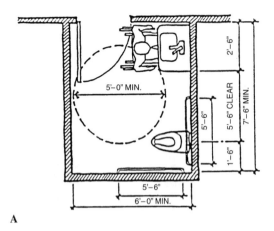

A

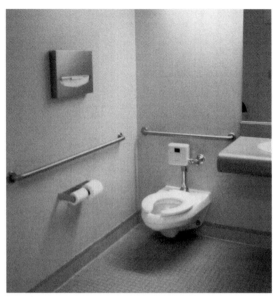

B

Figure 20-7. (A) An accessible unisex restroom requires a 60-in. wheelchair turning radius, as shown in this drawing. **(B)** The wall-hung sink in this unisex accessible restroom allows for a side approach to the toilet.

shaped handles to accommodate people with manual dexterity problems; a minimum maneuvering space of 18 in. on the latch side of the door; clear floor space within the restroom area providing a 60-in. turning radius to allow access to the accessible toilet and sink; accessible tap sets using levers, paddles, or electric eyes; a self-closing door; accessible interior locks in the form of slide bolts that can be activated with the heel of the hand; and grab bars (Figure 20-7).

In addition, certain changes were made in the existing restrooms. To accommodate people using the fitness center who could not stand while bathing, a transfer seat was added to one of the 36-sq. in. showers on the wall opposite the controls. The ideal solution is a roll-in shower, which is large enough to accommodate a wheelchair and has no curb. Because this requires a 30- × 60-in. stall, it was architecturally infeasible for the existing locker rooms. One lavatory sink was made accessible in each restroom, with the apron under the counter allowing 29-in. vertical knee clearance, insulated drain and hot water pipes, tap sets within proper reach range, the bottom of the mirror lowered to 40 in. AFF, and all operable parts of dispensers mounted no higher than 48 in. AFF.

One urinal in each men's room was lowered to have a rim height of 17 in. AFF.

Miscellaneous Elements

Elevators

Because elevators were already adequately sized to allow for maneuvering of a wheelchair, they were not considered a priority. However, the emergency telephone handset was fitted with a 29-in. cord, however, which was an inexpensive and simple retrofit. When funds become available, other changes will be made to meet the needs of those with visual disabilities. Audible signals sounding once for up and twice for down must be installed along with raised numbers and grade II Braille floor designations at 60 in. AFF on both jambs of the elevator hoistway. Similarly, grade II Braille must be added to the existing raised characters on the interior cab control panels. The adjustment of the elevator car to reduce the gap between the landing edge and the car platform, though not yet accomplished, could be achieved easily and inexpensively and should therefore not be delayed. The possibility

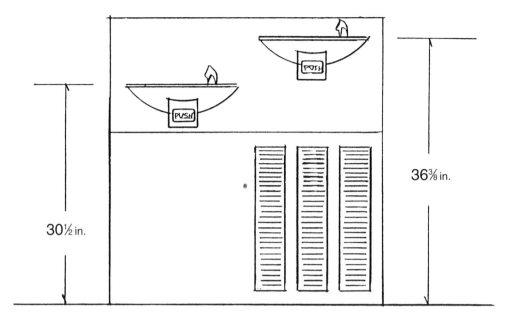

Figure 20-8. Drinking fountains offering both high and low spouts accommodate people who have difficulty stooping and people in wheelchairs, as well as short or tall people without disabilities.

of accidents resulting from the wide gap far outweigh the minor expense involved.

Drinking Fountains

The ADA mandates that half the drinking fountains (or a minimum of one) on each floor of a public building be accessible, with a spout no higher than 36 in. AFF, knee clearance for a wheelchair, and operable parts requiring neither grasping nor twisting (ADAAG, 1991, 4.15). Where architecturally and financially feasible, the combination high-low fountain should be installed because it provides easy usage by people of all heights as well as those using wheelchairs (Figure 20-8). Because this was a medium-priority item, paper cups were provided on site to achieve accommodation until units can be replaced.

Telephones

The public telephone in the third-floor lounge and one of the two in the cafeteria were lowered so that the highest operable part was no more than 48 in. AFF. Volume control was added to accommodate

people with hearing disabilities. Although volume control was necessary on the public phone in the cafeteria, it was an added convenience in the third-floor lounge. Because the lounge is used by employees only, it did not require the volume control because any employee needing an assistive device would already have one at his or her work station.

Alarms

The survey team recommended that visual alarms be installed for the benefit of people with auditory disabilities in restrooms, meeting rooms, hallways, lobbies, eating rooms, and all other common use areas, as required by ADAAG (1991).

Interior Signage

Signage for permanent rooms (such as the copy room, bathrooms, boiler room) and core stairs in the building was created using raised characters and grade II Braille. Signs are presently being affixed on the wall on the latch side of the door at 60 in. AFF rather than on doors, where they are virtually inaccessible to blind people when the doors are open.

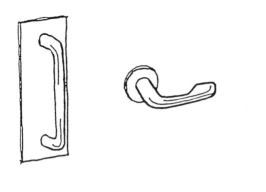

Figure 20-9. Three accessible door handles are, from left to right, a U-shaped pull bar, a lever handle, and a push bar.

Coat Rods

A section of each coat rod is to be lowered to 48 in. AFF to provide a comfortable reach range for people in wheelchairs and people of short stature.

Doors

All doors should be fitted with accessible handles as funds become available (Figure 20-9). Retrofitting should be done first for doors most used by employees or the general public.

Prioritizing Solutions

Although the survey team provided a prioritized list of the solutions described above, the decisions regarding the actual retrofit work were ultimately up to the client. They chose the logical first step of rendering the exterior accessible, a choice that matches the ADA priorities as well as the survey team's own conviction that the first step should be to remove barriers that keep people with disabilities from arriving at and entering a building. In the opinion of the survey team, however, once inside they should have addressed one of the most pressing problems: the lack of accessible bathroom facilities. For employees especially, having to travel around a 550,000-sq. ft building to use an accessible bathroom is inconvenient, time consuming, and demeaning. The funds allocated to the relocation of the Human Resources Center might have been better spent in retrofitting bathrooms or installing an accessible unisex restroom. Although the client was taking a major step toward compli-

ance with the law by moving Human Resources, the ADA expressly states that an alternative accommodation could be achieved by interviewing a prospective employee with a disability in an accessible area of the building. Retrofitting a bathroom for current employees might have been a more immediately beneficial use of funds.

Of the items that remain to be completed other than the bathrooms, the survey team would choose to replace the vending machines in the cafeteria and retrofit the salad bar, put visual alarms in bathrooms, and replace inaccessible signage in the building. Each of these design solutions would greatly reduce the remaining barriers in the building.

Evaluation

When retrofitting a facility to make it accessible, the first and foremost concern is the users. Will the changes suggested eliminate the barriers they are encountering? Will the safety of the users be increased? Fortunately for designers, references such as the ADAAG exist to make their decisions easier. These guidelines are based on years of research and practice; on the firsthand experiences of people with disabilities, some of whom are designers; and on the process of refinement and revision that has continued since the publication of the first standards in 1961 by the American National Standards Institute. Each revision is based on a better understanding of universal design; hence, each new version offers the designer state-of-the-art solutions that are better grounded in research and experience. ADAAG is by far the most thorough of these documents.

Even though it, too, is under constant revision, a designer who uses it can trust the solutions offered in its pages as long as they are used with sensitivity to the needs of people with disabilities. Not every technical solution to a barrier problem in the guidelines works well in every situation. The designer must always rely on personal experience as well as guidelines to be sure that his or her solutions are truly accessible.

With this in mind, the survey team can be reasonably confident that the design solutions offered to the client will in fact resolve the accessibility problems of this expansive building. An essential method of verification is to interview disabled users of the building. Several employees, all of whom are wheelchair users, agreed to be interviewed. The comments of one employee, L.K., represent a consensus. This person uses crutches as well as a wheelchair.

Before the retrofit work, L.K. experienced difficulties with barriers in a number of areas in the workplace. These are listed in Figure 20-10 and followed by a check mark (√) if the retrofit has been accomplished satisfactorily, an asterisk (*) if the retrofit or alternative accommodation did not work for L.K., or *NC* if the retrofit has not been completed yet. Comments made by L.K. follow in italics.

Of the 17 barriers that impeded L.K.'s access, 11, or 65%, were addressed. Of these, the nine retrofits produced positive results, but the alternative accommodations were less desirable. Overall, L.K. expressed satisfaction with the retrofit progress, reporting that it has become easier to travel to and through the facility and to perform on the job. Independence has also increased in several areas. L.K. also commented on a heightened sense of security because of a new policy, suggested by the survey team, that institutes a buddy system whereby employees with and without disabilities are paired to ensure evacuation in case of emergency. When asked to prioritize the retrofit of the remaining barriers, L.K. responded that restrooms should be the top priority, followed by the cafeteria, interior door opening force, and drinking fountains.

Conclusion

The process of interviewing people with disabilities is one of the best ways to become familiar with their needs. Although ADAAG provides tech-

nical solutions, there are certain pitfalls that are less likely to trip up the more experienced designer. For example, certain specifications, such as knee clearances or visual alarms, represent obvious needs. Other things are less obvious, though. Why is it acceptable for objects to protrude 4 in. from the wall when they are within the height range that might cause accidents? It is because blind people sweep their canes in an arc in front of their bodies to detect obstacles, and the arc formed by the cane necessarily keeps them a certain distance from walls. Guide dogs perform this function as well.

Sometimes ADAAG solutions do not work for all users. ADAAG offers *minimum* guidelines, meaning that they are geared to meet the needs of users in the middle range. Often, more stringent specifications would result in a more inclusive design. Clearly, the child in a wheelchair would not have the reach range of an adult, leaving items inaccessible despite the best of intentions on the part of the designer. The same holds true for adults with limited trunk or back mobility, whose reach may not extend to the 54 in. AFF allowable for a side approach. Similarly, L.K. indicated that interior doors were too heavy even though they had been adjusted to the recommended 5 lbf. In spite of these considerations, ADAAG still offers the best solution for a public place. In private spaces the needs of these individuals can be tailored more adequately.

Finally, ADAAG does not always specify everything there is to know. For example, paper towel dispensers must be placed within an acceptable reach range, but nowhere does the present edition of ADAAG (1994) indicate that the ideal location for a dispenser is beside the accessible sink. Propelling a wheelchair over to the paper towel dispenser is not easy with wet hands and the user has probably dripped water into his or her lap in the process as well as dirtied the hands again while wheeling.

All these examples point to the fact that technical solutions play an essential but limited role in achieving universal design. Although they are the designer's best resource for creating accessible features, they are not to be substituted for the awareness culled from experience. Universal design is at its best when technical solutions and sensitivity play complementary roles.

1. With accessibility symbol on ground, nondisabled people sometimes use accessible parking spaces. Need vertical signage. √

2. Built-up ramp at bank entrance impedes exit from car. √

3. Exterior doors too heavy. Need automatic openers. √

4. Interior doors too heavy. Need automatic openers. *NC*
   These should be placed at least on doors in critical areas.

5. Cafeteria tray and silverware dispensers out of reach range. √

6. Ice, water, and soda dispensers in cafeteria out of reach range. *NC*

7. Perimeter items on salad bar within reach range, but inside items inaccessible. *
   Staff assistance available, but creates dependence.

8. Dessert counter too high. *NC*

9. Bank teller windows too high. Must prepare transaction slips at own work station and reach up to teller. *
   Was not informed that transactions can take place at service desk. No signage indicating this alternative accommodation.

10. Nearest restroom to work station inaccessible due to sofa in entry vestibule. *NC*
    Only uses this restroom on days when physically able to use crutches rather than wheelchair. Nearest accessible restroom for wheelchair use is in another section of building.

11. Signage on door indicates that restroom with sofa is accessible when it is not; no signage indicating nearest accessible restroom. √

12. Sink in restroom is set too far back to reach tap set comfortably. √

13. Towel dispenser too high. √
    Placing a stack of towels on counter near sink is a simple solution if dispensers had not been lowered.

14. Mirror too high.

15. Drinking fountain closest to work station has spout too high. *NC*
    Must use accessible fountain in another section of building. Occasionally tries to fill glass with water to take back to work station, but difficult to maneuver wheelchair with full glass.

16. Telephone in third-floor lounge too high for forward approach, the only possible approach at that phone. √

17. Overhead flipper door cabinet within work station is too high to use. *NC*

Figure 20-10. An employee's (L.K.'s) list of barriers and retrofit evaluation. Comments made by L.K. follow in italics. (√ = retrofit has been accomplished satisfactorily; * = retrofit or alternative accommodation did not work for L.K.; *NC* = retrofit has not been completed yet.)

References

Kearney, D.S. (1992). *The new ADA: Compliance and costs.* Kingston, MA: R.S. Means Company.

U.S. Architectural and Transportation Barriers Compliance Board. (1990). *UFAS accessibility checklist.* Raleigh, NC: Barrier Free Environments.

U.S. Department of Justice, Office of the Attorney General. (1991). *ADA accessibility guidelines for buildings and facilities.* Washington, DC: Government Printing Office.

U.S. Department of Justice, Office of the Attorney General. (1994). *ADA accessibility guidelines for buildings and facilities, transportation facilities, and transportation vehicles.* Washington, DC: Government Printing Office.

Wilkoff, W.L., & Abed, L.W. (1994). *Practicing universal design: An interpretation of the ADA.* New York: Van Nostrand Reinhold.

Appendix 20-1

A Comparison of UFAS and ADAAG Survey Forms

The survey forms shown here are taken from the UFAS and ADAAG survey packets, which contain forms dealing with 21 and 29 topics, respectively. In general, ADAAG is a more sophisticated survey document. Although they both cover parking, elevators, toilet rooms, and other common building elements, ADAAG also includes such topics as transient lodging and transportation facilities. The following survey forms, each dealing with drinking fountains, are representative of the two documents. A comparison of the two demonstrates how they vary in their complexity and ease of use.

The UFAS form (Survey Form 4) was published in June 1990. It lists reference numbers and their associated technical requirements. For each of these, the surveyor can check off boxes indicating that the criterion has or has not been met or is not applicable. There is no room for comments on the form.

The ADAAG form (Survey Form 5), published in October 1992, is more comprehensive than that offered by UFAS, with more criteria per topic. Supplying both the reference number and an item label (i.e., 4.15.5[1] Fountains with Knee Space) expedites the surveying process and eliminates the need to read lots of technical requirements while searching for the appropriate item. Like UFAS, ADAAG displays the technical requirements and offers boxes to indicate whether or not they have been met. It also offers space for comments, allowing the surveyor to add necessary information that might reflect priorities for retrofitting, nontechnical information that would create a more sensitive design, and so on.

It is important to remember that both UFAS and ADAAG are scoping documents (i.e., where and how many) and are based on the American National Standards Institute A117.1 standards. Therefore, the item reference numbers are consistent throughout these documents.

UFAS Survey Form 4: Drinking Fountains and Telephones
Facility Name: _____
Drinking Fountains/Water Coolers
Fountain Location: _____
4.1.2(9) Drinking Fountains and Water Coolers: If drinking fountains are provided, then at least 50% but not less than one shall meet the following recommendations.

UFAS Section	Technical Requirements	Yes	No	NA
4.15.5(2)	If the unit is free-standing or built in and does not have a clear space beneath it, does it have a clear space along side it at least 30 × 48 in. which allows a wheelchair user to make a parallel approach?	❑	❑	❑
4.15.5(1)	If the unit is wall- or post-mounted, is there a clear knee space between the bottom of the apron and the ground that is at least 27 in. high, 30 in. wide, and 17 in. deep?	❑	❑	❑
4.4.1	If a wall-mounted drinking fountain has a bottom edge between 27 and 80 in. from the floor, does it project less than 4 in. into the pathway? (Wall-mounted fountains with bottom edges at or below 27 in. may project any amount as long as the required clear width of an accessible route of travel is not reduced.)	❑	❑	❑
	Is there an accessible path of at least 36 in. clear alongside the drinking fountain?	❑	❑	❑
4.15.2	Is the spout outlet no higher than 36 in. from the ground?	❑	❑	❑
4.15.3	Is the spout at the front of the unit, with a water flow parallel or nearly parallel to the front edge?	❑	❑	❑
	Is the water stream at least 4 in. high to allow the insertion of a cup under the stream?	❑	❑	❑
4.15.4	Are the controls located near the front edge?	❑	❑	❑
4.15.4; 4.27	Are the controls operable with one hand?	❑	❑	❑
	Are they operable without tight grasping, pinching, or twisting of the wrist?	❑	❑	❑

ADAAG Survey Form 5: Drinking Fountains
Use with the Minimum Requirements Summary Sheets and ADAAG.
See Minimum Requirements Summary Sheets I and J for special requirements that may be allowed in alterations and historic preservation. See also ADAAG 4.1.6 and 4.1.7.
Facility Name: _____
Fountain Location: _____

ADAAG Section	Item	Technical Requirements	Comments	Yes	No
4.1.3(10)(a), 4.15.1	Water fountains	Where there is only one drinking fountain on a floor, is there one accessible to wheelchair users in accordance with 4.15 (see below) and one accessible to persons who have difficulty bending or stooping (e.g., drinking fountains mounted at standard height or a water cooler)?		❏	❏
4.1.3(10)(b), 4.15.1		Where there is more than one drinking fountain on a floor, do 50% comply with 4.15 (see below)?		❏	❏
4.1.3(10)	Accessible route	Is the accessible drinking fountain on an accessible route?		❏	❏
4.15.5(2)	Clearance— fountains without knee space	If the unit is free-standing or built in and does not have a clear space underneath it, does it have a clear floor space alongside it at least 30×48 in. which allows a wheelchair user to make a parallel approach (see Figures 27(c) and (d))?		❏	❏
4.15.5(1)	Fountains with knee space	If the unit is wall- or post-mounted, is there a clear knee space between the bottom of the apron and the floor that is at least 27 in. high, 30 in. wide, and 17–19 in. deep (see Figures 27(a) and (b))?		❏	❏
		Does such a unit also have a clear floor space at least 30×48 in. perpendicular to the unit, allowing a forward approach?		❏	❏
4.4.1	Protruding objects	If a wall-mounted drinking fountain has a leading edge between 27 and 80 in. from the floor, does it project less than 4 in. into the pathway? (Wall-mounted fountains with leading edges at or below 27 in. may project any amount so long as the required clear width of an accessible route is not reduced.)		❏	❏
4.15.2	Spout height	Is the spout outlet no higher than 36 in. from the floor?		❏	❏

ADAAG Section	Item	Technical Requirements	Comments	Yes	No
4.15.3	Location	Is the spout at the front of the unit, with a water floor trajectory parallel or nearly parallel to the front edge?		❏	❏
	Water flow	If the fountain has a round or oval bowl, is the water flow within 3 in. of the front edge of the fountain?		❏	❏
		Is the water flow at least 4 in. high to allow the insertion of a cup under the flow?		❏	❏
4.15.4	Controls— location	Are the controls located on the front or the side near the front edge?		❏	❏
4.15.4, 4.27.4	Operation	Are the controls operable with one hand?		❏	❏
		Are the controls operable without tight grasping, pinching, or twisting of the wrist?		❏	❏
		Is the force required to operate the controls no greater than 5 lbf?		❏	❏

Index